BRAIN IMAGING IN
PSYCHIATRY

BRAIN IMAGING IN PSYCHIATRY

Shôn Lewis

BSc, MD, MPhil, MRCPsych
Professor of Psychiatry,
University of Manchester
Manchester

Nicholas Higgins

BA, MRCP, FRCR
Department of Radiology
Royal Free Hospital
London

b

**Blackwell
Science**

©1996 by
Blackwell Science Ltd
Editorial Offices:
Osney Mead, Oxford OX2 0EL
25 John Street, London WC1N 2BL
23 Ainslie Place, Edinburgh EH3 6AJ
238 Main Street, Cambridge
  Massachusetts 02142, USA
54 University Street, Carlton
  Victoria 3053, Australia

Other Editorial Offices:
Arnette Blackwell SA
  224, Boulevard Saint Germain
  75007 Paris, France

Blackwell Wissenschafts-Verlag GmbH
  Kurfürstendamm 57
  10707 Berlin, Germany

Zehetnergasse 6
A-1140 Wien
Austria

First published 1996

Set by Setrite Typesetters, Hong Kong
Printed and bound in Great Britain
at the University Press, Cambridge

The Blackwell Science logo is a
trade mark of Blackwell Science Ltd,
registered at the United Kingdom
Trade Marks Registry

DISTRIBUTORS

Marston Book Services Ltd
PO Box 269, Abingdon
Oxon OX14 4YN
(*Orders*: Tel: 01235 465500
            Fax: 01235 465555)

USA
Blackwell Science, Inc.
238 Main Street
Cambridge, MA 02142
(*Orders*: Tel: 800 215-1000
                 617 876-7000
          Fax: 617 492-5263)

Canada
Copp Clark Professional
200 Adelaide Street West, 3rd Floor
Toronto, Ontario
Canada, M5H IW7
(*Orders*: Tel: 416 597-1616
                800 815-9417
          Fax: 416 597-1617)

Australia
Blackwell Science Pty Ltd
54 University Street
Carlton, Victoria 3053
(*Orders*: Tel: 03 9347 0300
          Fax: 03 9349 3016)

A catalogue record for this title
is available from the British Library

ISBN 0-632-03647-8

Library of Congress
Cataloging-in-publication Data

Brain imaging in psychiatry
  [edited by] Shôn Lewis, Nicholas Higgins.
         p.   cm.
  Includes bibliographical references and index.
  ISBN 0-632-03647-8
  1. Mental illness—Pathophysiology.
  2. Brain—Imaging.
  I. Lewis, Shôn. II. Higgins, Nicholas.
  [DNLM: 1. Mental Disorders—pathology.
  2. Mental Disorders—physiopathology.
  3. Brain—pathology.   4. Brain—physiopathology.
  5. Diagnostic Imaging.   6. Psychiatry—methods.
  7. Psychopathology—methods.
  WM 141 B8137 1996]
  RC473.B7B734 1996
  616.89'0754—dc20
  DNLM/DLC
  for Library of Congress   96-6148

Contents

List of Contributors

H. B. Andrews MA, DM, MRCPsych, Department of Psychiatry, Sir Robert Kilpatrick Clinical Sciences Building, Leicester Royal Infirmary, Leicester LE2 7LX, UK

A. J. Bailey BSc, MD, MRCPsych, Department of Child Psychiatry, Institute of Psychiatry, De Crespigny Park, London SE5 8AF, UK

T. Baldeweg PhD, Department of Academic Psychiatry, Charing Cross & Westminster Medical School, St Dunstan's Road, London W6 8RP, UK

A. Burgess PhD, Mental Health Unit, Chelsea & Westminster Hospital, 369 Fulham Road, London SW10, UK

E. H. Burrows MRad, FRCR, Emeritus Consultant, Southampton University Hospitals, NHS Trust, Tremona Road, Shirley, Southampton SO16 6YD, UK

J. D. Cohen MD, PhD, Carnegie-Mellon University, Department of Psychology, Pittsburgh, PA 15213, USA

T. Cox FRCR, Department of Radiology, Maudsley Hospital, Denmark Hill, London SE5 8AF, UK

R. J. Dolan MD, MRCPsych, The National Hospital for Neurology and Neurosurgery, Queen Square, London WC1N 3BG, UK

G. M. Goodwin MA, DPhil, MRCPsych, MRC Brain Metabolism Unit, Royal Edinburgh Hospital, Morningside Park, Edinburgh EH10 5HF, UK

C. L. Grady PhD, Laboratory of Neurosciences, National Institute on Aging, National Institutes of Health, Bethesda, MD 20892, USA

J. Gruzelier PhD, Department of Academic Psychiatry, Charing Cross & Westminster Medical School, St Dunstan's Road, London W6 8RP, UK

J. N. P. Higgins BA, MRCP, FRCR, Department of Radiology, Royal Free Hospital, Pond Street, London NW3 2QG, UK

W. W. Hong PhD, Laboratory of Neurosciences, National Institute on Aging, National Institutes of Health, Bethesda, MD 20892, USA

M. S. Keshavan MD, MRCPsych, University of Pittsburgh, Department of Psychiatry, Western Psychiatric Institute and Clinic, 3811 O'Hara Street, Pittsburgh, PA 15213, USA

S. W. Lewis BSc, MD, MRCPsych, School of Psychiatry and Behavioural Sciences, University of Manchester, Manchester M20 8LR, UK

P. F. Liddle PhD, MRCPsych, Department of Psychiatry, University of British Colombia, Vancouver, V6H 326, Canada

P. K. McGuire BSc, MD, MRCPsych, Institute of Psychiatry, De Crespigny Park, London SE5 8AF; and MRC Cyclotron Unit, Hammersmith Hospital, DuCane Road, London W12 0HS, UK

M. J. Mentis MD, Laboratory of Neurosciences, National Institute on Aging, National Institutes of Health, Bethesda, MD 20892, USA

D. G. M. Murphy MD, MRCPsych, Department of Psychological Medicine, Institute of Psychiatry, De Crespigny Park, London SE5 8AF, UK

G. D. Pearlson MBBS, Department of Psychiatry and Behavioral Sciences, The Henry Phipps Psychiatric Service, 600 North Wolfe Street/Meyer 3-166, Baltimore, MD 21287-7362, USA

S. M. Pickman DCR, DMU, Royal Free Hospital, Pond Street, London NW3 2QG, UK

L. S. Pilowsky BSc, PhD, MRCPsych, Institute of Psychiatry, De Crespigny Park, Denmark Hill, London SE5 8AF, UK

A. D. Platts MBBS, FRCS, FRCR, Royal Free Hospital, Pond Street, London NW3 2QG, UK

A. R. Valentine MBBS, FRCR, Royal Free Hospital, Pond Street, London NW3 2QG, UK

P. W. R. Woodruff, Institute of Psychiatry, De Crespigny Park, Denmark Hill, London SE5 8AF, UK

Preface

It is a historical irony that psychiatrists are ambivalent about the brain. For most of the twentieth century, psychiatry has held to a dualistic approach, seeing the mind as its proper territory, the brain being a dangerously reductionist notion. However, progress in psychiatry has been inexorably from mind to brain and not the other way round. Recent classification systems reflect this, and the past 20 years have witnessed the rise and rise of biological psychiatry in research. Syndromes and symptoms previously thought of as 'functional' are ever more open to explanation in terms of brain dysfunction.

Modern brain imaging has played a central part in bringing about this change. Until the late 1970s, the living brain was well protected from clinical or scientific investigation, largely by virtue of its being inside a dense, hard box. The arrival of computerised X-ray tomography changed this overnight. This and subsequent brain imaging techniques have revolutionised diagnostic neurology. In psychiatry, its impact has been more gradual. Yet, over the past 15 years, computerised brain imaging has redrawn much of psychiatry's theoretical landscape, and started to influence clinical practice. This book reflects an increasing need to be aware of these techniques from many perspectives. What techniques are available to look at brain structure and function? What are their capabilities and their limitations? How do they work and what do they show? When are they indicated clinically and what are the risks, if any? What issues are important in designing research projects, or evaluating published research articles?

The arrival of computed tomography in the mid-1970s was the first of a cascade of new approaches to visualising the structure and function of the living brain. The architecture of the brain became the subject of the beautiful images of magnetic resonance (MR) imaging in the 1980s. Imaging regional brain function using high-resolution single-photon and positron emission tomography (SPET and PET) burgeoned during the 1980s. Not long prior to this the scientific dogma still held that, unlike other tissue, brain did not increase its local metabolism or oxygen consumption when working. The metabolic maps of regional brain activity produced with SPET or PET show how wrong this idea was and the notion of watching the brain think, both in health and disease, has become a reality. Imaging brain receptors is now possible, as is the imaging of aspects of brain biochemistry, using MR spectroscopy. Electroencephalographic three-dimensional (3-D) techniques and magnetoencephalography (MEG) track the tiny changes in electrical and magnetic fields which occur during brain activity and the new process of functional MR sees the localised changes in regional blood flow as they happen during perception and cognition.

The book is arranged conceptually in two parts. The first (Chapters 1–9) explains from first principles how the different brain imaging techniques work. The contributors are mainly radiologists. Burrows starts by setting the recent developments in historical context. Valentine then explores the principles and applications of computed tomography. Higgins and colleagues do the same for the more complex but more versatile technique of MR imaging. How these techniques help the understanding of normal brain anatomy is then examined in a chapter designed to be a neuroanatomy primer from the perspective of imaging. In the next chapter of this section, Lewis looks at principles of functional imaging, particularly SPET and PET, and discusses some of the challenges of image analysis. Keshavan and Cohen then examine the principles and findings of the two new MR techniques attracting so much attention: spectroscopy and functional MR. Brain electrical activity mapping and MEG have been less widely used but have potential for showing brain changes in real time, as they occur, and are explained by Gruzelier and colleagues, and Andrews. Pilowsky discusses the special application of SPET and PET to receptor imaging with radioligands, increasingly important in psychopharmacology and drug development.

The second part of the book (Chapters 10–16) looks in more detail at how brain imaging has illuminated the nature of what goes wrong in a range of psychiatric disorders. Schizophrenia is a classic illustration of how the understanding of the pathogenesis of a disorder has been transformed by the use of brain imaging. Woodruff and Lewis review the structural findings, discussing also the determinants of normal variation in brain structure, including alcohol use. Liddle takes further the story of functional imaging, focusing on schizophrenia, whose symptom clusters correlate with patterned abnormalities on PET, based largely on work

pioneered by his own team. Dolan and Goodwin review similar approaches to the understanding of affective disorders, where mood and cognitive symptoms each seem to have a signature in brain function. Pearlson reviews structural findings in the field of neuropsychiatry, looking at the effects of ageing and then reviewing the clinical correlates and radiological findings in the major dementias. Murphy and colleagues examine functional correlates. Neurotic disorders such as obsessive compulsive disorder, as well as childhood developmental disorders, have also revealed abnormalities on brain imaging. The fields are reviewed by Maguire, and Bailey and Cox, respectively.

The field is growing ever more quickly. The understanding of mechanisms in psychiatric disorders, as well as the clinical management of patients, has changed as a result of brain imaging and will change further as the power of these tools is enhanced further by integrating approaches from allied fields of neuropathology, neuropsychology, pharmacology and molecular biology. Clinicians and academics need to understand the possibilities, the limitations, the risks and the future of the new imaging technology.

We gratefully acknowledge Professor Nieuwenhuys for agreeing reproduction of some of his figures.

Shôn Lewis
Nicholas Higgins

1: A Brief History of Brain Imaging

E. H. Burrows

Discovery of X-rays

Fate ordained that a century ago W.C. Röntgen (Fig. 1.1), a hitherto obscure teacher of physics at a provincial German university, would identify a new form of radiation which was to revolutionise medical practice. Academic physicists had been experimenting with the passage of electrical currents across vacuums since the 1880s, when Sir William Crookes, the Victorian prince of science, built a glass tube for this purpose. It is clear that in the decade before Röntgen performed his experiments and published his results (Röntgen, 1896) countless scientists in England, Europe and America, including Crookes, had generated X-rays without their realising it, but none could challenge the discovery he made in October 1895 of the invisible rays which are generated when cathode rays are driven against an object, such as the wall of a glass tube. He named these radiations 'X-rays' and this term is still used in Britain, although in Germany, America and elsewhere they are usually called 'roentgen rays'.

Röntgen is unlikely himself to have realised the medical significance of his discovery during his experiments. He photographed his wife's left hand and wedding ring (Fig. 1.2), but simply because her hand was an object readily available and an excellent experimental model with which to test different densities, including metal, bone and skin. The man who recognised the potential benefits of X-rays for mankind was a Viennese journalist, Z.K. Lecher, who disseminated the news telegraphically round the world within hours of receiving it (Burrows, 1986). It was a journalistic scoop, and soon cartoons appeared in *Punch* (Fig. 1.3).

Röntgen's work ranks in pure science as one of the high points of the nineteenth century; Faraday's discovery of electromagnetism is another. But it owed its instant and universal acclaim to the perception by surgeons of the value of X-rays in clinical localisation. They realised at once that they now possessed a means of siting fragments of metal and perhaps also glass and wood trapped in the soft tissues of an extremity. No such injury was ever a minor matter before antibiotics because of the risk of infection, which prior to X-ray localisation was often the penalty of surgical removal. It is also important to remember that Röntgen announced his discovery to a medical world that was ripe to receive and ready to exploit any innovation (Burrows, 1994). Lister's aseptic technique had just opened the door to abdominal surgery, and a contemporary neurologist hopefully declared, 'the dura may be no more inviolable than the peritoneum'. Leading clinical localisers were Hughlings Jackson, who first associated what he called 'a special type of epilepsy' (Jacksonian attacks) with superficial lesions of the hemisphere, and William MacEwan, the Glasgow surgeon who linked post-traumatic hemiplegia to a surgically curable condition, subdural haematoma. Such men viewed X-rays as an ally. Soon surgically minded neurologists embraced X-rays to promote more accurate intracranial diagnosis.

Röntgen made his experiments with a tabletop set consisting of a fragile glass tube, an underpowered coil and a wet battery (Fig. 1.4). In most British cities, a modification of this primitive apparatus, locally built by an amateur enthusiast, was usually adequate to localise fragments of

1

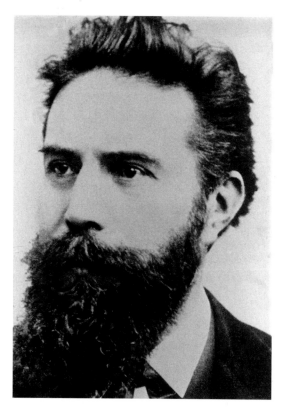

Fig. 1.1 W.C. Röntgen (1845–1923).

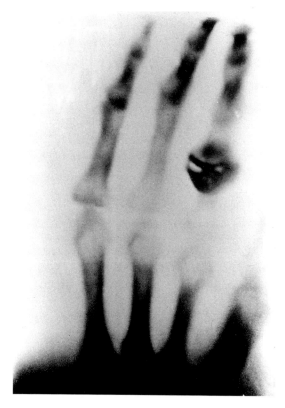

Fig. 1.2 The first human radiograph. The left hand and wedding ring of Frau Bertha Röntgen, photographed by her husband in November 1895.

metal in fingers or toes (exposure time, 10 minutes!). In 1897 a portable kit was available to the British Army and radiographs were made of fractures and bullet wounds on the battlefield. More robust machinery soon followed for the limbs and the skull.

Skull radiography

Suddenly the world possessed a reliable method of siting an intracranial bullet and of identifying a closed fracture of the skull and locating its position in the right or the left side of the vault, thereby providing the surgeon with the preoperative information he requires. The focal bone changes of meningioma and calcific deposits in brain tumours, each representing about 10% of the total, could now be recognised. Within a decade, characteristic excavations of the skull

base were identified, such as pituitary adenomas and cranial nerve tumours like acoustic neuroma, as was the picture of hydrocephalus and acromegaly. In 1906 the first textbook of skull radiography (neuroradiology) appeared in Germany. An early English *cause célèbre* had been the case of Mrs Eliza Hartley of Nelson, Lancashire, who was shot in the head by her husband during a domestic quarrel in April 1896, only 4 months after Röntgen announced his discovery. The bullet lodged in her brain. Arthur Schuster, the German-born professor of physics at Manchester and an acquaintance of Röntgen, rigged up a set at Mrs Hartley's bedside and took a radiograph which localised the bullet (Fig. 1.5).

Skull radiography only ever had a limited relevance in intracranial diagnosis. But even senior

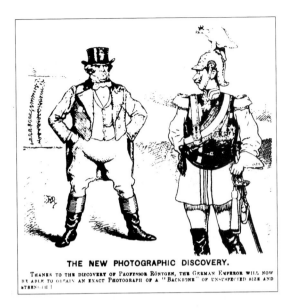

THE NEW PHOTOGRAPHIC DISCOVERY.

THANKS TO THE DISCOVERY OF PROFESSOR RÖNTGEN, THE GERMAN EMPEROR WILL NOW BE ABLE TO OBTAIN AN EXACT PHOTOGRAPH OF A "BACKBONE" OF UNSUSPECTED SIZE AND STRENGTH

Fig. 1.3 Cartoon in *Punch*, 25 January 1896. The caption alludes to Röntgen's discovery in order to express British resentment at the Kaiser's intervention in colonial affairs.

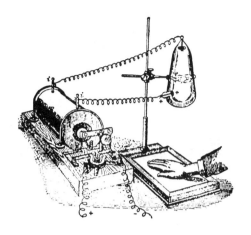

Fig. 1.4 Röntgen's tabletop apparatus for generating X-rays. The items were: a glass vacuum tube excited by an induction (Rühmkorff) coil with mechanical interrupter, connected to a battery (not shown). The patient's hand rests on a light-tight box probably containing an ordinary photographic dry plate. The exposure time would have been about 10 minutes!

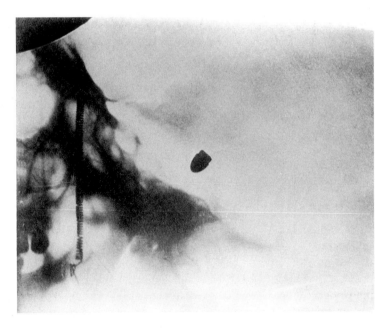

Fig. 1.5 Bullet at the base of the brain. This is a radiograph of Professor Schuster's simulated model, which he made by fixing a bullet within a dry skull, in order to determine the required exposure for a radiograph of Mrs Elizabeth Hartley's head in Lancashire in April 1896.

radiologists may be surprised to discover, from the safe vantage point of the modern imaging era, how remarkably small this impact ever was. In 1991 the author reviewed the skull radiographs of 200 patients, all of whom had lesions of the brain which had been proved by appropriate investigation in a British neurosurgical centre. Of these 200, 122 (61%) showed no abnormality of their skull radiographs; these included 57 tumour cases. Even more unhelpful was the fact that in the remaining 78 patients, i.e. the abnormal 39%, the abnormalities were academically interesting but not practically useful in the patient's management. The abnormal radiological signs included fracture, pineal displacement and evidence of generalised raised intracranial pressure, but in not a single case did their presence obviate the need for brain scanning or angiography, which are the investigations on which the management decisions nowadays depend. The introduction of computed tomography (CT) sounded the death-knell of skull radiographs in neurological management, and for the past 20 years their use has been confined to accident and emergency departments as an increasingly questionable screening test of serious head injury.

Air studies (pneumography)

In 1887, when Lister's nephew, Victor Horsley, successfully removed a tumour from the spinal canal of one of Sir Ernest Gowers's patients, it is said that the eminent neurologist stood by the surgeon's side, and told him as he pointed, 'If you cut there, Horsley, you should find the trouble.' Gowers, as a result of his careful clinical examination, had been able accurately to indicate the level of the tumour (Bull, 1961). Such exceptional anecdotes serve perhaps more to emphasise the unreliability of clinical localisation and its inadequacy as a basis for scientific neurosurgery. Without more direct and visual evidence of the site and size of the lesion the surgeon expects to remove, success was likely to remain elusive. Thus the neurosurgeons became the principal seekers of some kind of preoperative investigation that could show them what they needed to see.

The story starts in 1918 at the John Hopkins Hospital, Baltimore, among the coterie of talented doctors, including Osler, Halsted and the neurosurgeon Harvey Cushing, who had founded

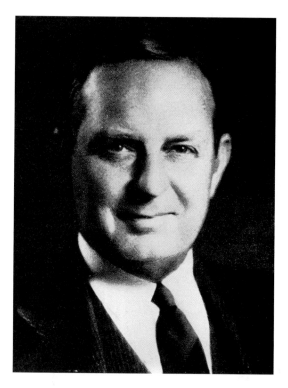

Fig. 1.6 Walter Dandy, the Baltimore neurosurgeon who was the begetter of intracranial pneumography.

the school of medicine there 30 years previously. Walter Dandy (Fig. 1.6), Cushing's first assistant in 1918, widened the scope of the burr-hole technique, which was then the standard method of identifying extracerebral haematomas, to provide more diagnostic information by means of skull radiography. This he did by injecting air into the cerebral ventricles through a brain needle, and then making radiographs (*ventriculography*) (Dandy, 1918). A year later he injected the air through a lumbar puncture needle (*encephalography*), thus avoiding preliminary burr-hole surgery for diagnostic purposes.

Dandy recalled that he simply applied to the cranial cavity a remark made by Halsted on a ward round, apropos a radiograph of the abdomen, that normal gas in the large bowel 'seems to perforate the bone'. He would also have known of the case of the New York drayman described by

Luckett (1913), whose skull radiographs revealed air-filled ventricles after a severe head injury. Luckett's was a prelude to other similar cases complicating penetrating skull fracture encountered during the First World War, which lard the contemporary European literature. Dandy's discovery helped to launch modern brain surgery, because intracranial pneumography was accurate enough to image the majority of operable space-occupying lesions, and the incidence of negative exploratory craniotomies due to erroneous clinical localisation immediately fell. In 1925 Dandy reported on 500 pneumograms with only three deaths — 'it is less dangerous than exploratory craniotomy, and it frequently gives more information', he wrote.

However, one survey in the 1920s gave ventriculography a detection rate of only about 30%. This unreliability arose from a failure to manipulate the injected air into the third ventricle, aqueduct of Sylvius and fourth ventricle, which consequently were not imaged. The reason was simple: the Americans had failed to devise a proper pneumographic technique which would have yielded a much higher success rate. This required special X-ray apparatus (which did not then exist), and a rigid technical protocol. Both the apparatus and the protocol were developed in Stockholm.

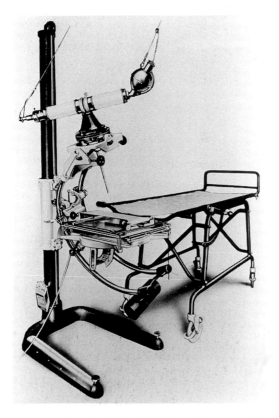

Fig. 1.7 Early Schönander skull table with patient trolley. This apparatus gave reality to Erik Lysholm's technique of precision pneumography.

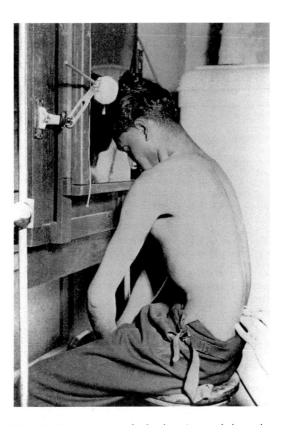

Fig. 1.8 Correct position for lumbar air encephalography. The seated patient had his chin tucked in, in order to ensure that the small increments of air passed into the fourth ventricle. After about 50 ml was introduced, the needle was withdrawn and the patient was placed on an X-ray table, and this air was utilised to examine various parts of the ventricular system in turn.

Erik Lysholm, a Swedish radiologist, provided the catalyst for Dandy's discovery. He designed an X-ray apparatus for precision radiography of the skull, which operated on the then novel principle that the X-ray tube moves around a sphere and the central ray can always be directed at the centre of the sphere (Lysholm, 1931). A Stockholm engineer, Georg Schönander, built the prototype machine and his company held the monopoly for 40 years (Fig. 1.7). Lysholm also developed a technique of ventriculography and lumbar encephalography (Fig. 1.8) to use with Schönander's skull table (Lysholm *et al.*, 1935). It was based on the precept that the ventricular pathways of the brain must be studied systematically, segment by segment, using the same small volume of air and making two or three radiographs of each segment. During examination of each segment, the X-ray tube is moved but not the patient's head, so that the air in the brain remains undisturbed. Upon completion the air is moved to the next segment by careful repositioning of the patient's head, and the process is repeated (Fig. 1.9).

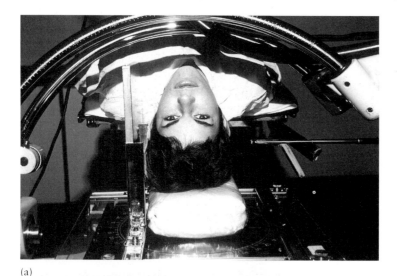

(a)

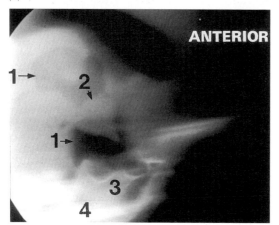

(b)

Fig. 1.9 Hanging-head autotomogram—a pneumographic technique used to demonstrate a suprasellar mass deforming the third ventricle. (a) The patient was positioned supine with her head extended down to rest on the padded tabletop, with a chin-strap sufficiently loose to enable her to rotate her head as if saying 'No' during the exposure. (b) Lateral tomogram of midline structures. 1. Gas–fluid levels in the third ventricle (top) and basal cisterns (bottom) are orientated 'vertically' because of the position of the head when the film was taken. 2. Crescentic deformity of the elevated anterior third ventricle produced by the midline suprasellar mass. 3. Pituitary fossa showing forward excavation—the so-called J-sella deformity associated with optic pathway glioma. 4. Clivus.

Lysholm's precision pneumography gave optimal results, and enabled all but the smallest and most infiltrative brain tumours to be imaged for neurosurgeons. In the decades following 1935 generations of radiologists made the pilgrimage to Stockholm to learn their trade and to purchase a Schönander skull table, which became the international hallmark of high-quality neuroradiology. Ventriculography became a standard preoperative investigation in patients with papilloedema or other clinical evidence of raised intracranial pressure. Fractional pneumoencephalography also became the stock-in-trade of the neurologist for confirming non-surgical syndromes caused by atrophic or congenital brain lesions. As these techniques were refined, Dandy's early mortality disappeared, but morbidity remained high; all ventriculography patients require their heads to be shaved for burr-hole surgery, and most encephalography patients used to be laid low for several days by headache. The introduction of CT scanning in the 1970s totally abolished the need for pneumography; and the proliferation of CT facilities probably raises ethical objections nowadays to the use of pneumography as a primary diagnostic measure.

Angiography

Dandy stimulated others, and in the 1920s attempts were made to outline the brain by utilising his principle—namely, making skull radiographs after the injection of a contrasting substance. The victor's palm went to Egaz Moniz, a Portuguese neurologist who trained in Paris under Babinski (Fig. 1.10). Moniz was a figure larger than life, a man with a Renaissance cloak over his shoulders. After returning to Lisbon in middle life, he had a career in politics, serving as ambassador in Madrid and as the foreign minister of his country. When the Portuguese dictatorship came, Moniz resumed his medical career, which went from strength to strength; in 1949 he was awarded a Nobel Prize for medicine.

Moniz had two methods in mind: (i) to opacify the brain itself through intravenous or parenteral

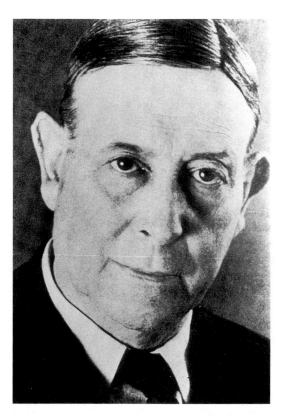

Fig. 1.10 Egaz Moniz (1874–1955), the Portuguese pioneer of angiography, who performed the first successful carotid angiogram in 1927.

injection; and (ii) to inject a radio-opaque substance into the cerebral arteries. He failed in the first method and succeeded in the second. The technique of intra-arterial injection was then already known, neosalvarsan having been injected into the carotid artery in the treatment of brain syphilis; therefore the problem was not that of needling the carotid artery. The difficulty was to find a substance to inject that would produce an X-ray image which was safe. Moniz adopted a trial-and-error approach with salts of lithium, strontium, iodine and bromine; and finally he chose iodine on account of its higher atomic weight and thus greater radiographic density. Sodium iodide 25% was satisfactorily tolerated, and this solution was injected into the carotid

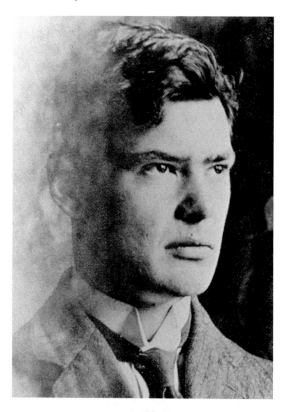

Fig. 1.11 Norman Dott, the Edinburgh neurosurgeon. In 1937 he was the first surgeon successfully to ligate an intracranial aneurysm after its localisation by angiography.

after surgical exposure of the artery in the neck. Only upon the ninth attempt, in a 20-year-old man with a pituitary tumour, was the technique a success. In July 1927 Moniz presented his discovery to the Neurological Society of Paris (Moniz, 1927). Four years later he recorded 90 cases (180 angiograms), with two deaths, in his book, *Diagnostic des Tumeurs Cérébrales et épreuve de Encéphalographie Arterielle.*

Moniz begat a school of angiography in Lisbon which swiftly disseminated the new technique around the world—notably to Spanish America and Mexico, whence it passed to the United States. His work also stimulated Norman Dott (Fig. 1.11), an Edinburgh surgeon who returned home in 1933 after a neurosurgical training with Cushing. In that year Dott became the first surgeon in the world to ligate an intracranial aneurysm after its localisation by angiography. The case was the eighth of the 17 aneurysms he described to the Edinburgh Medico-Chirurgical Society. His first seven observations predated Moniz's book, but case 8 was a 23-year-old woman with a left oculomotor palsy who complained of increasingly severe headaches. Dott suspected a leaking aneurysm, and feared that a rupture was imminent. 'We therefore made an arterial radiogram of the left internal carotid artery and its branches. This showed a round aneurysmal sac, about 7 cm in diameter, attached by a narrow neck to the inferior aspect of the circle of Willis at the mouth of the posterior communicating artery' (Dott, 1933). Thanks to the visual help afforded by the angiogram, Dott was able to apply a ligature to the neck of the aneurysm, and the patient's oculomotor palsy and headaches receded. She was cured.

Dott was to pioneer more than the angiography of brain aneurysms. He launched their surgical treatment upon his own country and the world, and thereby substantially consolidated neurosurgery. But this process was retarded by the reluctance of most surgeons to perform cut-down carotid angiography, because of the technical difficulty of the procedure and its unpleasant side-effects. Sodium iodide was now replaced by thorium dioxide (Thorotrast), despite fears of using a radioactive substance. In 1932 Almeida Lima, an acolyte of Moniz, came to London and carried out the first cut-down carotid angiogram at the National Hospital, Queen Square.

The next major advance came after the end of the Second World War. Iodine-containing contrast media such as Abrodil were developed to replace Thorotrast; and apparatus for rapid serial angiography reached the market. As had been the case with pneumography before the war, technical advances and investigative protocol became the preserve of the Scandinavians, and their radiologists and apparatus-makers were to maintain a monopolistic lead in the field of cerebral angiography for the next 25 years. In 1951 Engeset, the radiologist who worked with Torkildsen in Oslo, reported on 2000 angiograms performed with Abrodil, many of these by percutaneous injection. In that year, the Swedish neurosurgeon Norlén came to London to discuss 44 angiographically proved aneurysms that had been treated by direct assault. At the same time, James Bull, back from Stockholm to be assistant radiologist at the National Hospital, Queen Square, described over 1000 successful percutaneous cerebral angiograms; his article was one of the first modern monographs of intracranial arterial diseases (Bull, 1950).

The need for someone with the ability to inject each of the four cerebral arteries in the neck safely and confidently helped to spawn the modern neuroradiologist 40 years ago. When image intensification brought safety to catheter studies in the 1960s, transfemoral arteriography replaced the four-needle technique and the need for such skills diminished. A string of improvements coinciding with the advent of catheter angiography ensured that the decade of the 1960s was the high noon of cerebral angiography. These advances included ultrafast serial angiography, magnified and subtracted images, and more concentrated but less toxic iodine agents.

Perversely, the central role of angiography in intracranial diagnosis thereafter receded. The new scanning techniques, apart from being non-invasive, have proved to be more reliable in the diagnosis of mass lesions, by revealing their specificity and site better. With mass lesions no longer an indication, angiography now has a more limited use as a primary investigation, notably in demonstrating berry aneurysms. It also remains an important way of providing the surgeon with preoperative information in cases of arterial occlusion and in demonstrating the blood supply and drainage of mass lesions in certain sites. For these reasons and because of the indispensability of the catheter technique in therapeutic embolisation, brain angiography has an assured future.

Scintigraphy

This was the first successful brain imaging tech-nique utilising an energy source other than X-rays. Radionuclide imaging involves introducing an appropriate radioactive substance into the patient's body, and then counting the photons (gamma rays) emitted from the part to be examined. The favoured isotope for the brain is ^{99m}Tc-pertechnetate, given preferably by intravenous injection (half-life only 6 hours). The original apparatus was the *rectilinear scanner* with a single-photomultiplier head, which moved back and forth across the brain orthogonally to make the count, like a lawnmower cutting the grass. It was superseded by H.A. Anger's *gamma camera*, which contains an array of photomultipliers and remains stationary during the count, like taking a portrait photograph (Fig. 1.12).

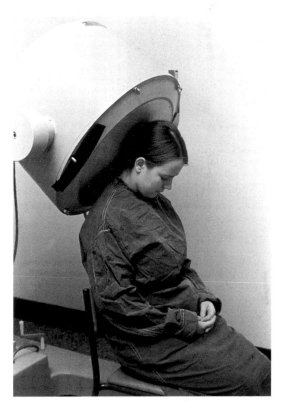

Fig. 1.12 Scintillation (gamma) camera. The patient is correctly positioned against its detectors for a posterior scintigram of the brain.

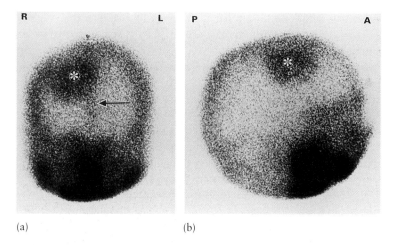

(a)   (b)

Fig. 1.13 Right parasagittal meningioma (asterisk) shown by frontal (a) and right lateral (b) scintigrams made with a gamma camera. Physiological uptake in the superior sagittal (arrow) and sigmoid sinuses provide anatomical window-frames which are useful for topographical localisation of brain lesions. R, Right; L, left; P, posterior; A, anterior.

Apparatus refinements included the *section scanner*, which can count selected slices of tissue. Devised by D.E. Kuhl in the early 1960s, this apparatus uses the tomographic principle by utilising two or more detector heads fitted to the scanner. (Tomography is the radiation technique which provides an image of a slice of tissue at a chosen level.) The acronyms ECAT (emission computer-assisted tomography) and SPECT or SPET (single-photon emission computed tomography) are now applied to section scanning. Although scintigraphic slicing yields superior information, SPET has proved to be no clinical match for CT and magnetic resonance (MR) scanning. Another advance is the positron camera, which is a refinement of the gamma camera permitting positron emission tomography (PET). Two opposed detectors are used to count the emissions of a positron-emitting radionuclide such as fluorine-18. The potential benefit of PET lies not as a competitor to routine CT or MR scanning but in functional studies by mapping areas of brain activity.

The gamma camera was the standard clinical tool for intracranial diagnosis in the early 1970s. It helped radiologists and their clinical colleagues come to terms with the new world of 'non-invasive' imaging. It was a safe and reliable screening method which, until swept aside by CT and MR imaging (MRI), gave results which were often adequate for surgical management. For example, it provided sufficient information for surgeons to perform biopsies and to remove tumours or subdural haematomas without recourse to additional pneumography or angiography. The background radiation present in the venous sinuses provides useful topographical orientation for accurately siting lesions ('hot spots') (Fig. 1.13). Scintigraphy has a 90% diagnostic accuracy in detecting hemispherical lesions (Burrows, 1972). However, surgeons point to the shortcoming which eliminates scintigraphy as a 'one-stop' preoperative test, namely, its failure to image the cerebral ventricles, and thereby to indicate the effect of a lesion on the brain.

Computerisation

To the brain-imager, the year 1970 is the equivalent of the historian's 1914: it was the year that the old order collapsed and disappeared. Computed techniques swept away conventional neuroradiology for ever. The finality of this change was reflected in the conference jokes at that time—1970 marked the changeover from BC (before computerisation) to AD (after digitalisation). Of all the marriages arranged after 1970 between computers and medicine, that with X-ray tomography was the first and it remains by far the most successful. CT is the greatest advance in clinical diagnosis of the brain since Röntgen's discovery.

Computed tomography (CT)

Moniz spoke of body organs as being 'mute', and by this he meant that they were unresponsive or inaccessible to imaging. His own efforts and those of others such as Dandy were directed at breaching this barrier through introducing radio-opaque substances into the skull. What Moniz and others failed to explore was the possibility of improving the picture of the X-ray beam emerging from the patient's head. This is what the computer link achieved, yielding an immensely enhanced image on a television screen, which could never be accomplished with photographic emulsion.

Godfrey Hounsfield was an electronics engineer in the central research laboratories of Electrical and Musical Industries (EMI) Ltd. London, who in the 1960s was engaged in pattern recognition experiments in the music industry. While neither a physicist nor a doctor, he perceived the diagnostic potential of image computerisation more clearly than others. In 1967 he set out to solve the practical difficulties, and within a year he had built a tabletop model which could scan sections of human brain (Hounsfield, 1973). Four years later the prototype EMI brain scanner was installed at Atkinson Morley Hospital, Wimbledon (Fig. 1.14), and in October 1971 the first patient was examined there (Fig. 1.15). James Ambrose, the neuroradiologist working with Hounsfield, announced the discovery at the annual meeting of the British Institute of

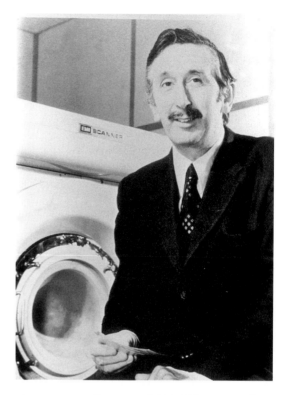

Fig. 1.14 Sir Godfrey Hounsfield, British inventor of computed tomography (CT), photographed in 1970 beside the world's first CT scanner. Designed only to examine the brain, Hounsfield's EMI scanner cradled the patient's head in a water-filled bathing cap during the examination.

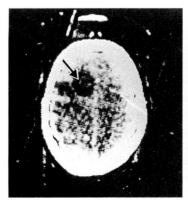 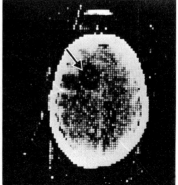

Fig. 1.15 The first clinical CT scan, 1971. The patient had a cystic glioma of the left frontal lobe (arrow). (Convention was that slices were displayed as if viewed from the top.) Left image made with 160 × 160 matrix, right image with 80 × 80 matrix.

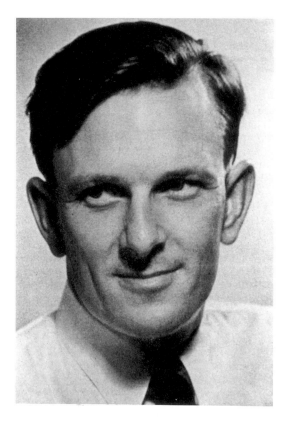

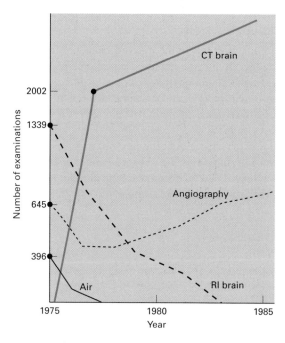

Fig. 1.17 The impact of computerisation. This graph shows the dramatic effect upon conventional neuroradiological practice of installing a CT scanner. Figures from the Wessex Neurological Centre, Southampton, in 1975–85. RI, radionuclide imaging; air, air encephalography.

Fig. 1.16 Professor Allan Cormack, Cape Town physicist and fellow Nobel Prizewinner with Hounsfield, who validated the theoretical basis of CT scanning.

Radiology on 19 April 1972 (Ambrose, 1973), and in 1974 he and a colleague reviewed their first 650 patients (Paxton & Ambrose, 1974).

Hounsfield shared a Nobel Prize with the scientist who validated the theoretical basis of the CT method. He was Allan Cormack, a professor of physics in Boston with an interest in X-ray absorption coefficients for use in radiotherapy (Fig. 1.16). Cormack, while still working in Cape Town, had the idea of using energy loss data to determine the variable density of matter, and he proved that this method was feasible (Cormack, 1963). Hounsfield acknowledged that he would not have been able to get his model to work without Cormack's theoretical solutions.

The impact of CT scanning in 1970 was imme-diate, and during the past 25 years demand for it has remained overwhelming. It was the clinicians' loss of confidence in conventional tests, such as skull radiography, pneumoencephalography and scintigraphy, which destroyed their viability. If the demands for CT could have been met imme-diately, their use would have atrophied even faster (Fig. 1.17): the flat peak of the CT curve reflects the clinical rationing imposed by the inadequate provision of CT scanners in the United Kingdom.

Magnetic resonance imaging (MRI)

MRI, the third non-invasive imaging method and the one to prove the most successful for imaging the brain, involves examining the patient in a mag-netic field. The germ of the idea was the paper of an American academic chemist published in the scientific journal *Nature*, in which he described a new imaging technique derived from the interaction of two magnetic fields (Lauterbur, 1973). The method was developed from an analytical technique used by chemists since the late 1940s, called *nuclear magnetic resonance*. Although early hopes were dashed that MRI would provide a means of differentiating cancer cells, its future was assured after the finding at the University of Nottingham that the MRI of anatomical detail was possible based purely on the measurement of water content (Mansfield *et al.*, 1980).

References

Ambrose, J. (1973) Computerised transverse axial scanning (tomography): Part 2. Clinical application. *Br. J. Radiol.* **46**, 1023–47.

Bull, J.W.D. (1950) Cerebral angiography. *Postgrad. Med. J.* **26**, 156–63.

Bull, J.W.D. (1961) History of neuroradiology. *Br. J. Radiol.* **34**, 69–84.

Burrows, E.H. (1972) False-negative results in brain scanning. *Br. Med. J.* **1**, 473–6.

Burrows, E.H. (1986) *Pioneers and Early Years: A History of British Radiology.* Colophon Press, Alderney, CI, p. 14.

Burrows, E.H. (1994) The imaging quarter: Stanley Graveson Memorial Lecture, Southampton, 9 October 1991. *Southampton Med. J.* **10**, 32–7.

Cormack, A.M. (1963) Representation of a function by its line integrals, with some radiological applications. *J. Appl. Phys.* **34**, 2722–7.

Dandy, W.E. (1918) Ventriculography following the injection of air into the cerebral ventricles. *Ann. Surg.* **68**, 5–11.

Dott, N.M. (1933) Intracranial aneurysms: cerebral arterio-radiography: surgical treatment. *Edinburgh Med. J.* **40**, 219–40.

Hounsfield, G.N. (1973) Computed transverse axial scanning (tomography): Part 1. Description of system. *Br. J. Radiol.* **46**, 1016–22.

Lauterbur, P.C. (1973) Image formation by induced local interaction: examples employing magnetic resonance. *Nature* **242**, 190–1.

Luckett, W.H. (1913) Air in the ventricles of the brain following a fracture of the skull. *Surg. Gynecol. Obstetr.* **17**, 237–40.

Lysholm, E. 1931 Apparatus and technique for roentgen examination of the skull. *Acta Radiol.* suppl. **12**, 1–120.

Lysholm, E., Ebenius, B. & Sahlstedt, H. (1935) Das Ventriculogramm. *Acta Radiol.* suppl. **24**, 1–75.

Mansfield, P., Morris, P.G, Ordidge, R.J., Pykett, I.L., Bangert, V. & Coupland, R.E. (1980) Human whole body imaging and detection of breast tumours by NMR. *Phil. Trans. Roy. Soc. London* **B289**, 503–10.

Moniz, E. (1927) L'Encéphalographie artérielle, son importance dans la localisation des tumeurs cérébrales. *Rev. Neurol. (Paris)* **2**, 72–90.

Moniz, E. (1931) *Diagnostic des Tumeurs Cérébrales et épreuve de Encephalographie Arterielle.* Masson, Paris.

Paxton, R. & Ambrose, J. (1974) The EMI scanner: a brief review of the first 650 patients. *Br. J. Radiol.* **47**, 530–65.

Röntgen, W.C. (1896) On a new kind of rays. (Translation by Arthur Stanton.) *Nature* **53**, 274–6.

2: Computed Tomography

A. R. Valentine

Introduction

Tomography (from the Greek, *tome*, section) is the radiographic technique of isolating a plane of interest in a subject by blurring out adjacent planes. An X-ray tube moves above the patient in one direction and the film beneath the patient in the other. Only objects in the same plane as the fulcrum about which this apparatus turns are projected 'in focus' on to the X-ray film. Everything else is blurred out in proportion to its distance from this plane (Fig. 2.1).

Computed tomography (CT) uses a very narrow beam of X-rays so that only the plane of interest is irradiated (Fig. 2.2). The emergent X-ray beam impinges on a radiation detector system which records how much it has been reduced in intensity (attenuated) by intervening tissue. These data are converted into digital form, making them amenable to computer processing, and from them an image is reconstructed. CT has become the most generally accepted term to denote this technique, although synonyms have abounded, including computerised axial tomography, computerised transmission tomography and computer-assisted tomography. The development of CT technology proved to be one of the major innovations in modern medicine and its use proved revolutionary, particularly in the context of imaging for neurological disease, although here magnetic resonance imaging (MRI) has subsequently replaced it as the prime modality.

The physical basis of computed tomography

A CT examination yields a series of sectional images, usually transverse to the long axis of the subject, which reflect the radiographic densities of tissues in the plane of scanning. The operation involves data acquisition, data processing and image presentation. Data acquisition is the function of the scanner gantry, which houses both the X-ray source and detector system. Data processing involves the calculation of radiographic density for each point in the tissue section from the raw data accumulated by the radiation detectors. Image presentation refers to the way in which these numerical data are converted into a diagnostically meaningful image.

CT images have become a familiar diagnostic tool and it is easiest to consider the way in which the image is presented first, before looking at the acquisition and processing of the data from which it is derived.

Image presentation

The CT image represents a grey-scale depiction of radiographic densities across a 'slice' of tissue irradiated by the rotating X-ray tube. This slice has a finite thickness set partly by the requirements of the particular study being undertaken (usually 5–10 mm for brain examinations) and a finite resolution set by physical limitations on detector size and other factors. Each slice is divided into a matrix (grid) of cubes ('voxels'). Measurements are made of the average radiographic density of all the tissue contained in each small cube.[1] Early CT machines used an 80×80 matrix. Modern scanners use a 512×512 matrix.

---

[1] Or rather cuboid, since all sides are not equal.

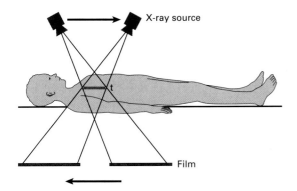

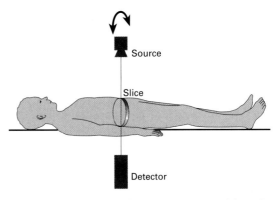

Fig. 2.1 Plain-film tomography. During a long exposure the X-ray source moves in one direction and the film in the other. Everything in the plane about which they pivot (for example, the trachea, t) remains in focus, but structures more anterior or posterior are blurred.

Fig. 2.2 A narrow beam of radiation is projected through the plane of interest (e.g. transverse, upper abdomen) and the intensity of the emerging radiation measured by a detector. An image of the whole slice is built up by multiple readings from multiple projections.

The width of each voxel is set by the size of the matrix and the depth by the thickness of the slice. The radiographic density of each voxel is represented in the final image by its two-dimensional equivalent, the picture element, or 'pixel' (Fig. 2.3).

The radiographic density calculated for each voxel depends on the mixture of tissue it contains. Bone is very radiodense, air radiolucent and brain intermediate. Standardisation of density measurements is achieved by assigning a CT number to each voxel according to its calculated radiodensity relative to water:

$$\text{CT number} = 1000 \cdot (\mu_x - \mu_{water})/\mu_{water},$$

where μ_x is the radiodensity (or attenuation coefficient, see below) of tissue x. Water has a CT number of 0, air -1000. Tissues denser than water have positive values, tissues less dense have negative values, in a range that usually encompasses CT numbers from -1000 to about $+3000$, where dense bone is approximately $+2000$. In deference to the inventor of CT (Hounsfield, 1973) this measurement range is called the Hounsfield scale and its units of measurement Hounsfield units (HU). Each pixel is allocated a shade of grey according to the CT number assigned to its voxel equivalent, with black indicating low density and white high density.

'Window' width and 'window' levels

The range of radiodensity found in human tissue covers a large proportion of the Hounsfield scale

Fig. 2.3 (a) Each section is divided into a finite number of blocks, called voxels, whose length and breadth are functions of the tissue matrix and the field of view. Voxel depth is determined by slice thickness. (b) The average radiodensity of each voxel is represented by its corresponding pixel.

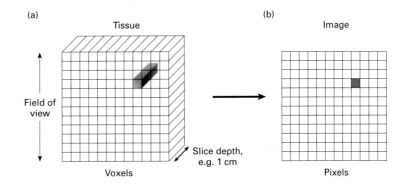

from air to cortical bone, and yet the range of densities found within an area of interest (for example, the brain) may be very narrow. The human eye is capable of discriminating only a limited number of shades of grey between black and white, which means that, in the absence of any manipulation of the measurement scale, contrast between tissues in an area of interest may not be appreciated. The measurement scale can be manipulated, however, a process called 'windowing'.

The term 'window' refers to the actual range of radiographic densities represented by the grey scale. In the brain, the bulk of normal tissue is encompassed by CT numbers from 0 (cerebrospinal fluid (CSF)) to 39 (grey matter) with white matter in between at 32. Reducing the number of HU represented in the grey scale produces visible contrast between normal anatomical structures and allows detection of subtle differences in density due to pathological change (Fig. 2.4). Plaques of demyelination, for example, usually cause only a minimal diminution in radiodensity compared with normal white matter, and these have to be represented by visually appreciable shades of grey for detection.

The brain is usually viewed at a window width of about 80 HU, with the central point on the grey scale at about 30. This latter point is referred to as the window level, whose value is also crucial to optimum visualisation of normal anatomy and pathology. At these settings, grey and white matter occupy median shades of grey, grey matter lighter than white matter, and CSF appears dark (Figs 2.4 & 2.5). Any tissue with a CT number equal to or less than −10 (e.g. fat or air) will appear black. Any tissue with a CT number equal to or greater than +70 (e.g. blood, calcium or bone) will appear white. Clearly, tissues lying on either side of the grey scale range cannot be distinguished from each other purely on the basis of their brightness. This depends on other observations such as location and morphology. Where necessary window levels and window widths can be adjusted, or precise measurements made of the average density over a small area defined by a cursor on the viewing console.

Different window widths and window levels are used in different parts of the body. In the petrous temporal bone, where contrast in the image is between air (−1000) and dense bone (+2000), very wide windows are used.

Partial-volume effect

The CT image is made up of square pixels, each

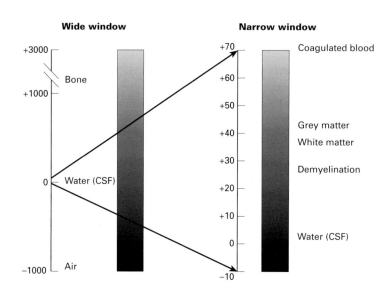

Fig. 2.4 Narrowing the window width allows structures which have only small differences in radiodensity between them to be detected on the CT image. Typically the brain is viewed at a window width of about 80 units, centred around 30. All tissues with a CT number greater than 70 will appear white and all tissues with a value less than −10 will appear black.

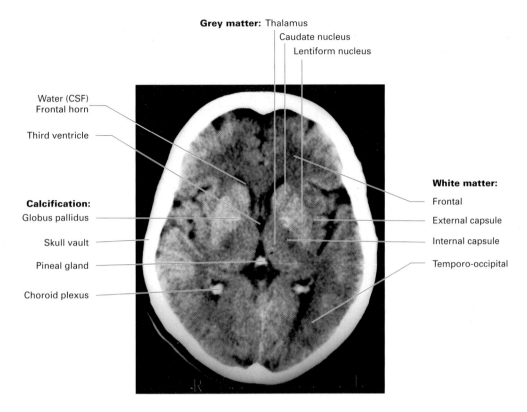

Grey matter: Thalamus
Caudate nucleus
Lentiform nucleus

Water (CSF)
Frontal horn

Third ventricle

White matter:

Frontal

Calcification:

Globus pallidus — External capsule

Skull vault — Internal capsule

Pineal gland — Temporo-occipital

Choroid plexus

Fig. 2.5 Physiological densities in CT scanning at a window width of 80 units centred at 30.

of which has been allocated a CT number according to the radiodensity of tissue in its corresponding voxel (Fig. 2.3). Often, however (and increasingly with thicker sections), more than one tissue will be present in any voxel and the CT number will represent an average of their radiodensities. This phenomenon is referred to as the partial-volume effect or volume averaging. In the brain, volume averaging may be seen in relation to the ventricular system, for example, when the uppermost parts of the bodies of the lateral ventricles project into the slice containing the corpus callosum and corona radiata, producing a localised, but ill-defined, reduction in the average radiodensity. Review of adjacent slices usually resolves any difficulty in interpretation. Calcium is very dense and relatively small amounts will make a considerable difference to the average radiodensity of a voxel (Fig. 2.6).

Partial-volume averaging can never be avoided entirely because every scan is of finite thickness. It can be minimised with thin sections and fine matrices but at a cost of increased radiation dose and reduced contrast resolution.

Spatial resolution and contrast resolution

Spatial resolution refers to the ability of a system to distinguish two small high-contrast objects separated by only a small distance. It is determined by numerous factors, which include scanner geometry, reconstruction algorithms and display parameters. There must be a pixel of different value on either side of the pixel containing the object for resolution to be possible. Modern scanners can separate high-contrast objects less than 0.5 mm apart. This is still inferior to plain film resolution, which is about 10 times better than CT.

(a)

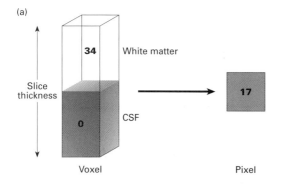

(b)

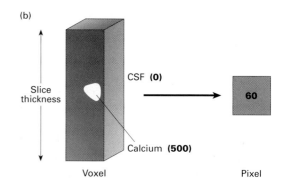

Fig. 2.6 Partial-volume averaging (voxel turned on its side compared with Fig. 2.3). (a) Equal contribution to the voxel by CSF (0 HU) and white matter (34 HU) averages to 17 HU. (b) The averaging effect of a small extreme radiodensity.

Contrast resolution refers to the minimum density difference required between an object and its environment before it can be detected. It is a measure of the sensitivity of a technique in distinguishing between objects of similar radiographic density. For an object to be detectable it must produce a sufficient difference in the locally absorbed radiation to raise (or lower) the recorded CT number above (or below) the expected level of statistical variation between voxels. Anything that reduces the normal statistical variation—increased radiation dose, increased voxel size—will improve contrast resolution (the latter affecting spatial resolution adversely). CT hugely outperforms plain radiography here. A 10% difference in density is required to distinguish an object from its surroundings on plain film, but objects with density differences of less than 0.5% can be discriminated on CT (Curry *et al.*, 1990).

Image reformatting

The orientation of the plane of scanning can be varied within limits dictated by scanner geometry and patient compliance. The ability to tilt the scanner gantry gives some flexibility, and in many patients coronal scans can be acquired directly, using this facility and either scanning with the patient prone and the neck extended, or supine in a 'head-hanging' position. Where this is impossible, or where sagittal views are required, images must be reconstructed from data acquired in the axial plane. This process is known as reformatting.

Scans can be reformatted in any plane. The best-quality reformatted images will be derived from narrow-section axial scans performed with no interslice gap, and the patient will have had to remain motionless throughout the acquisition of data. Spatial resolution in reformatted images is never as good as in images acquired directly.

Absorption of radiation in tissue (attenuation)

Before describing the acquisition and processing of data, it is worth looking for a moment at the way in which X-rays behave when they impinge on tissue and what it is we are trying to measure. The term radiodensity has been used in the preceding paragraphs, but it is actually shorthand for 'attenuation coefficient'.

Different tissues are distinguished on a radiograph or CT image because they exhibit differences in their ability to absorb radiation. Similarly, pathological change becomes detectable when it causes an alteration in a tissue's X-ray-absorbing power. The ability of a particular tissue to absorb radiation is largely dependent on electron density and is described by its linear attenuation coefficient, μ. If a parallel beam of radiation of intensity I_0 is incident on a block of tissue of thickness x, then the intensity of the radiation that emerges from the other side of the block (I) is given by the equation:

$$I = I_0 \cdot \exp(-\mu x),$$

where e is a constant (= 2.718), the base for the natural logarithm. This is an exponential function (Fig. 2.7). If a given thickness of absorber (x) reduces the intensity of the emergent radiation by a half, then twice that thickness will reduce its intensity by half again. The thickness of absorber required to reduce the intensity of the emergent radiation by a given percentage depends on the value of its attenuation coefficient, μ. The attenuation coefficient can be calculated if I, I_0 and x are known.

If two tissues of equal thickness but with differing attenuating coefficients (μ_1 and μ_2) are placed in the path of the radiation beam such that the radiation beam has to pass through them both, then the intensity of the emergent radiation is dependent on the attenuation coefficients and thicknesses of each (Fig. 2.8). The equation becomes:

$$I = I_0 \cdot \exp-(\mu_1 + \mu_2)x.$$

The attenuation coefficients, μ_1 and μ_2, cannot be calculated from the attenuating affects of the tissues on a single beam of radiation, but can be calculated if two beams of radiation are directed on to the tissues from different directions. In CT the entire tissue section is divided into a matrix of equal components (voxels, Fig. 2.3), commonly 512×512, and the attenuation coefficient must be calculated for each one before assigning it a CT number. This means that 261 144 separate attenuation coefficients have to be measured, requiring repeated measurements of transmitted radiation (I), following irradiation from multiple different directions.

Data acquisition (CT apparatus)

The earliest CT scanner employed an X-ray tube

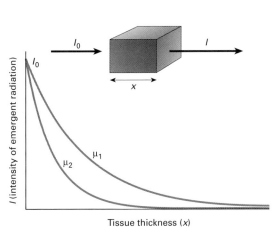

Fig. 2.7 The linear attenuation coefficient (μ) is a measure of the absorbing power of a particular tissue. The attenuation coefficient of a block of tissue of thickness x can be calculated by measuring the intensity of the emergent beam of radiation if the intensity of the incident radiation (I_0) and x are known. μ determines the slope of the graph (the graphs for two tissues with different attenuation coefficients are drawn).

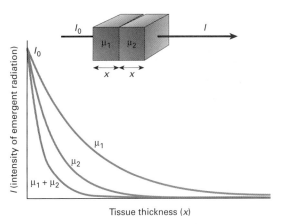

Fig. 2.8 When a tissue section is divided into blocks (voxels) of equal thickness, the intensity of the emergent beam is dependent on the sum of the individual attenuation coefficients of each block. Calculating each attenuation coefficient requires more than one equation, which is generated by irradiating tissue from different aspects and measuring the intensity of the emergent beam each time. The larger the matrix (more voxels), the greater the number of attenuation coefficients to be calculated and the greater the number of measurements that have to be made.

and a radiation detector held opposite each other in a rigid frame. The patient's head was placed between them. The tube emitted radiation, reduced by filters to a narrow 'pencil' beam. The radiation detector was shielded so that it would only detect unscattered radiation in the line of the radiation beam. The tube and detector passed across the patient's head (translation), transverse to the long axis, making a series of exposures covering the whole width of the head. Then the frame holding the tube and detector was rotated by 1° (rotation) and the process repeated. This was continued until 180 passes had been made at increments of 1° (Fig. 2.9).

The translate–rotate movements of the first scanners were retained in the second generation of CT scanners, which used a fan beam of X-rays irradiating a short bank of detectors. This allowed more samplings per translation and a larger index of rotation, with a concomitant reduction in scanning time.

Modern scanners have produced further improvements in image quality and scanning speed. Third-generation scanners employ a rotate–rotate system, in which a fan-beam X-ray source is coupled with an arc array of detectors, but where the width of the beam is sufficient to cover the entire field of view, eliminating the requirement for translation of the X-ray tube. Data can therefore be acquired during a continuous rotation. Fourth-generation scanners employ a rotating X-ray tube and a complete circle of stationary detectors positioned within the gantry. This is called a rotate–stationary system.

Spiral/helical CT

More recently, the use of slip-ring technology has increased the speed of CT data acquisition. In conventional CT, the power source reaches the tube through a cable, which restricts its movement, and after each 360° rotation the machine has to stop, reverse direction and unwind the cable. By conducting the power through two rings which brush against each other, continuous rotation is made possible and data can be acquired as a continuous spiral (helical) slice while the patient is slowly moved through the gantry aperture on a motorised table. These data require some additional computer processing in order to present images of contiguous parallel slices but examination times are measured in seconds rather than in minutes.

X-ray tubes and detectors are bulky and heavy. Image data may be acquired in fractions of a second by eliminating the necessity to move them around the patient. X-rays are produced when high-velocity electrons strike a tungsten target. This is what happens inside an X-ray tube. If the

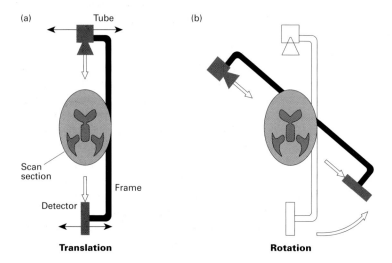

Fig. 2.9 Early CT scanner with one X-ray tube and one detector. The detector was attached to the tube by a rigid frame. (a) The detector took readings of the emergent radiation intensity as the tube moved across the head. (b) After each pass the frame was rotated by 1° and the process repeated. (Forty-fifth rotation depicted.)

X-ray tube in the scanner gantry is replaced by a ring of tungsten, then a beam of electrons generated outside the scanner can be directed around the ring, using magnetic deflecting coils. Changing the direction of the electron beam requires no moving parts. X-rays generated in the target ring are directed on to the subject and measurements made by an array of stationary detectors in the usual way. Ultrafast CT scanning of this capability, however, is more appropriate to cardiac studies than neuroradiology, as image quality is not optimal.

Data processing

The mathematics involved in the production of a sectional image from the intensity of transmitted (narrow-beam) radiation has been understood for many years (Radon, 1917). The problem has been simply that of the enormous data load. A matrix of 512 × 512 contains 261 144 voxels. Working out their attenuation coefficients requires a minimum of 261 144 calculations of the type already described:

$$I = I_0 \cdot \exp -(\mu_1 + \mu_2 + \cdots + \mu_{261144})x.$$

Such problems have had to await the development of modern computing before they could be tackled, and, even here, a variety of mathematical 'short cuts' have had to be employed in order to reduce the time between data acquisition and image production.

'Iterative' (repetitive) reconstruction is a well-known mathematical device for estimating the composition of a matrix containing a large number of variables, where more exact methods have become too cumbersome to be of practical use. This was the technique applied in the first CT scanner. It involves asking the computer to guess at the composition of the final image, and then to start adjusting this estimate in line with the measured data. Usually, the first assumption is that all points on the image matrix will have the same CT number. This estimated image is then repeatedly corrected to fit in with detector readings from each translation in turn. Every correc-

tion introduces errors that affect the validity of the previous calculation, but when the whole cycle is repeated, estimated values for the image matrix tend towards a solution that satisfies all projections within acceptable limits. Many cycles (iterations) may have to be completed before this stage is reached, and the earliest images took several hours to reconstruct.

'Back-projection' was first applied to image reconstruction in nuclear-medicine scanning (Kuhl & Edwards, 1963, 1968). As before, for every line irradiated, a single attenuation value is calculated from the detector readings which represents the sum of all the attenuating objects in the path of the radiation beam. In back-projection reconstruction this value is projected back across the width of the image matrix towards the radiation source. Each point in the image, along the projected ray, is given the attenuation value of the whole ray (Fig. 2.10). As the number of projections increases, the image of an object becomes more accurate, although background 'noise' generated by this technique is considerable.

A modified form of back-projection is the method of reconstruction in commonest use today. Here back-projected rays are mathematically adjusted (often by a process of Fourier transformation (Shepp & Logan, 1974)), by the addition of negative values at their edges, to increase the sharpness of the objects displayed by their sum (Brooks & DiChiro, 1975).

Image storage

The reconstructed image is displayed on a viewing console, where adjustments can be made to the window level and window width for optimum diagnostic quality. Two views at different settings may be necessary to present all the relevant information. Raw data (detector readings) are temporarily stored on a hard magnetic disc, but once satisfactory images have been obtained they are discarded because of the large amount of disc space they occupy. Image data (voxel CT numbers) are retained and may be transferred to magnetic

(a)

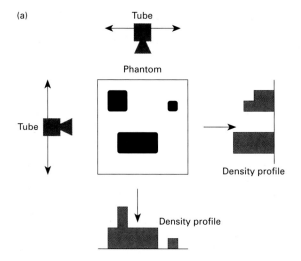

(b)

Tube

Tube

Phantom

Density profile

Density profile

Image

Fig. 2.10 Back-projection method of image reconstruction demonstrated on an X-ray 'phantom' containing three objects. (a) During scanning each translation (two shown) produces a profile of density readings representing the sum of all the attenuating objects in the field of view. (b) The computer projects each density profile back on to the image along the axis from which it was derived. Only two projections shown, but, as data from each translation are added to the reconstructed image, the image becomes an increasingly accurate representation of the objects in the phantom. 'Noise' in the image derives from regions where the back-projected rays indicate a density reading but where there is no object. (NB. Dark = high density here.)

diskette, magnetic tape or an optical disc. Hard copy is recorded on X-ray film by a camera.

Procedure in cranial CT

Scanning procedure

Each study is initiated by positioning the patient carefully in the scanner gantry and performing a projection radiograph, named variously by different manufacturers as a topogram, scannogram or scout view. This image, which resembles a conventional radiograph, is achieved by moving the patient steadily through the gantry aperture while pulsed X-ray exposures are made with the X-ray tube and detectors stationary (Fig. 2.11). Cursor lines are then applied to the image to delineate the desired scan planes, these being limited by a maximum gantry tilt of + or –30° in most CT scanners.

Modern machines allow slice widths from 1 or 2 mm up to 8 or 10 mm. The field of view can be reduced, or 'targeted', over an area of interest, producing smaller voxels with the same matrix size, thereby increasing spatial resolution, though with the penalty of some loss of contrast resolution.

Scanning protocols

The CT examination will vary depending on the clinical problem under investigation. All CT machines have a number of scanning options (protocols) for different clinical problems, but these can be modified, if necessary, as results emerge. A standard cranial scan produces contiguous scans with a slice width of 8–10 mm, from the foramen magnum to the vertex. This slice width gives good contrast resolution at an acceptable radiation dose and adequate spatial resolution, providing reasonable sensitivity in the detection of parenchymal abnormality. An increase in spatial resolution and a reduction in the partial volume phenomenon may be obtained

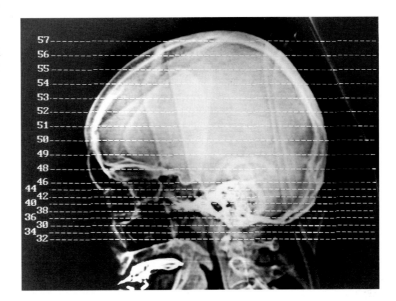

Fig. 2.11 Scanned projection radiographs, 'scout view'. Planes of sections examined in a full cranial study. Note that narrower slices are employed in the posterior fossa compared with the supratentorial compartment.

by reducing the slice width to 3 to 5 mm but there is a penalty in reduced contrast resolution. This is fairly standard practice in the examination of the posterior fossa.

Routine cranial CT is usually performed parallel to the radiographic baseline (external auditory meatus to outer canthus of the eye). If the posterior fossa is under particular suspicion, tilting the gantry may reduce artefact. Gantry tilt may also be used to bring the neuro-ocular plane fully into the scan field for optic-nerve and chiasmal studies.

The pituitary region may be examined with contiguous axial scans (usually 2 mm thick), followed by reformatting in the sagittal and coronal planes, or by direct coronal scanning from the outset. The clinical picture may give a clue as to the underlying pathology and therefore the technique likely to be most useful: the suspicion of a pituitary microadenoma, for example, would be best explored by direct coronal scanning using thin slices, while a clinical presentation indicating chiasmal compression suggests a substantial suprasellar component, in which case axial scanning and reformatting are probably more versatile, not least because satis-

factory sagittal and axial images cannot usually be generated from coronal images.

Anatomical regions with inherent high radiographic contrast can be studied with high spatial resolution techniques, as, for example, in the paranasal sinuses and petrous temporal bones where the main tissue interfaces involve bone, air and soft tissue. For the middle and inner ear, slice thicknesses as small as 1 mm give very good spatial resolution. At the craniocervical junction, bone, CSF and soft tissue interface, and, although thin slices may be required for adequate definition of the bony anatomy and to allow detailed reformatting, contrast resolution must be preserved to distinguish the neuraxis from CSF.

Intravenous contrast material in cranial CT

The use of intravenous contrast material is intended to increase the sensitivity of CT in the detection of abnormality, and sometimes to improve the specificity of diagnosis. Iodine is the constituent element providing radiographic contrast in the agents used in routine practice, the relationship between iodine concentration in tissue and attenuation value being linear. A concentration of 1 mg iodine/ml increases tissue attenuation by about 25 HU (Gado *et al.*, 1975).

Enhancement of tissue is potentially biphasic, with an early rapid peak predominantly reflecting intravascular contrast density and a subsequent phase predominantly reflecting extravascular contrast (Kormano & Dean, 1976). Most enhanced scans are obtained during the second phase, which may persist for several hours. The brain is protected by the blood–brain barrier, which, under normal conditions, prevents contrast material from leaving the vascular compartment. Disease processes which disrupt the blood–brain barrier allow contrast to pass into the extravascular space, and this is detectable at CT as pathological enhancement.

Enhancement of normal intracranial structures is seen where the blood–brain barrier does not exist, i.e. in the dura mater, choroid plexus, posterior pituitary gland and pituitary stalk, as well as in arterial and venous structures. Intracranial lesions which are primarily 'extra-axial', such as pituitary tumours, meningiomas and cranial-nerve neuromas, have no blood–brain barrier and may enhance due to a combination of inherent vascularity and extravascular passage of contrast.

Intravenous contrast is frequently used to elucidate plain-scan abnormalities, i.e. to increase the specificity of abnormal features. An enhanced scan may allow a more convincing differentiation of tumour from surrounding oedema when compared with the plain scan. The multifocal nature of a tumour may only be appreciable after contrast injection. The presence of loculation in an abscess or remote further lesions may, similarly, only be apparent after intravenous contrast. Infection of an extracerebral collection may be suggested by intense enhancement of membranes.

Occasionally, it is reasonable to administer contrast before commencing the examination, for example, in the search for pituitary microadenoma, or in the follow-up of established lesions such as abscess or metastatic disease, although the risk of confusing calcification, blood and enhancement then arises.

Limitations of CT

Even with the fast scan times of modern machines (1–5 s) patient immobility is a requisite and the restless or uncooperative patient may require sedation or general anaesthesia. CT scan images are subject to degradation by artefact from metallic foreign bodies such as neurosurgical clips, metallic plates and dental amalgam. Other artefacts are a product of data acquisition, e.g. from 'beam hardening' due to a heterogeneity in the energy of incident radiation, or partial-volume averaging, others a product of the method of data processing, and yet others due to malfunctions in these operations.

As in plain-film tomography, patient compliance and scanner geometry set limits on the number of possible scanning orientations. Axial sections can be reformatted in sagittal, coronal or oblique orientations but the value of these images is limited by the loss of spatial resolution.

Any CT scan represents a compromise between what is an acceptable radiation dose to the patient and the best possible image quality, with contrast and spatial resolution suffering if radiation exposure is to be limited. Image aesthetics should be a secondary consideration.

CT compared with MRI

The development of CT continues, even while MRI becomes increasingly widely available, and inevitably there will be some overlap in the indications for their use. Clearly, with its vastly superior soft-tissue discrimination, MRI offers distinct advantages over CT in brain imaging. However, some questions are addressed equally well by either modality and there are others where CT has an advantage over MRI. CT provides high-quality images of bone and a good assessment of bone destruction or erosion. Similarly, calcium is easily seen on CT but is represented, with less sensitivity, as signal void on MRI. Acute haemorrhage is represented by high density within a few hours on CT, and acute subarachnoid haemorrhage or haemorrhagic change in a subacute infarct may be obvious on CT where it is invisible on MRI.

These considerations ensure that a role in neuroradiological diagnosis will remain for CT, even apart from its use in imaging patients who, for various reasons, cannot be imaged by MRI. Indeed, CT is sometimes useful following MRI to further elucidate the nature of an abnormality.

References

Brooks, R.A. & DiChiro, G. (1975) Theory of image reconstruction in computed tomography. *Radiology* **117**, 561–72.

Curry III, T.S., Dowdey, J.E. & Murry, R.C. (1990) *Christensen's Physics of Diagnostic Radiology*, 4th edn, pp. 314–17. Lea & Fabiger, Philadelphia.

Gado, M.H., Phelps, M.E. & Coleman, R.E. (1975) An extravascular component of contrast enhancement in cranial computed tomography. *Radiology* **117**, 589–93.

Hounsfield, G.N. (1973) Computerized transverse axial scanning (tomography): part 1. Description of the system. *Br. J. Radiol.* **46**, 1016–22.

Kormano, M. & Dean, P.D. (1976) Extravascular contrast material: the major component of contrast enhancement. *Radiology* **121**, 379–82.

Kuhl, D.E. & Edwards, R.Q. (1963) Image separation radioisotope scanning. *Radiology* **80**, 653–62.

Kuhl, D.E. & Edwards, R.Q. (1968) Reorganizing data from transverse section scans of the brain using digital processing. *Radiology* **91**, 975–83.

Radon, J. (1917) On the determination of functions from their integrals along certain manifolds. *Berichte uber die Verhandlungen der koniglich Sachsischen Gessellschaft der Wissenschaften zu Leipzig. Mathamatisch – Physische Klasse* **69**, 262–77.

Shepp, L.A. & Logan, B.F. (1974) The Fourier reconstruction of a head section. *IEEE Trans. Nucl. Sci.* **NS21**, 21–43.

3: Principles of
Structural Magnetic Resonance Imaging

J. N. P. Higgins, A. D. Platts and S. M. Pickman

Prologue

FLASH, FLAIR, FISP and FSE. Spin–echo, double echo, gradient echo and inversion recovery. Magnetic resonance imaging (MRI) has spawned a language, arcane at best, which disorientates and disheartens the newcomer. This chapter is written for the newcomer. Its aim is to present the fundamental principles of MRI using accepted physical models, but otherwise with the minimum use of analogy, and with the minimum of mathematics.

The text is divided into four parts. First, the phenomenon of nuclear magnetic resonance (NMR) is described in detail, an understanding here being pivotal to a proper understanding of what follows. Next, there is a description of the mechanism by which the magnetic resonance (MR) signal (the product of NMR) is transformed into an image. Again this is covered in some depth, because a grasp of this process facilitates an understanding of the imaging sequences described later. Thirdly, commonly used imaging sequences are presented which illustrate the principles outlined in the first two sections. Fast imaging techniques are discussed briefly, introducing some of the different approaches to the problem of how to reduce scanning time. Finally, there is a brief discussion of some of the more practical aspects of MRI. Special functional applications such as blood oxygen-level-dependent (BOLD) and NMR spectroscopy are discussed in Chapter 6.

Many texts discuss NMR in terms of quantum physics, with atoms being depicted as having to occupy one or other of two discrete energy levels. For the non-physicist this often means that the starting-point for an explanation of basic principles is an idea which is only partially understood. This approach is not a requirement, however, and an intuitive grasp of MRI can be developed using classical physics as the basis of discussion. This is the approach adopted here.

Introduction

Plain radiography and computerised tomography (CT) are based on the capacity of organic tissue to absorb X-rays in proportion to tissue (electron) density. In the former, an image is formed when X-rays are transmitted through the subject on to a photographic plate. In the latter, an image is calculated from data acquired when X-rays are transmitted on to radiation detectors.

MRI is based on the ability of organic tissue, placed in a magnetic field, to absorb energy from radio waves, and then re-emit it, in proportion to the mobile hydrogen ion concentration. Two processes have to be explained. First, what happens when radio waves impinge on organic tissue, i.e. the nature of NMR, and, second, how the product of this reaction (radio waves) is transformed into an image.

Nuclear magnetic resonance

The warming that occurs when an object is exposed to infrared radiation is a matter of common observation. In the presence of a magnetic field, however, certain elements will also absorb energy from radiation at the radio frequency (RF) end of the electromagnetic spectrum. The energy absorbed can be detected because, when the external source of radiation is turned off, energy is released again, which can be picked up by a radio receiver (Fig. 3.1). The basis of this process is an interaction between radio waves and atomic nuclei, called *nuclear magnetic resonance* (Bloch *et al.*, 1946; Purcell *et al.*, 1946).

The term 'resonance' is used because the frequency of the radiation to which these elements are subjected is critical. NMR will only occur at a frequency which corresponds to the natural frequency of the element in the magnetic field and, moreover, the natural frequency of the element dictates the frequency of the radiation which is re-emitted.

The behaviour of tuning-forks forms a useful mechanical analogy. If a vibrating tuning-fork is held next to a stationary tuning-fork, the second tuning-fork will pick up energy from the first, as long as their pitches are identical. The sound waves which are incident on the stationary tuning-fork must correspond to its natural frequency before they will cause it to resonate. There will be no energy exchange and no resonance if their pitches are different. The sound (energy) emitted by the second tuning-fork will be heard if the first is silenced (Fig. 3.2).

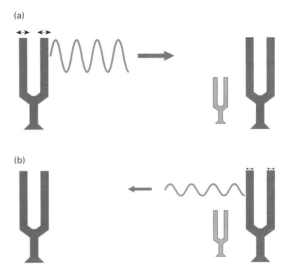

Fig. 3.2 (a) A stationary tuning-fork will start to resonate if held next to a vibrating tuning-fork of the same pitch. (b) The sound emitted by the second tuning-fork can be heard if the first is silenced and will be of the same frequency (pitch) as the first, but of lower amplitude.

Nuclear physics

What happens to atoms in a magnetic field and what does it mean to talk about them having a natural frequency?

The hydrogen ion comprises a single proton with a positive charge, spinning on its axis. Now, a fundamental law of physics states that a moving electrical charge is always accompanied by a magnetic field. A spinning charge therefore creates a magnetic field, which conforms to a magnetic dipole, which can be thought of as a tiny bar magnet with a north and south pole. This magnetic dipole is called a *magnetic moment* because of the way it is formed, and it represents a vector force whose strength and direction can be denoted by the length and orientation of an arrow (Fig. 3.3).

Any nucleus whose rotational movement creates a magnetic movement will be affected by an external magnetic field. In MRI, hydrogen is the most important, firstly, because of its abundance in organic tissue and, secondly, because it has a large magnetic moment relative to

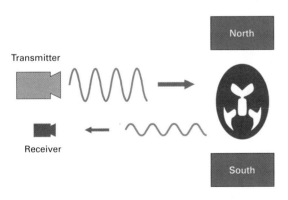

Fig. 3.1 Electromagnetic radiation will be absorbed by tissue in a magnetic field as long as its frequency is the same as the natural frequency of elements in the magnetic field. When the transmitter is turned off, the receiver will detect a returning signal of lesser amplitude but identical frequency.

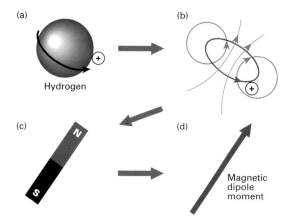

Hydrogen

Magnetic
dipole
moment

Fig. 3.3 (a) The hydrogen ion spins on its own axis. (b) A moving charge is always associated with a magnetic field (light grey lines) and a charge which moves in a circle creates a magnetic dipole (c). This is represented by an arrow (d) denoting its strength and orientation, and is called a magnetic dipole moment.

its mass, making it especially susceptible to a magnetic field. Further discussion in this text, therefore, is based on the hydrogen ion (a single proton), and the term 'proton' is used as a synonym for the hydrogen ion, rather than referring to the individual particles that make up larger atoms.

The net magnetisation vector

Hydrogen ions can be represented by arrows denoting the strength and direction of their magnetic moments. Normally these magnetic moments are aligned randomly in space and tissue has no overall magnetisation. However, in a magnetic field they experience a force analogous to that experienced by a compass needle, and a proportion of them become orientated along the lines of force of the magnetic field. The result is an induced magnetisation in tissue in the direction of the magnetic field, equal to the sum of the hydrogen ions which have changed their orientation in response to it. This magnetisation can also be represented by an arrow and is called the *net magnetisation vector* (NMV) (Fig. 3.4).

At rest, the orientation and strength of the NMV represents the stable, low-energy state which develops in tissue placed in a magnetic field, and to which tissue returns (still in a

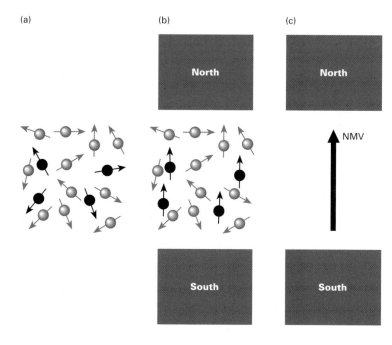

Fig. 3.4 (a) Protons are randomly orientated in the absence of a magnetic field. (b) A few protons (black) align themselves in response to a magnetic field, giving tissue a net magnetisation (c). NMV, net magnetisation vector.

Table 3.1 Mobile hydrogen ion concentration.

Tissue	H⁺ concentration
CSF/most pathology	High
Fat/grey matter	↓
White matter	Low
Cortical bone	Very low

magnetic field) after it has been disturbed. Only a small proportion of hydrogen ions respond to the magnetic forces acting upon them but nevertheless it is these ions that make up the NMV and which ultimately are responsible for the MRI signal. The size of the NMV (and hence the MRI signal) is dependent on the strength of the magnetic field, since the larger the magnetic field the greater the number of protons that will be induced to orientate along it.

The induction of magnetisation in tissue placed in a magnetic field is dependent upon the presence of hydrogen ions that can respond to the forces which act upon them, i.e. it is dependent upon the presence of *mobile* hydrogen ions. Hydrogen ions that are fixed in a rigid lattice (in bone, for example) will not contribute to magnetisation. Organic tissue is inhomogeneous and different regions will contribute different amounts towards the NMV of the whole organism, depending on the local concentration of hydrogen ions and their relative mobility. MRI, on an elementary level, is about detecting these differences and theoretically the simplest image would be equivalent to a map of mobile hydrogen ion concentrations, as defined by local magnetisation densities across a selected region (Table 3.1).

Precession and the Larmor equation

Only protons which have realigned along the magnetic field and which contribute to the NMV need be considered further. The remainder can be disregarded because their random orientation means they cancel out each other's effects (Fig. 3.4).

The alignment of these protons is, in reality,

more complex than has been suggested above. Rather than orientating exactly along the lines of magnetic force, their individual magnetic moments actually rotate (or wobble) about them, in the same way that the axis of a spinning-top rotates about the line of gravitational force (Fig. 3.5). This movement is called *precession* and it is the frequency of this movement that defines the natural frequency of protons in a magnetic field, and hence the frequency of electromagnetic radiation that will cause resonance.

The frequency of precession (ω) is proportional to the strength of the external magnetic field (B_0) and the simple formula that describes their relationship is known as the Larmor equation:

$$\omega = \gamma \cdot B_0,$$

where γ is the constant of proportionality called the *gyromagnetic ratio*, whose value depends on the element being observed, and where ω is measured in radians/s and B_0 is measured in tesla (T).

When the frequency of precession is measured in megahertz (MHz) (i.e. million cycles/s), the

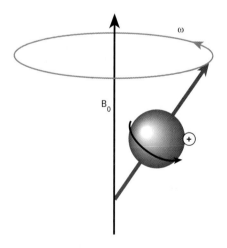

Fig. 3.5 In a magnetic field, protons (and their magnetic moments) 'wobble' around the lines of magnetic force (B_0) —a movement called precession. The frequency (ω) of this movement refers to the rate at which the magnetic moment turns about B_0.

(a)   (b)   (c)

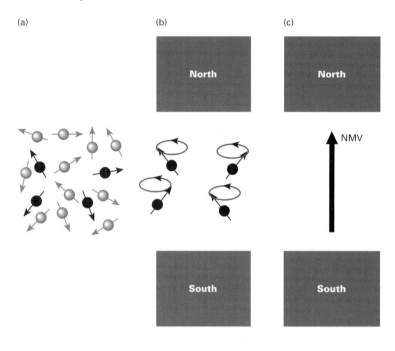

Fig. 3.6 The NMV is the sum of the longitudinal components of magnetisation of magnetic moments that reorientate in response to the external magnetic field. The remainder can be ignored. It is unaffected by the precessional motion of individual magnetic moments because they precess out of phase (see text), cancelling out any component of magnetisation in the transverse plane.

constant of proportionality changes, ω becomes f, but the relationship between precessional frequency and the magnetic field is unaltered. The equation becomes

$$f = (\gamma/2\pi) \cdot B_0.$$

The gyromagnetic ratio (divided by 2π) for hydrogen is 42.57 MHz/T, which means that the precessional frequency of hydrogen at 1.5 T, for example, is 63.86 MHz.

At rest, the orientation of the NMV is not affected by the precessional motion of individual magnetic moments because, although they precess at the same frequency, they are not in phase (see below) and any component of magnetisation in the transverse plane is cancelled out (Fig. 3.6).

Longitudinal and transverse magnetisation

The magnetic strength of a compass needle cannot be estimated unless it is displaced from its north/south orientation and a measurement taken of the force it exerts in trying to return to equilibrium. In the same way, the longitudinal magnetisation of tissue in a magnetic field cannot be measured directly. The equilibrium position must first be disturbed by tilting the NMV out of the longitudinal plane so that a component of magnetisation appears in the transverse plane, which can be detected.

Individual magnetic moments precessing around the axis of an external magnetic field will have components of magnetisation in both the longitudinal and transverse planes. The longitudinal component remains static whilst the transverse component rotates at the precessional frequency (Fig. 3.7a). The NMV, however, is the sum of all these individual magnetic moments and, unless disturbed, remains orientated along the lines of magnetic force. There is no *net* magnetisation in the transverse plane because, at any single moment, for every proton angled to one side of the magnetic field there will be another angled to the other side cancelling its effects in that plane (Figs 3.6 & 3.7b). Net transverse magnetisation will only appear if individual protons can be made to precess in phase, and this is achieved through the use of RF radiation.

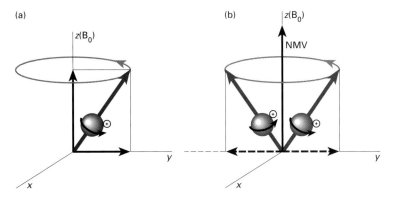

Fig. 3.7 (a) Individual magnetic moments have components of magnetisation (black arrows), longitudinal (*z*) and transverse (*y*) to the direction of the external magnetic field (B₀). The transverse component rotates around the longitudinal axis at the precessional frequency. (b) At equilibrium, however, the transverse components of magnetisation cancel (broken arrows), whilst their longitudinal components summate to form the net magnetisation vector. The NMV does not precess (two protons only shown). NB. Magnetic moments are drawn as if they arise from the same origin in order to show how their vectors summate. In reality, they are scattered throughout tissue, as shown in Fig. 3.6b, and it is helpful to remember this when considering how the MR signal decays (see text).

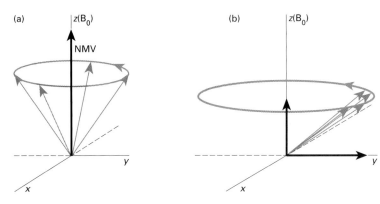

Fig. 3.8 Phase. (a) At equilibrium, magnetic moments (four shown) which have reorientated in response to the external magnetic field occupy all positions around the path of precession—they are 'out of phase'—and there is no net component of magnetisation transverse to the external magnetic field. (b) Electromagnetic radiation at the Larmor frequency throws precessing nuclei into phase, giving a net component of magnetisation (black arrow) in the transverse) (*xy*) plane. Longitudinal magnetisation is diminished by this process (see text) and the NMV (not drawn) is tilted away from the longitudinal axis.

Phase (transverse magnetisation)

The term *phase*, as applied to magnetic moments, refers to their position relative to each other on a 360° path around the axis of precession. At equilibrium, they are 'out of phase', being orientated in all positions around this circular path (Figs 3.6 & 3.8a). Electromagnetic radiation at the *Larmor frequency* upsets this equilibrium (see below) by forcing magnetic moments to orientate in the same direction relative to the axis of precession, i.e. to precess in phase (Fig. 3.8b). This is an unstable situation, but for a short time, before they move out of phase again, their vectors summate to produce a net component of magnetisation in the transverse plane, which can be measured.

Phase coherence (i.e. in-phase precession) and transverse magnetisation are inseparable. The greater the degree of phase coherence, the larger is the component of magnetisation in the transverse plane.

Resonance

The mechanism by which RF radiation induces protons to precess in phase and the manner in which they return to equilibrium go to the heart of the NMR experiment. These reactions are difficult to conceptualise, and with this in mind the following account has been divided into two parts: one simplified (but not simple), the other more comprehensive. The first account is designed to provide the newcomer with a working knowledge of basic principles, the second to satisfy the curiosity of those who have already had some exposure to the subject. This latter section would be better left to a second reading.

Resonance 1

A short pulse of RF radiation has two simultaneous effects on tissue in a magnetic field. It induces, first, a loss of magnetisation in the longitudinal plane and, second, the development of magnetisation in the transverse plane. It accomplishes this by tilting the NMV from a longitudinal into a transverse orientation. Two factors must apply before this can occur. First, the RF pulse must be at the Larmor frequency and, second, it must be incident on tissue at right angles to the direction of the magnetic field (Fig. 3.9).

The term 'electromagnetic radiation' describes the propagation of energy by a combination of oscillating electric and magnetic fields. RF radiation is associated with a magnetic field, and it is this field which exerts the destabilising force on the NMV. As already discussed, the NMV is a product of precessing magnetic dipoles but does not itself precess in the magnetic field induced by the main magnet. However, when a new magnetic force, induced by RF radiation, is superimposed at right angles to the main magnetic field, the NMV starts to precess around it. Precession about this axis rapidly turns the NMV towards the transverse plane and, if the RF radiation is turned off when the magnetisation vector has tilted by 90°, then longitudinal magnetisation will have disappeared and there will be maximum magnetisation in the transverse plane (Fig. 3.9).

Once the RF radiation has been turned off, the transversely orientated NMV starts to precess about the main magnetic field at the same rate as its constituent magnetic dipoles, i.e. at the Larmor frequency. Any magnetic vector rotating across lines of magnetic force must induce electromagnetic radiation, which will have an amplitude proportional to its size and a frequency equal to its frequency of rotation. This is the MR signal.

Resonance 2

How does the RF pulse cause the NMV to tilt into the transverse plane? Or, put another way, why does the NMV precess into the transverse plane about the magnetic field created by the RF radiation, if it was not precessing around the magnetic field created by the main magnet? Or, put another way, how can RF radiation cause the individual magnetic dipoles all to tilt in the same direction, when at equilibrium they are all at different phases of their precessional cycle, i.e. how is phase coherence generated out of phase incoherence?

How can the vector sum of two magnetic fields at right angles to each other (main magnetic field and RF field) cause the NMV to align completely with the second, especially when the second magnetic field is so much smaller than the first? Why does the RF radiation have to be at the Larmor frequency?

The answers to these questions can be found by looking at the behaviour of the individual magnetic moments that make up the NMV, and seeing how they respond to RF radiation.

Fig. 3.9 Nuclear magnetic resonance 1. (a) At equilibrium the NMV does not precess and is orientated along the main magnetic field (B_0). (b) Radio-frequency radiation is applied at right angles to B_0, exerting an additional magnetic force (B_{RP}, here drawn along the x axis) about which the NMV must precess. (c) If the radio-frequency radiation is turned off when the NMV has tilted by 90°, then longitudinal magnetisation will have disappeared and there will be maximum magnetisation in the transverse plane. Now precessional movement starts about the longitudinal axis, giving rise to the MR signal. (d) The strength of the MR signal is proportional to the size of the component of magnetisation in the transverse plane (thin black arrow on the y axis), and this fades as the NMV 'relaxes' back into equilibrium.

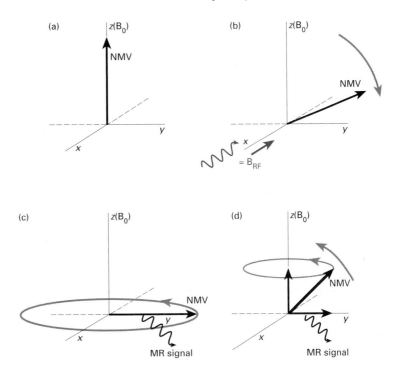

Remember that the phenomenon is one of resonance, where a small force (RF radiation) applied rhythmically can have large effects.

NMR is best observed using rotating coordinates. This may seem confusing at first, but it is a very effective device for reducing complex movements into simpler components. Think of it as stepping on to a fairground roundabout to get a proper look at the behaviour of the carnival horses. From this perspective their movements appear simple (up and down) because rotational movement relative to the ground can be ignored. Back on solid ground the insight gained through this adventure makes everything easier to understand.

Stationary coordinates in three dimensions are defined by three axes. The x and y axes represent coordinates at right angles to each other in the transverse plane. The z axis is at right angles to them both in the longitudinal plane. The z axis corresponds to the direction of the external magnetic field (and by convention is drawn as a vertical line, even though in most MRI scanners the orientation of the external magnetic field is

actually horizontal) (Fig. 3.10a). In a system of rotating coordinates the z axis is unchanged, but the x and y axes rotate about the z axis and are renamed the x' and y' axes.

In a coordinate system rotating at the precessional frequency, the x' and y' axes rotate about the z axis at the same speed as the precessing hydrogen ions which make up the NMV. *From this perspective*, therefore, these ions appear stationary (you have stepped on to the roundabout, Fig. 3.10b). They will seem to be behaving as if there were no magnetic field (since protons must precess in a magnetic field), representing instead merely a number of magnetic dipoles whose orientation happens to be such that their vector sum is aligned along the z axis. If a magnetic force is applied at right angles to the z axis (e.g. the x' axis) now, the magnetic dipoles (and the NMV they comprise) will respond as if it were the only magnetic force acting upon them and they will start to precess around it (Fig. 3.10c).

How is it possible to create a magnetic force

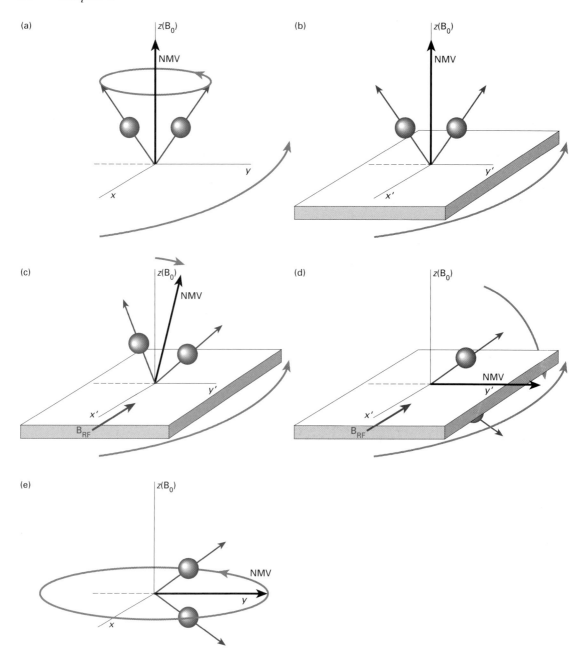

Fig. 3.10 Nuclear magnetic resonance. Radio-frequency radiation creates a magnetic field at right angles to the longitudinal axis (e.g. along the x' axis), which causes protons comprising the NMV to rotate (about x') into the transverse plane. (For simplicity only two protons are shown, but of course the NMV in (a) is the product of millions of magnetic dipoles spread out evenly along the path of precession. Work through the figures to see how the individual dipoles depicted respond to radio-frequency radiation. Then imagine how dipoles at other points on the precessional path would behave. See how the result would be a cone of dipoles tilted on its side with the NMV in its centre. Phase coherence generated in this way does not mean that all dipoles point in exactly the same direction, merely that their sum, the NMV, has been turned at right angles to the external magnetic field, B_0.)

that acts at right angles to the longitudinal (z) axis in a constant direction within a system of rotating coordinates? Only by creating a force that, in fact, rotates around the z axis exactly in time with the x' and y' axes, i.e. at the precessional frequency. Any form of electromagnetic radiation (including radio waves) carries its own oscillating magnetic field, and electromagnetic radiation at the precessional frequency will create just such a force if it is incident on tissue at right angles to the longitudinal axis.

What happens next to hydrogen ions *in this system of rotating coordinates* when this transverse magnetic force is applied, i.e. when the RF transmitter is switched on? As already stated, they start to precess around the new force, but, crucially, because the axis of precession has been turned into the transverse plane, there is immediately an imbalance between the number of protons angled to one side of the *new (x')* axis of precession and the number angled to the other, which is equal to the number of protons that comprised the original NMV in the longitudinal plane (Fig. 3.10c). In other words, relative to the x' axis, protons start their precessional movement in phase and the degree to which they are in phase, and hence the size of net magnetisation at right angles to the x' axis, equals the size of the original longitudinal magnetisation vector.

Although this magnetisation is at right angles to the magnetic force induced by the RF radiation, at first it is still longitudinal to the static external magnetic field and therefore cannot be measured. Before any significant dephasing can occur, however, precessional movement about the x' axis quickly turns protons away from their orientation around the z axis (Fig. 3.10c), and if the RF radiation is turned off when the NMV has turned by 90° (90° RF pulse), there will be maximum net magnetisation in the transverse plane (Fig. 3.10d).

The situation in stationary coordinates at the end of a 90° RF pulse ('pulse' because it is short-lived) (Fig. 3.10e) is similar to the situation in rotating coordinates at the beginning of the RF pulse (Fig. 3.10c). Immediately, protons start to precess around the external magnetic field again, but now there is a component of magnetisation in the transverse plane caused by an excess of protons orientated to one side of the longitudinal axis (Fig. 3.10e). These protons are in phase as they revert to precessing around the z axis, and the degree to which they are in phase, and hence the size of net magnetisation in the transverse plane, is equal to the size of the original longitudinal magnetisation vector. Now, this transverse magnetisation can be measured.[1]

In summary, a short burst of RF radiation at the Larmor frequency has been used as a device to tilt the NMV from a longitudinal orientation into the transverse plane. The original magnetisation vector is the result of an excess of hydrogen ions orientated along an external magnetic field. This is converted into an excess of hydrogen ions

[1] In the quantum approach to MR the 90° RF pulse deposits just enough energy in tissue to cause half the excess of protons orientated parallel to the magnetic field (low energy state, Fig. 3.4) to turn antiparallel (high energy state). Longitudinal magnetisation is thus abolished. Figure 3.10e equates with this position, with an equal number of protons orientated above and below the transverse plane. What the classical approach, encapsulated in Fig. 3.10, shows in addition is how these protons have been thrown into phase.

Fig. 3.10 *continued* (a) Stationary coordinates. At equilibrium the magnetic dipoles precess around the external magnetic field and the NMV is aligned along the z axis. (b) Rotating coordinates. x' and y' turn around the z axis at the precessional frequency, making the dipoles which comprise the NMV appear stationary. (You have stepped on to the roundabout.) (c) Rotating coordinates. Magnetic dipoles (and the NMV) respond to a magnetic force in the transverse plane (grey arrow along the x' axis) by starting to precess around it, and after a short time (d) the NMV will have turned into the transverse plane. (e) Stationary coordinates. The RF pulse can be turned off when the NMV has tilted by 90° into the transverse plane. Simple precessional movement then reasserts itself about the external magnetic field (z axis). Protons (or magnetic dipoles) are in phase by an amount proportional to the size of the original, longitudinally orientated NMV and there is magnetisation in the transverse plane.

angled to one side of the longitudinal axis compared with the other, i.e. converted into phase coherence. This transverse magnetisation equals the size of the original NMV.

It should now be easier to understand the whole interaction from the perspective of stationary coordinates (Fig. 3.11). Before the RF pulse, the NMV is aligned with the external magnetic field. RF radiation causes the NMV to tilt towards the transverse plane about an axis (x' axis) that is itself rotating in the transverse plane at the precessional frequency of hydrogen in the external magnetic field. The rate at which the NMV tilts about x', on the other hand, is dependent on the precessional frequency of hydrogen in the magnetic field created by the RF radiation (Fig. 3.10c). This field is several orders of magnitude smaller than the external magnetic field, and therefore the rate at which the NMV tilts towards the transverse plane is slow (see the Larmor equation) compared with the rate at which the axis about which it is tilting is rotating. The result

is that, under the influence of the RF radiation, the NMV performs a spiralling motion towards the transverse plane, which terminates when the RF pulse is turned off.

The MR signal and dephasing

The transverse magnetisation that develops following a 90° RF pulse is the vector sum of protons that are precessing in phase around the lines of force of the external magnetic field (Fig. 3.10e). Therefore, this vector must also rotate around the same axis at the precessional frequency. A magnetic vector rotating through lines of magnetic force produces electromagnetic radiation whose amplitude is proportional to its size and whose frequency equals its frequency of rotation. This emitted electromagnetic radiation is what constitutes the MR signal, with an amplitude dependent on the amount of magnetisation in the transverse plane and a frequency equal to the frequency of precession (Fig. 3.12).

What happens to transverse magnetisation and the MR signal at the end of a 90° RF pulse? It fades, as tissue returns to the stable, low-energy state, present before it was disturbed. Importantly, however, this is achieved not simply by a reversal of the movements just described. The creation of transverse magnetisation was brought

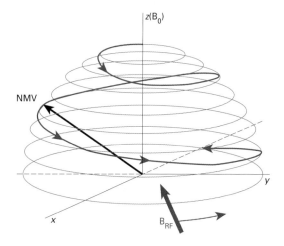

Fig. 3.11 Stationary coordinates. Under the influence of the RF pulse, protons precessing about the z axis due to the external magnetic field (B_0) are forced also to precess about an axis which itself is rotating at the precessional frequency in the xy plane (thick grey arrow) due to the magnetic field created by the RF radiation. The NMV therefore performs a spiralling motion towards the transverse plane.

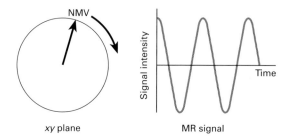

Fig. 3.12 Once the NMV has been tipped into the transverse plane, it rotates at the precessional frequency through perpendicular lines of force created by the external magnetic field. This produces electromagnetic radiation with a frequency equal to the frequency of rotation. Its amplitude (intensity) is equal to the size of the NMV. This is the MR signal.

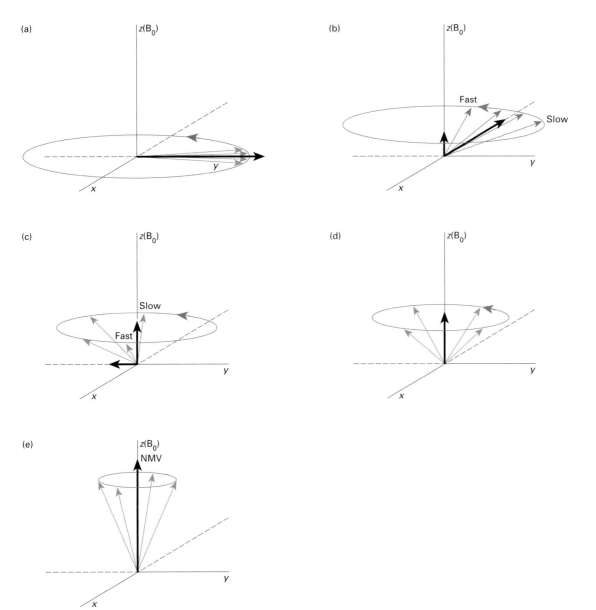

Fig. 3.13 Dephasing and the return to equilibrium (relaxation) following a 90° RF pulse. Stationary coordinates. The NMV is shown, split into its longitudinal and transverse components since it is the transverse component that gives the MR signal. Four magnetic dipoles contributing to the NMV are drawn. (a) At the end of the RF pulse the NMV lies in the transverse plane. There is no longitudinal magnetisation. Protons are in phase, causing the NMV to rotate about the z axis at the precessional frequency. (This figure equates with Fig. 3.10e, but dipoles are drawn here pointing in the same direction and in the same transverse plane, for reasons of clarity.) (b) Longitudinal magnetisation begins to regrow (black arrow on the z axis) as protons start to reorientate along the axis of B_0. Transverse magnetisation (black arrow in the xy plane) diminishes as individual magnetic moments comprising the NMV move out of phase owing to small differences in their rate of precession. (c) Dephasing is rapid compared with the rate of reorientation along B_0. (d) Therefore transverse magnetisation (and the MR signal) is lost before longitudinal reorientation is complete. (e) Longitudinal magnetisation continues to grow as tissue relaxes back into its resting state.

about by tilting the NMV into the transverse plane. In the restoration of equilibrium, however, transverse magnetisation diminishes independently of, and much more rapidly than, the rate at which longitudinal magnetisation reappears. The explanation for this lies in *dephasing*.

At the end of the RF pulse, protons are in phase (Figs 3.10e & 3.13a). In a uniform magnetic field they should continue to precess at the same rate and at first sight there would seem to be no reason for them to move out of phase. However, even in a perfectly uniform external field, spinning magnetic moments generate their own small magnetic fields, leading to inhomogeneities in the magnetic field within tissue. The precessional frequency of hydrogen ions throughout tissue, therefore, does not conform to a single value but occupies a range of values on either side of that calculated from the known external parameters. This means that immediately after the 90° pulse some protons comprising the transverse magnetisation vector will precess faster and others slower than the calculated rate (Fig. 3.13b). The result is a rapid loss of transverse magnetisation as protons move out of phase (Fig. 3.13c,d), a process which is exacerbated by imperfections in the external magnetic field (which are inevitable).

Longitudinal magnetisation begins to reappear immediately after the cessation of RF radiation but takes considerably longer to return to its resting state than transverse magnetisation takes to disappear. Protons that are responsible for transverse magnetisation may have moved completely out of phase but this does not mean they have returned yet to their original orientation relative to the longitudinal plane, and longitudinal magnetisation continues to grow until they do (Figs 3.13d,e & 3.14).

Free induction decay

The loss of transverse magnetisation and accompanying decay of the MR signal just described are called *free induction decay*. It is the pattern observed when tissue is allowed to 'relax' into its equilibrium position without being disturbed by

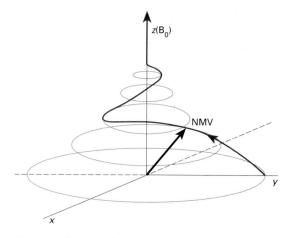

Fig. 3.14 The strength and orientation of the NMV depend on the extent to which protons are in phase (transverse component) and their orientation relative to the external magnetic field (longitudinal component). Following a 90° RF pulse, the NMV reorientates with a spiralling motion (at the precessional frequency) but approximates to the *z* axis rapidly as protons move out of phase and then continues to lengthen into its resting value (see Fig. 3.13).

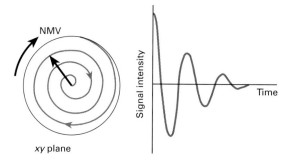

Fig. 3.15 Free induction decay. The MR signal decays with transverse magnetisation. Frequency remains constant.

further RF pulses (Fig. 3.15). Loss of signal is less rapid with more complex imaging sequences (e.g. spin–echo) which can compensate for dephasing due to inhomogeneities in the external magnetic field, leaving only the effects of magnetic field inhomogeneites generated in tissue by the protons themselves (see below).

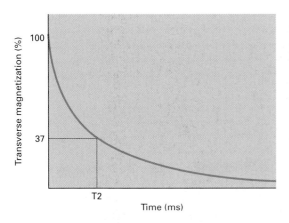

Fig. 3.16 T2 relaxation curve. Transverse magnetisation diminishes exponentially following a 90° RF pulse, a process called 'spin–spin' or T2 relaxation (but see text for discussion on T2*). The relaxation rate is defined by the T2 constant, which is the time taken for transverse magnetisation to diminish by 63% from its initial value.

Tissue relaxation / T1 and T2 curves

Relaxation is the term used to describe the return of tissue magnetisation to its resting state at the end of the RF pulse. As described in the preceding paragraphs, this involves two components of magnetisation, which relax independently of each other. The rate at which these components return to their resting state is a defining quality of tissue in a magnetic field and means that the MR signal is dependent upon, not just mobile hydrogen ion concentration, but also two other physical properties: T1 relaxation, which defines the rate at which longitudinal magnetisation reappears, and T2 relaxation, which defines the rate at which transverse magnetisation disappears. Tissue characterisation in MRI (as far as it goes) is based on these parameters (Bydder *et al.*, 1982; Crooks *et al.*, 1982b; Bottomley *et al.*, 1984, 1987).

T2 relaxation (spin–spin relaxation)

Transverse magnetisation is lost as a result of proton dephasing. Energy is transferred between protons, causing some to precess faster and others slower than the expected rate of precession. The rate at which transverse magnetisation diminishes

(relaxation rate) depends on the physical environment in which protons find themselves, and so varies according to the tissue being studied. A typical T2 relaxation curve is drawn in Fig. 3.16. It is an exponential function defined by the time taken for transverse magnetisation to fall to 37% of its initial value, a time constant referred to as the T2 value. Images which depend on T2 differences between tissues to provide contrast are said to be T2-weighted.[2]

T1 relaxation (spin–lattice relaxation)

'Spin' is a reference to rotating protons. 'Lattice' is a term for the tissue matrix in which these protons are situated. T1 relaxation refers to the gradual reorientation of protons in the direction of the external magnetic field, and the accompanying regrowth of longitudinal magnetisation. It involves giving up energy to the lattice, and occurs more efficiently in some tissues than in others. It is independent of the extent to which protons are in phase.

Recovery of longitudinal magnetisation is also an exponential process (Fig. 3.17) and the 'T1 value' of a particular tissue is a time constant describing the time taken for 63% of longitudinal magnetisation to reappear. Tissues with moderate T1 values (e.g. brain) recover longitudinal magnetisation more quickly than tissues with long T1 values (e.g. cerebrospinal fluid (CSF)). Imaging sequences have been devised which take advantage of these differences to provide image contrast (see below).

---

[2] The 'true' T2 value of a particular tissue is a theoretical value that would be found in a perfectly uniform external magnetic field. Dephasing in these circumstances would only be due to magnetic field inhomogeneites inherent in the tissue being observed. However, imperfections in the external magnetic field cause a more rapid dephasing and earlier loss of transverse magnetisation. The truncated T2 value in this situation (acquired, for example, from free induction decay, Fig. 3.15) is referred to as T2*. Establishing a 'true' T2 curve requires more complex pulse sequences (spin–echo) which compensate for imperfections in the external magnetic field (see below).

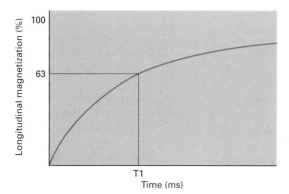

Fig. 3.17 T1 relaxation curve. Longitudinal magnetisation increases exponentially from zero following a 90° pulse, a process called 'spin–lattice' or T1 relaxation. The relaxation rate is defined by the time taken for magnetisation to regain 63% of its resting value, the T1 constant.

Image formation

For imaging purposes, the fact that tissue can be induced to give off RF radiation is of no value unless its origin can be defined in space. Then, given that this can be achieved, the strength of this emitted radiation (signal) must vary between different tissues in order to provide contrast on an image. The MR image is essentially a map of signal strengths across a defined section of tissue. Each point on the image corresponds to a small volume of tissue within the section being scanned and is assigned a level of brightness according to the strength of the RF radiation emitted from its tissue equivalent. As already discussed, the MR signal is dependent on the behaviour of hydrogen ions in a magnetic field and this means that signal strength at any particular point on an MRI section will be affected by the local hydrogen ion concentration.

In common use are MRI sequences that yield an image largely dependent on hydrogen ion concentration, called 'spin' or 'proton density' scans. However, in nearly all MR images, signal strength is dependent, not only on the hydrogen ion concentration, but also on the effects of T1 and

T2 relaxations on transverse magnetisation. The weight attached to each of these parameters can be varied by using different imaging sequences but the effects of none of them can be excluded entirely. Herein lies the complexity of MRI, to which must be added the effects of flow, 'chemical shift' and other 'artefacts' (Babcock *et al.*, 1985; Bellon *et al.*, 1986).

This section describes briefly how the origin of the MR signal is defined within a block of tissue and how T1 and T2 differences between tissues can be used to generate image contrast. The techniques used to construct images which are weighted towards one or other of these parameters, or towards hydrogen ion concentration, will be described in the next section.

Location of the source of signal/gradient fields

Up to now the discussion of MR has assumed that tissue is placed in a uniform magnetic field, and this is exactly what happens when a patient is placed in an MRI scanner. However, in a uniform magnetic field the application of RF radiation at the precessional frequency will cause an MR signal to be emitted from all parts of the sample simultaneously, with nothing to distinguish the contribution of one area from that of another. What is required is a method of exciting protons in a small segment of tissue so that the strength of the emitted radiation can be referred back to its source (Lauterbur, 1973). *Gradient magnetic fields*, generated by accessory coils situated inside the main magnetic field, are the means by which this is achieved.

There are three gradient fields, orientated at right angles to each other along the coordinate axes already described. (The *z* axis lies along the line of the uniform external magnetic field — usually horizontal. The *x* and *y* axes lie in the transverse plane — *x* axis horizontal, *y* axis vertical.) They act in two ways. Firstly, as just suggested, they limit the volume of tissue excited by the RF pulse to a single narrow section and (since this is not enough), secondly, they qualitatively alter

(a)

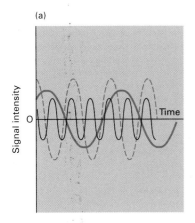

(b)

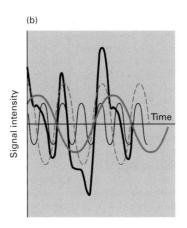

(c)

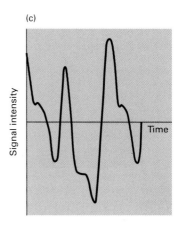

Fig. 3.18 Under the influence of the gradient magnetic fields, each point on a thin section of tissue excited by the RF pulse emits radiofrequency radiation with a unique amplitude, frequency and phase. Amplitude equates to the signal strength at a given point; frequency and phase are determined by the *x* and *y* coordinates respectively. The MR signal emitted by the tissue section is the sum of these waves, and image reconstruction involves the process of identifying the individual components. (a) The individual components of an MR signal. Thin black trace, high frequency; thick grey, low frequency; broken line, high amplitude; thin black, low amplitude. Phase is judged by the position of each wave in its cycle relative to the origin, O. (b) The components combine to produce a composite signal (thick black). (c) The radio-frequency receiver coil only sees the composite signal. Fourier transformation is used to calculate the amplitude, phase and frequency of the sine waves of which it is comprised (a) and hence the spatial information contained within it.

the emitted signal according to its site of origin within the selected slice (Kumar *et al.*, 1975; Edelstein *et al.*, 1980). The MR signal is thus changed from a simple, exponentially decaying, sine wave, with no spatial information (Fig. 3.15), into a signal with a highly complex waveform which is the sum of multiple sine waves of varying amplitude, phase and frequency containing the spatial information encoded by the gradient fields (Fig. 3.18).

Slice-select gradient coil (z axis)

The slice-select coil superimposes a small magnetic field gradient, orientated in the same direction as the main magnetic field, causing a gradual increase in its strength along its length of action. Obeying the Larmor equation, the precessional frequency of hydrogen therefore also increases along the length of the tissue sample while the coil is operative (Fig. 3.19). If RF radiation, *at a single frequency*, is applied now, it will only excite resonance in protons at a particular point along

the *z* axis where the frequency of precession corresponds. The term 'slice-select' is used because at this stage there is no field gradient along the *x* or *y* axes and the frequency of precession across any given transverse section remains uniform. An RF pulse will therefore cause resonance in all protons across a particular transverse slice of tissue. What is more, since the strength of the magnetic field at any position along the *z* axis is known, the precessional frequency of hydrogen in any transverse plane can be predicted and the frequency of the RF pulse set to excite resonance in that plane (Fig. 3.19).[3]

The slice-select gradient coil is switched on only during the application of the RF pulse.

Phase-encoding gradient coil (y axis)

With the cessation of the RF pulse, protons in the

---

[3] In fact, for technical reasons the frequency of the RF pulse is kept constant and slice selection is made by varying the origin of the gradient field on the *y* axis (Fig. 3.19).

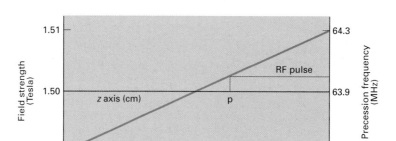

Fig. 3.19 Slice-select gradient. Superimposition of a small magnetic-field gradient along the axis of the uniform external magnetic field (*z* axis, drawn horizontally) causes the magnetic-field strength to increase gradually along the length of the sample. The precessional frequency of hydrogen therefore also increases along the length of the sample. RF radiation at a certain frequency will therefore excite all protons in a transverse slice of tissue defined by a point (p) along the *z* axis.

slice of tissue defined by the slice-select gradient start to emit the MR signal. The frequency of this signal is governed by the strength of the stable, uniform, external magnetic field, now that the slice-select gradient field has been turned off. Before it is read by the radio receiver coil, however, another gradient magnetic field is applied from front to back (the *y* axis). Immediately the frequency of precession across the section changes from a single value to a range of values increasing uniformly along the *y* axis in line with the new magnetic field gradient. Protons begin to move out of phase as those precessing at a faster rate at one end of the *y* axis move ahead of those precessing more slowly at the other end. After a short time the *y* axis gradient coil is turned off and protons in the selected slice revert once more to a single precessional frequency, but now there is a permanent gradation of phase along the *y* axis created during the brief period in which the phase-encoding gradient was active (Fig. 3.20). This phase gradation is dependent on the strength of the gradient field and the length of time it is applied and, since these variables are known, the source of the MR signal can be calculated in relation to the *y* axis.

The phase-encoding gradient is switched on after the application of the RF pulse and turned off before the signal is read by the receiver coil.

Frequency-encoding gradient coil (x axis)

Sometimes referred to as the 'read-out' gradient, the frequency-encoding, gradient-field coil is switched on during the period when the receiver coil is reading the MR signal. It acts at right angles both to the main magnetic field and to the direction of the phase-encoding gradient, creating a magnetic gradient from side to side. Again, hydrogen ions, which were precessing at a uniform rate once the phase-encoding gradient had been turned off, start to precess at a rate proportional to the increasing magnetic field along the *x* axis. If the RF receiver coil reads the MR signal while the frequency-encoding coil is active, then instead of seeing a signal with a single frequency it will detect an MR signal made up of a range of frequencies, where the frequency of its individual components marks their origin in relation to the *x* axis (Fig. 3.21). The phase gradation already imposed on the MR signal in the *y* axis direction is unaffected because no further magnetic gradient has been applied along the *y* axis.

Image reconstruction

All pictures have a finite resolution. It is not possible to measure the signal from individual

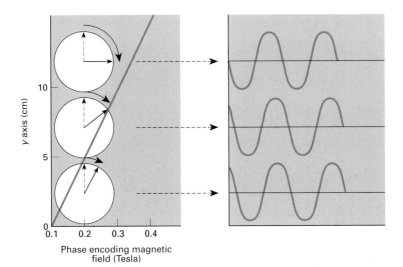

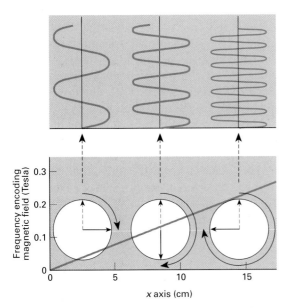

Fig. 3.20 Phase-encoding gradient. A phase difference along the y axis is created by the phase-encoding gradient because during the short period active protons at one end of the y axis rotate through a greater distance than those at the other end. This difference persists when the gradient field is turned off (unbroken arrow, and start of sine waves), marking the origin of individual components of the MR signal along the y axis. Broken and unbroken arrows represent positions of magnetic dipoles before and after the application of the phase-encoding gradient. The magnetic field gradient depicted is actually superimposed on the main magnetic field.

Fig. 3.21 Frequency encoding gradient. Unlike the phase-encoding gradient, the frequency-encoding gradient is applied whilst the MR signal is being read. A frequency gradation is therefore superimposed on the MR signal according to its origin relative to the x axis. The magnetic field gradient depicted is actually superimposed on the main magnetic field.

hydrogen ions. Instead, each slice of tissue is divided equally into small blocks and measurements are taken of the MR signal emitted by each block. The number of blocks in a section determines the quality of the final image and the number of measurements that have to be made along the frequency- and phase-encoding axes. A large (or fine) matrix gives high spatial resolution, a small (or coarse) matrix low spatial resolution. The MR signal emitted by each block is then allocated a level of brightness on the image according to its strength.

Detailed discussion of the way in which spatial information is derived from the MR signal is beyond the scope of this text (see Further reading). Briefly, what the receiver coil sees following an excitation of tissue by an RF pulse is a highly complex signal, comprising the sum of multiple sine waves of different amplitude, frequency and phase, containing the spatial information necessary to form an image (Fig. 3.18c). Working out the composition of these components (Fig. 3.18a) is not possible from a single excitation. Instead, this information is accumu-

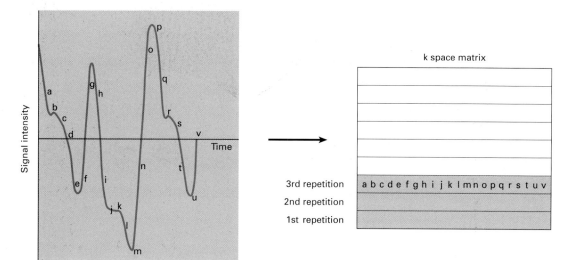

Fig. 3.22 The k space. Measurements taken from the MR signal are stored in a line of a mathematical matrix called 'k space'. Each repetition is performed with a different phase-encoding gradient, producing a different MR signal and a new set of measurements for the next line of the k-space matrix. The third repetition is shown.

lated gradually, using repeated pulses of RF radiation, each repetition adding to the sum of knowledge about a particular slice of tissue. The MR signal is sampled at regular intervals (Fig. 3.22) and the measurements stored in a mathematical matrix called the 'k space' (Tweig, 1983). Each repetition provides data for a line of k space and when k space is full the requisite number of excitations will have been completed. The process by which these data are then resolved into component amplitude, frequency and phase values, and hence into an image, is known as Fourier transformation (Wood, 1992).

Why are repeated excitations required to form an image? Because of the number of variables[4] to be computed. Each repetition is performed with a stepwise increase in the strength of the phase-encoding gradient, which changes the phase gradation in the y axis direction and alters the configuration of the MR signal. Each line of the k-

space matrix is therefore filled with a series of measurements made from a different MR signal, but containing the same (though unknown) variables. The image is calculated by combining the data from all the repetitions. (Decoding the MR signal in this way can be compared to solving a problem by simultaneous equations: two unknown variables require two equations; 256 unknown variables—typical tissue matrix size—require 256 equations.)

The need for multiple excitations explains why MRI can be a lengthy process. The time interval between each excitation is known as 'time to repetition' (TR) and is set according to image requirements (see below). It cannot be shortened to speed up data collection without qualitatively altering the image. With long TR sequences and large matrices (e.g. 512 × 256), several minutes may elapse before an image is formed.

Generation of image contrast

The dependence of the MR signal on mobile hydrogen ion concentration is explained by the nature of the NMR interaction. So-called 'proton-density' images provide useful demonstrations of anatomy. However, the power of MRI comes from its ability to improve soft-tissue contrast by enhancing other tissue characteristics that reflect

---

[4] A variable here refers to the signal strength to be assigned to each block of tissue within the tissue matrix.

the local physical environment, namely T1 and T2 relaxation times. Contrast between tissues whose mobile hydrogen ion concentrations are similar can be accentuated by taking advantage of differences in T1 or T2 values (Tables 3.2 & 3.3). Such images are said to be T1- or T2-weighted, the term 'weighting' serving as a reminder that these are not pure T1 or T2 images (any more than a proton-density image is pure), merely that T1 or T2 effects on the MR signal are predominant in the generation of image contrast.

Contrast weighting towards T1 or T2 relaxation values is achieved by timing the collection of data to coincide with the period when the relaxation curves of the relevant soft tissues are optimally separated. For T1-weighted images, spin–echo sequences that use a short TR (e.g. 500 ms) will highlight differences in T1 relaxation values (Fig. 3.23). For T2-weighted images, a long TR (e.g. 2500 ms) first minimises T1 differences by allowing enough time for tissues with both long and short T1 values to relax fully (Fig. 3.23).

Then a long TE (time to echo, when the signal is read, e.g. 100 ms) allows T2 differences to evolve (Fig. 3.24). (These concepts will become clearer in the discussion on imaging sequences below.)

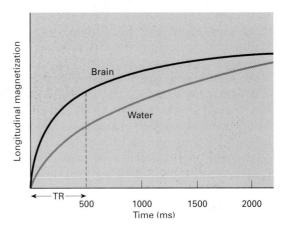

Fig. 3.23 T1-weighted image. Longitudinal magnetisation of brain (medium-length T1) recovers more quickly than that of water (long T1). If the MR signal is read when the relaxation curves are widely separated (e.g. using a TR of 500 ms), T1 differences will affect image contrast. (If the MR signal is read later (e.g. using a TR of 2500 ms, longitudinal magnetisation will have recovered in both tissues and image contrast will depend on mobile hydrogen ion concentration.)

Table 3.2 T1 values and signal intensities in soft tissue on a T1-weighted image.

Tissue	T1 constants	Signal intensity
CSF	Long	Low
Pathology (most)	↓	↓
Grey matter		
White matter		
Fat	Short	High

Table 3.3 T2 values and signal intensities in soft tissue on a T2-weighted image.

Tissue	T2 constants	Signal intensity
CSF	Long	High
Pathology (most)	↓	↓
Grey matter		Low
White matter		
Fat	Short	Moderate*

*Complete T1 relaxation, a high proton density and complex T2-relaxation processes usually give fat a moderately high signal on T2-weighted sequences.

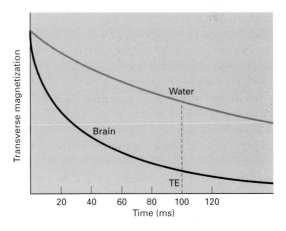

Fig. 3.24 T2-weighted image. Following excitation by an RF pulse, brain tissue loses its transverse magnetisation (and signal) more quickly than water. Delaying reading the MR signal (e.g. TE of 100 ms) accentuates this difference and image contrast is determined by T2 values.

Three-dimensional (3-D) volume imaging

Spatial encoding in MRI is usually carried out by the means described above. Imaging in different planes is accomplished by mixing the applications of the gradient fields. Coronal scans, for example, are acquired using the *x* axis gradient for slice selection and the *y* and *z* gradients as phase- and frequency-encoding gradients.

Another way of acquiring spatial information is with *3-D volume imaging*. Figure 3.19 depicts the slice-selection process but is oversimplified in that the RF pulse is not at a single frequency but occupies a narrow band of frequencies. The selected slice, therefore, is not infinitely thin but has a thickness dependent on the range of frequencies in the RF pulse and the steepness of the slice-select gradient. The narrower the range of frequencies, or the steeper the gradient, the thinner the slice. In 3-D volume imaging the slice-selection step is performed with a very shallow gradient so that the RF pulse excites the entire volume of tissue to be imaged at once. Both the *z* axis and the *y* axis gradient fields are then applied simultaneously to give phase encoding from head to toe and front to back. Frequency encoding occurs along the *x* axis during the reading of the signal in the normal way. Decoding the signal requires an extra step (3-D Fourier transformation) and image acquisition takes longer because the number of repetitions must be multiplied by the number of phase-encoding steps performed along the *z* axis.

These constraints confine the technique to 'fast' imaging sequences but data on a block of tissue are produced which can then be viewed, subsequently, in any plane. Spatial resolution varies according to the plane of section chosen, depending on the number of phase- or frequency-encoding steps performed along the different axes (Frahm *et al.*, 1986).

Magnetic resonance imaging sequences

Repeated tissue excitations are required to produce an image. Each RF pulse is followed by a short delay before the MR signal is read and a further delay before the cycle is repeated. The time interval between RF pulses and the interval between each RF pulse and the reading of the MR signal are critical in determining the extent to which mobile hydrogen ion concentration, T1 or T2 values affect image contrast. The terms 'pulse sequence' or 'imaging sequence' refer to the timing of these events, including the timing of any additional RF pulses designed to enhance or modify the MR signal.

A wide range of imaging sequences tends to intimidate the non-specialist. Most, however, are amenable to explanation with reference to the principles already outlined. The following section opens with a description of *partial-saturation* and *saturation-recovery* sequences, which, although rarely used now, are easily understood and introduce concepts that can be applied to other imaging sequences. *Spin–echo* sequences form the backbone of MRI and will be discussed in some detail. The idea of image weighting towards T1 or T2 values will become clearer in this discussion, as will the difference between T2 and T2*. *Inversion-recovery* sequences are in frequent use and form the basis of a fat-suppression sequence. Fast scanning techniques will be discussed briefly. A set of scans illustrating the appearance of the brain in commonly used imaging sequences are collected in the Appendix at the end of the chapter (Figs 3.A1–3.A5).

Saturation recovery and partial saturation

These are the simplest forms of tissue excitation. An RF pulse is transmitted whose strength and duration are just enough to tilt the NMV by 90° into the transverse plane—a '90° RF pulse'. The MR signal is read immediately, before it has a chance to decay. The cycle is then repeated for all the phase-encoding steps. In the saturation-recovery sequence, the time between each repetition of the RF pulse is long enough (e.g. TR of 2500 ms) for longitudinal magnetisation to recover in most tissues before each excitation (Fig. 3.25). This means that the MR signal emitted per

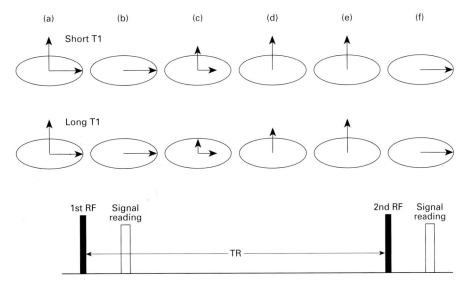

Fig. 3.25 Saturation-recovery sequence (proton-density scan). Following a 90° RF pulse, the NMVs are tilted into the transverse plane (b). Transverse magnetisation (and MR signal) fades, and longitudinal magnetisation reforms, at rates dependent on each tissue's T2* and T1 values respectively (c–e). With a long repetition time (TR), even tissues with long T1 values recover full longitudinal magnetisation within each pulse cycle (e). Relaxation rates, therefore, do not affect signal strength (f). Signal strength is dependent on hydrogen ion concentration. Two tissues are shown, one with a short T1, the other with a long T1.

unit volume of tissue, when the magnetisation vector is deflected, is dependent on the mobile hydrogen ion concentration.

In the partial-saturation sequence, TR is shorter (e.g. 400 ms). Tissues with short T1 values recover full longitudinal magnetisation before the next RF pulse but those with long T1 values do not—they remain partially saturated. Therefore, with the second and subsequent RF pulses, tissues with long T1 values have smaller longitudinal magnetisation vectors available for tipping into the horizontal plane and their MR signal is reduced (Figs 3.23 & 3.26). Tissues with long T1 values will appear dark next to those with short T1 values. In other words, T1 weighting is superimposed on the image of mobile hydrogen ion concentration.

Spin–echo sequences

The widespread clinical application of spin–echo imaging comes from its ability to produce T2-weighted images in addition to proton-density and T1-weighted images. Most brain pathology causes a relative lengthening of T1 and T2 values, partly because of an increased water content. Abnormal areas may therefore be hidden, on T1-weighted scans because of a diminution in MR signal. On T2-weighted scans, however, tissues with long T2 values give a strong signal and stand out brightly from their surroundings (Bailes *et al.*, 1982).

In a spin–echo sequence, the NMV is first tilted into the transverse plane by a 90° RF pulse. Then, instead of reading the signal immediately, as in a saturation-recovery or partial-saturation sequence, a short period of time is allowed to elapse (e.g. 10 ms) before another RF pulse (twice as long or twice as strong) is transmitted which tilts the NMV through a further 180°. This 'refocusing' RF pulse briefly restores the MR signal, which up to now has been fading rapidly (Fig. 3.15), by bringing protons back into phase. The signal is read when it reaches its 'refocused' peak (e.g. after another 10 ms) (Fig. 3.27).

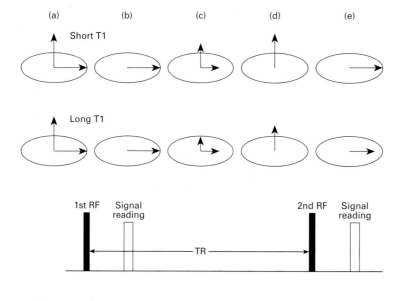

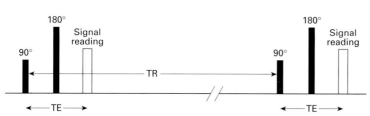

Fig. 3.26 Partial-saturation sequence (T1-weighted scan). With a short repetition time (TR), tissues with long T1 values will not recover longitudinal magnetisation fully before the next excitation (d) and, following the second and subsequent RF pulses, their MR signal will be reduced (e).

Fig. 3.27 Spin-echo sequence. Each cycle consists of a 90° RF pulse followed after an interval by a 180° refocusing RF pulse. The signal is read when the echo created by the refocusing pulse is maximal. TE, time to echo from the 90° pulse, is set by the timing of the refocusing pulse (see Fig. 3.28).

Understanding how spin–echo imaging works demands a brief return to basic principles. The strength of the MR signal is proportional to the amount of magnetisation in the transverse plane. Following a 90° RF pulse, this magnetisation decays as protons precessing around the longitudinal axis move out of phase (Fig. 3.13). Dephasing is due to two factors, the first a result of interactions between precessing nuclei (spin–spin, or T2 relaxation) and the second a result of inhomogeneities in the external magnetic field, which means that protons in one part of the same slice of tissue precess at a different rate from protons in another part.[5] The loss of signal observed is rapid and referred to as free induction decay (Fig. 3.15).

In the same way that different T1 (longitudinal) relaxation rates are used to distinguish between tissues on T1-weighted images, the rate of T2 (transverse) relaxation can be used to differentiate between tissues on T2-weighted images, but the loss of MR signal observed in free induction decay is more a measure of magnetic field inhomogeneity than a reflection of a tissue's innate physical properties. Such decay is governed by a different (much shorter) time constant, $T2^*$, and is known as $T2^*$ relaxation. True T2 relaxation can only be measured if the effects of magnetic field inhomogeneities are removed, and this is achieved by the refocusing pulse.

Dephasing due to spin–spin interactions is random. It cannot be recovered and represents the true T2 relaxation we want to measure. Dephas-

[5] The magnetic gradients used in reconstructing the image themselves cause a reduction in the amplitude of the MR signal by dephasing, but where appropriate this can be minimised by judicious use of compensatory gradients (Smith & Ranallo, 1989).

ing due to magnetic field inhomogeneities is not. Protons at any given point in the selected tissue plane will always precess at a rate determined by the local magnetic field, including any field inhomogeneity. Some will precess faster than the average and some more slowly. A 180° RF pulse applied as the MR signal is fading flips the NMV by 180°. It ends up in the same (*xy*) plane, but the phase of all the individual magnetic dipoles that make up the NMV is reversed. Faster protons now find themselves behind (in terms of phase) slower protons. Their speed of precession

is unchanged, however, because each still occupies the same point in the tissue slice and each is still subjected to the same magnetic field, including any inhomogeneity. Transverse magnetisation (and the MR signal) starts to reappear as faster protons catch up slower protons, and is maximal at the instant they are in phase again (Fig. 3.28).

The term 'echo' refers to the reconstituted MR signal after the 180° refocusing pulse. The moment of maximum rephasing, when the strength of the echo is greatest, is the moment magnetic field inhomogeneites have been compen-

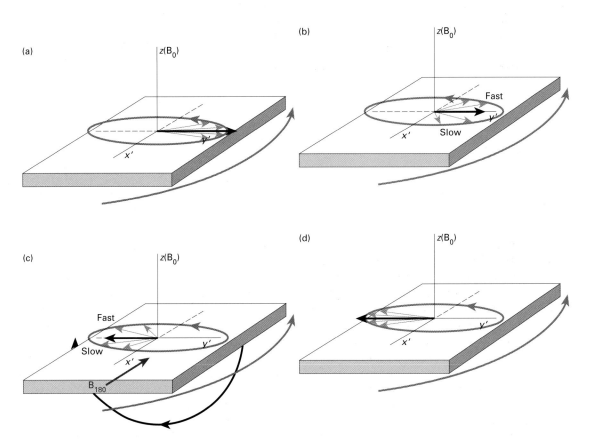

Fig. 3.28 The refocusing RF pulse looked at from the perspective of a coordinate system (*x'*, *y'*) rotating at the precessional frequency (cf. Fig. 3.13, and see discussion in text under heading Resonance 2). (a) The 90° RF pulse tilts the NMV into the *xy* plane. (b) Dephasing starts immediately as some magnetic dipoles move ahead of the average speed of precession and others fall behind.

(c) Application of a 180° pulse turns the shrinking NMV about the *x'* axis until it comes into the *xy* plane again (black arc) but now faster protons find themselves behind slower ones. (d) The NMV re-forms when these protons catch up and come (briefly) into phase again. Regrowth of longitudinal magnetisation is not shown because it is small in the time-scale of these reactions.

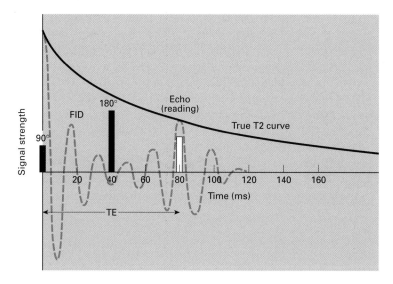

Fig. 3.29 True T2 relaxation curve. Transverse magnetisation and the MR signal fade by free induction decay (FID, broken grey line). A 180° refocusing pulse restores the signal to a maximum at TE (equal to twice the interval from the 90° to the 180° pulse). Reading the echo at this moment gives a signal intensity which is dependent on residual transverse magnetisation, diminished only by true T2 relaxation. Other points on the true T2 curve could be plotted by changing the time of the 180° pulse.

sated for. The strength of this signal is dependent on the residual transverse magnetisation, diminished only by pure spin–spin interactions, i.e. true T2 relaxation. To pick up this signal, the receiver coil must read the echo at an interval after the 180° pulse exactly equal to the interval between the 90° pulse and the 180° pulse (Fig. 3.29). Reading the signal too early or too late will result in the detection of a signal of lesser amplitude owing to dephasing from T2* effects.

Other readings can be obtained at different times after the 90° RF pulse by changing the timing of the refocusing pulse, as long as the echo is read at the correct interval. A plot of the TE after a 90° RF pulse against signal strength gives the true T2 curve (Fig. 3.29). The T2 value of a particular tissue is the time taken for signal intensity at a given TE (i.e. refocused transverse magnetisation) to fall to 37% of its initial value. Note that with long TEs signal strength becomes very small.

Imaging with spin–echo

Depending on the interval between 90° RF pulses (TR) and the interval between each 90° pulse and reading the echo (TE), spin–echo sequences can be T1-, T2- or proton-density-weighted.

*T1-weighted spin–echo sequences
(short TR, short TE)*

A short TR (e.g. 400 ms) ensures that only tissues with short T1 values recover longitudinal magnetisation between repetitions. Transverse magnetisation following the 90° pulse is therefore greater in short-T1 tissues, and the image becomes T1-weighted, similar to a partial-saturation sequence. The 180° refocusing pulse is applied soon after each 90° pulse, a short TE (e.g. 10–20 ms) ensuring that T2 differences between tissues do not have time to develop an impact on image contrast (Figs 3.30 & 3.A5).

*Proton-density spin–echo sequences
(long TR, short TE)*

A long TR (e.g. 2000 ms) allows a more complete recovery of longitudinal magnetisation in tissues with long T1 values. Transverse magnetisation after each 90° pulse, therefore, is less affected by T1 relaxation rates and becomes more dependent on mobile hydrogen ion concentration, similar to a saturation-recovery sequence. A 180° refocusing pulse is applied soon after the 90° pulse and the signal is read before T2 differences become operative (short TE, e.g. 10–20 ms). The image is

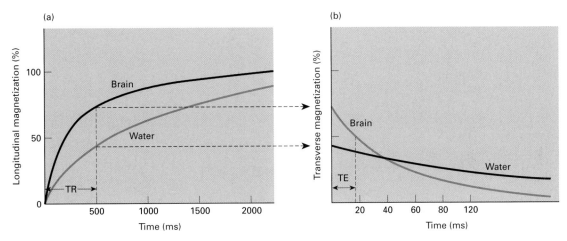

Fig. 3.30 T1-weighted spin–echo sequence (short TR, short TE). (a) A short TR emphasises T1 differences between tissues. (b) A short TE minimises the effects of different T2 relaxation rates. Image contrast is mainly dependent on T1 values. Brain gives moderate signal, water low. Transverse magnetisation equates to signal strength if corrections are made for the mobile hydrogen concentrations in the different tissues.

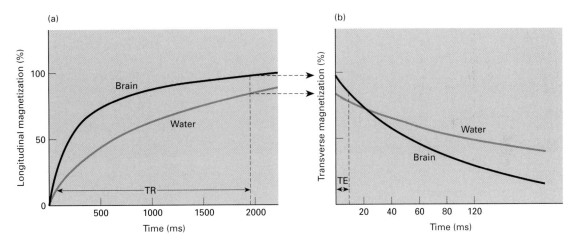

Fig. 3.31 Proton-density spin–echo sequence (long TR, short TE). (a) A long TR reduces the effects of T1 differences on the MR signal. (b) A short TE minimises the effects of T2 differences.

referred to as a 'proton-density' or 'spin-density' image (Fig. 3.31).

T2-weighted spin–echo sequences (long TR, long TE)

A long TR (e.g. 2000 ms) reduces the effects of T1 differences between tissues, as for a proton-density scan, but this time the refocusing pulse is applied after a delay, allowing T2 differences between tissues to have an effect on echo strength (long TE, e.g. 120 ms). The image becomes T2-weighted (Fig. 3.32).

'Double-echo' spin–echo (long TR, short and long TEs)

There is no reason why more than one refocusing pulse should not be used in each pulse cycle. After

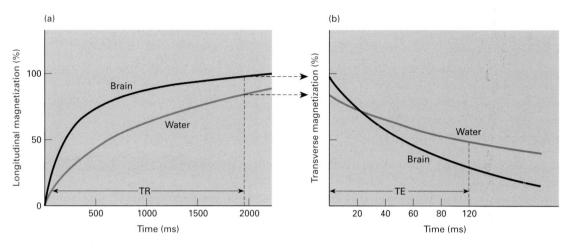

Fig. 3.32 T2-weighted spin–echo sequence (long TR, long TE). (a) A long TR minimises T1 differences. (b) A long TE maximises T2 differences.

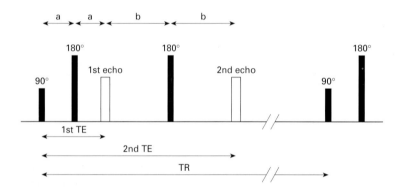

Fig. 3.33 Double-echo, spin–echo sequence. Two echoes give long and short TE images with a long TR. The timing of the second refocusing pulse determines the time of the second echo. Times a and b indicate intervals between pulses and echoes.

the first rephasing, a second echo can be induced with a second 180° refocusing pulse by exactly the same mechanism as the first. The interval between the first echo and the second refocusing pulse will equal the interval between this pulse and the second maximal rephasing (Fig. 3.33). Again, this is the moment when T2* effects are cancelled out, and should dictate the time at which the echo is read. The second TE is still measured from the time of the 90° pulse, because this is the period that dictates the strength of the signal and the amount of true T2 weighting (Fig. 3.29).

In a double-echo sequence TR is long and each 90° pulse is followed by two 180° refocusing pulses. The first is early, giving a short TE and a proton-density image. The second is delayed, giving a long TE and a T2-weighted image. A single examination thus yields two sets of images, adding considerably to its diagnostic value, without any prolongation of scanning time.

In theory more than two echoes could be collected in the same pulse sequence but as TE becomes longer the strength of the echo diminishes, owing to true T2 relaxation (Fig. 3.29). This becomes a problem with heavily T2-weighted images, where a very long TE (e.g. >150 ms) gives a signal that is increasingly difficult to distinguish from background noise.

*T2 curves and tissue contrast
at long TR values*

The exponential nature of the relaxation process means that full recovery of longitudinal magnetisation takes about five times the T1 value. Water (or CSF) has a very long T1 constant (1500 ms at 1.5 T) and may not recover full longitudinal magnetisation, even at quite long values of TR, i.e. values commonly used in the generation of the double-echo images (because prolonging TR leads to unacceptably long scanning times—see below). This makes little difference to the appearance of a heavily T2-weighted image (Fig. 3.32) but with the proton-density scan (Fig. 3.31) small differences in TE can cause striking alterations in image contrast. Thus, CSF, which, in fact, has a higher mobile hydrogen ion concentration than brain (Table 3.1), can appear dark on a proton-density scan where TE is very short (T1 effects impinging on the image). In proton-density scans with a slightly longer TE, T2 effects augment signal from CSF relative to brain, and the two tissues may become indistinguishable. At longer values of TE, CSF becomes bright.

Expected signal intensities (per unit volume) in different tissues, at different values of TE for a given TR, can be estimated from the T2 relaxation curves, if their origins on the *y* axis are adjusted for proton density (Figs 3.34, 3.A1 & 3.A2).

Inversion-recovery sequences

An inversion-recovery sequence starts with an RF pulse which turns the net magnetisation vector through 180°. This does not produce a signal immediately, because no magnetisation is created in the transverse plane. The inverted NMV shrinks to zero along the *z* axis, and then reasserts itself in the positive direction as individual magnetic dipoles begin to reorientate along the axis of the external magnetic field. The MR signal is generated by a subsequent 90° pulse, which tilts the relaxing magnetisation vectors into the transverse plane (Fig. 3.35).

The parameters which determine image con-

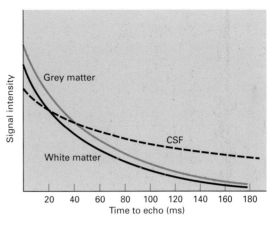

Fig. 3.34 Signal strength and T2 relaxation curves at a fairly long TR (e.g. 2000 ms). Each curve takes its origin on the *y* axis, depending on the length of TR and its proton density per unit volume. CSF has reduced signal at the origin because of incomplete longitudinal relaxation within the given TR. Both grey and white matter show complete T1 relaxation at this TR, but grey matter has a higher proton density than white matter. The T2 constants of grey and white matter are similar; that of CSF is prolonged. With lengthening values of TE, signal intensity becomes increasingly dependent on the T2 relaxation rate, i.e. the image becomes T2-weighted. At a short TE (often the first echo of a double-echo sequence, the so-called 'proton-density' scan), CSF may have the same signal intensity as white or grey matter.

trast on an inversion-recovery sequence include the TR, now represented by the interval between 180° inverting pulses at the beginning of each pulse cycle, and the inversion time (TI), which is the time between the inverting pulse and the 90° pulse. Usually the free induction decay which follows the 90° pulse is manipulated by another 180° pulse (for the purpose of refocusing, as in spin–echo), adding another variable, TE (Fig. 3.36).

Clearly, with three sequence parameters to exploit, quite complex images can be generated with contrast dependent on different mixtures of T1, T2 and proton-density weighting. The strength of the inversion-recovery sequence, however, derives from its ability to magnify T1 differences between tissues, and in practice these sequences are designed with one of two aims in

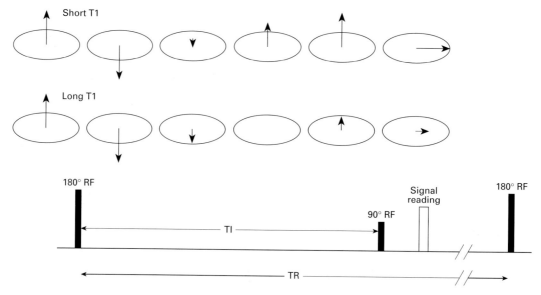

Fig. 3.35 Inversion-recovery sequence. A 180° RF pulse inverts the NMVs. Longitudinal magnetisation reasserts itself along the *z* axis according to each tissue's T1 constant. The interval, TI, before the 90° pulse dictates the extent to which T1 differences affect image contrast. A shorter TI than the one depicted would completely eliminate signal from the tissue with the longer T1 value.

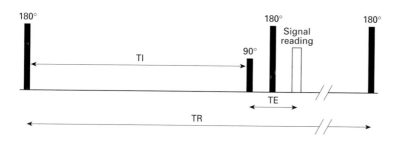

Fig. 3.36 Inversion-recovery with spin–echo sequence. When an inversion-recovery sequence is followed by spin–echo, TE is kept short so as not to mix any T2 effects with the strong T1 weighting (but see STIR sequences, Figs 3.38 and 3.39).

mind. The first is the generation of images with high contrast between grey and white matter. The second is the production of fat-suppression images.

In pursuit of the first aim, TR is kept long, because T1-dependent image contrast is developed by adjusting TI. TE is kept short, so as not to confuse the picture with any T2 weighting. Image contrast between grey and white matter may be very strong if the 90° pulse is applied close to the moment when their NMVs pass through the *xy* plane (Figs 3.35 & 3.37). Such scans are referred to as being heavily T1-weighted (Fig. 3.A3).

Fat suppression by inversion recovery (STIR)

A very short T1 and a high proton density gives fat high signal on T1- and proton-density-weighted scans and even moderately high signal on T2-weighted scans. Outside the brain, high signal from fat can provide useful contrast against low-signal 'space-occupying' pathology on T1-weighted scans (Teresi *et al.*, 1992). More subtle lesions, on the other hand, may not be seen, and on T2-weighted scans, where pathology typically gives increased signal, contrast is reduced if there is adjacent fat.

Inversion-recovery sequences can be used to

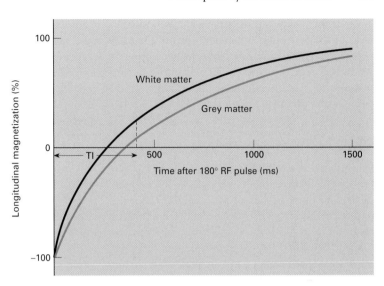

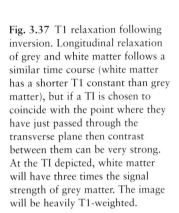

Fig. 3.37 T1 relaxation following inversion. Longitudinal relaxation of grey and white matter follows a similar time course (white matter has a shorter T1 constant than grey matter), but if a TI is chosen to coincide with the point where they have just passed through the transverse plane then contrast between them can be very strong. At the TI depicted, white matter will have three times the signal strength of grey matter. The image will be heavily T1-weighted.

reduce or eliminate signal from fat if the TI is shortened to coincide with the moment when the longitudinal magnetisation vector of fat is crossing the *xy* plane (Bydder & Young, 1985). This sequence—*short-TI inversion recovery*—is called STIR. The resulting image might be called T1-weighted, since contrast is dependent on differences in longitudinal relaxation rates. However, signal intensities are reversed compared with the usual T1-weighted scan because the 90° pulse

catches the magnetisation vectors of tissues other than fat whilst they are still inverted. This means that tissues with long T1 values, having a greater residual (inverted) magnetisation, will give stronger signals (Fig. 3.38). Water (or CSF), for example, appears bright on this 'T1-weighted' image and, since an increase in water content is a feature of much pathology, pathological lesions are also conspicuous by their high signal.

The power of the STIR sequence is enhanced by

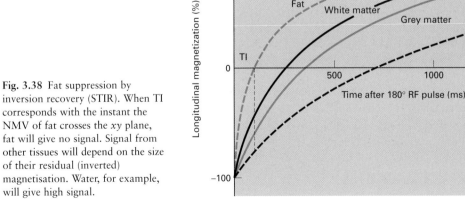

Fig. 3.38 Fat suppression by inversion recovery (STIR). When TI corresponds with the instant the NMV of fat crosses the *xy* plane, fat will give no signal. Signal from other tissues will depend on the size of their residual (inverted) magnetisation. Water, for example, will give high signal.

an elegant touch when the refocusing pulse which follows the 90° pulse is timed to give a long TE before the signal is read. Now T2 weighting is combined with the 'inverse' T1 weighting, giving water and tissue pathology very high signal compared with other tissues (Figs 3.39 & 3.A4).

Effect of intravenous contrast material

Gadolinium is a paramagnetic substance that can be given intravenously if it is attached to diethylenetriaminepenta-acetic acid (DTPA). Its paramagnetic properties cause a shortening of both T1 and T2 relaxation times in adjacent tissue. This shortening causes some loss of signal on T2-weighted images but increased signal on T1-weighted images. In the brain, gadolinium will penetrate areas where there is damage to the blood–brain barrier (e.g. active plaques of demyelination), making these regions very bright on T1-weighted scans.

Fast imaging techniques

The time taken to acquire an MR image has obvious disadvantages. Limiting factors are the TR (e.g. 2000 ms), the number of repetitions (e.g. 256) and then the number of the times the whole cycle is repeated (number of averages, e.g. four)

for best possible image quality. Optimal use of scanning time is made by acquiring data on all slices in a volume of tissue at the same time in an overlapping way (Crooks *et al.*, 1982a), so that, while waiting 2000 ms between the first and second excitations on the first slice, the next slice receives its first excitation and so on. This means that, depending on the length of TR, a variable number of slices can be imaged without prolonging the length of the examination. Nevertheless, the constraints above still apply and fast scanning techniques have been developed to try and overcome them (Haacke & Tkach, 1990).

Two examples illustrate different approaches to the problem: gradient-echo imaging and fast spin–echo imaging.

Gradient-echo imaging

One way to reduce the imaging time is to reduce the TR. This can be done, without changing image weighting, by reducing the amount the longitudinal magnetisation vector is deflected at the beginning of each pulse cycle. A spin–echo sequence begins with a 90° pulse. Gradient-echo sequences begin with a shorter RF pulse that deflects the NMV by only 30°, for example. The term *flip angle* refers to the angle of deflection of the NMV away from the *z* axis. Longitudinal

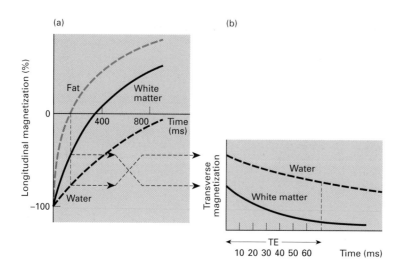

Fig. 3.39 Each cycle of a STIR sequence includes a 180° refocusing pulse (see Fig. 3.36) after the 90° pulse. If this is timed to give a long TE, T2 effects combine with 'inverted' T1 effects to give water a very high signal compared with other tissues (b).

magnetisation recovers more quickly and a shorter TR can be used for a given contrast weighting. Magnetisation in the transverse plane following each RF pulse is reduce (compared with that following a 90° pulse) but nevertheless can still be detected and amplified.

More of a problem is that, following the first pulse of a cycle, echoes for a proton-density or T2-weighted scan cannot be collected in the usual way by a refocusing pulse. Phase refocusing requires a 180° pulse and, although in normal spin–echo the effect of a refocusing pulse on the recovering longitudinal magnetisation can be ignored (Fig. 3.28), if the NMV has only been flipped by 30° then it will be inverted by a 180° pulse and TR will have to be prolonged in order to allow the magnetisation vectors to recover. The advantages of a small flip angle will be lost.

This problem is overcome by using the gradient coils along the frequency-encoding axis to perform a partial rephasing of the signal. Signal decay is by T2* effects because magnetic field inhomogeneites are not compensated for and 'T2-weighted images' are, in fact, T2*-weighted images. (See Further reading for more detailed discussion.)

Fast spin–echo imaging

In fast spin–echo imaging a different approach is used. TRs are not changed but instead the number of repetitions is reduced (Hennig *et al.*, 1986; Jolesz & Jones, 1993).

In the usual double-echo spin–echo imaging sequence, two echoes are collected following each 90° RF pulse, one for a proton-density and the other for a T2-weighted scan. In fast spin–echo imaging multiple echoes are created by multiple refocusing pulses at very short intervals, but, rather than each echo providing data points for separate images (of a single slice), each echo is performed with a different phase-encoding gradient and contributes new spatial as well as contrast information. Since multiple phase-encoding steps can be performed within a single repetition, the number of repetitions can be reduced. As might be expected, the contrast on these images reflects a mixture of the proton density and T2 weighting seen on conventional spin–echo.

The practice of MRI

Equipment

MRI requires the subject to be placed in a strong, uniform, static magnetic field. Additional gradient magnetic fields are used to locate the origin of the MR signal. An RF transmitter excites resonance. A receiver detects the emitted signal, and a computer reconstructs the image.

Static magnetic field

The static magnetic field can be generated in three different ways.

Permanent magnet: A permanent magnet is built from blocks of ferromagnetic material whose magnetism has been induced during manufacture by exposure to a magnetic field. Magnetic-field strength in these machines is low (up to about 0.3 T) and runs perpendicular to the bore of the gantry, and therefore perpendicular to the long axis of the patient. Running costs are low, merely a matter of keeping the blocks of ferromagnetic material at a constant ambient temperature by means of a small heating coil. Fringe fields (magnetic fields that extend beyond the bore of the magnet) are small.

These magnets cannot be switched off, and if a large object becomes attached it has to be pulled off by a winch.

Resistive magnet. The magnetic field in a resistive magnet is created by passing a current through a coil. Power consumption is heavy, and the heat generated while the magnet is in operation requires an extensive cooling system. Again, magnetic-field strength is limited, usually to about 0.3 T. These machines can be switched off in an emergency or when not in use.

Superconducting magnet. The limitations on field strength found with resistive magnets can be overcome by using 'superconducting' materials in the main field-induction coils. These materials have virtually no resistance at very low temperatures (about −263°C), which means that, once a current is induced in them, it will run almost indefinitely. In other words, a very large magnetic field can be generated (usually not more than 1.5 T for MRI) with virtually no electrical power. Running costs remain fairly high, however, because of the power required to run the refrigeration plant. Liquid helium (−269°C) is used as a coolant.

In a superconducting magnet, the magnetic field is horizontal, along the long axis of the patient. Fringe fields are large, increasing the danger from metallic objects inadvertently brought into the scanning room. The magnet remains operative even when the scanner is not in use. In an emergency, the coolants can be released and, with the consequent loss of superconductivity, current ceases to flow and the magnetic field disappears. This process is called a 'quench', and restarting the magnet after a quench is both expensive and time-consuming.

Gradient-field coils

Gradient-field coils are positioned inside the main magnetic-field coils and are of a configuration designed to alter the strength of the magnetic field in a linear fashion, along the different coordinate axes. Current is passed through them at critical moments, allowing the location of the MR signal to be defined in space, as discussed earlier.

Transmitter and receiver coils

A wide variety of different coil shapes can be positioned around or close to the part being scanned in order to maximise the signal-to-noise ratio. Often the same coil is used to transmit the RF pulse and to receive the MR signal. The coils must be positioned in such a way as to induce (or detect) an oscillating magnetic field at right angles to the main magnetic field.

The computer

The computer stores data and converts the MR signal into an image by a process called Fourier transformation.

Scanning procedure

Having an MRI scan is not an unpleasant procedure. The patient lies comfortably on a couch and the receiver coil is positioned over the area of interest. To image the brain, the coil is positioned over the head, fitting about as closely as a motor-cycle helmet. The patient is motored on the couch into the tunnel of the scanner, and when settled the examination is begun. A complete study normally takes 30–40 min, during which time a number of imaging sequences, each lasting several minutes, may be performed. The patient must remain completely immobile whilst each sequence is in progress; any movement will degrade image quality. The gradient coils vibrate against the side of the scanner during an acquisition, producing a knocking noise from which experts can guess at the type of sequence being performed.

When a patient is referred for MRI, the radiologist has an almost limitless series of options in his choice of scan sequences, and furthermore the area of interest can be imaged in any plane. Coronal scans can be angled perpendicular to the Sylvian fissure to show the temporal lobes in their best cross-section. The optic chiasma is elegantly demonstrated in a tilted axial plane. Any scan sequence can be used in any plane.

Scanning protocols depend upon the clinical problem, but in practice usually follow fairly standard lines. The brain is usually imaged in the axial plane first, using a double-echo sequence to give 'proton-density' and T2-weighted images. The axial plane is chosen more for its familiar appearance than for any superiority in demonstrating pathology. Further imaging depends on the findings of the first study and usually includes scans in different planes or with different weighting to resolve any uncertainty. Intravenous contrast may be given to show areas of pathologically increased vascularity or breakdown of the blood–brain barrier.

Choice of imaging modality, CT versus MRI

When MRI was first introduced into the imaging armamentarium it was compared with CT, with any benefit offset by the scarcity and expense of the technique. MRI scanners are now widely available and costs have fallen, so it seems reasonable now to consider MRI, with its superior soft-tissue contrast resolution, its multiplanar imaging capability and general lack of artefact and biological hazard, to be the preferred method of imaging intracranial disease.

MRI is unable to demonstrate dense bone, however, protons being too tightly constrained within the crystalline matrix to resonate, and is quite insensitive to calcification within lesions. CT is therefore valuable in demonstrating bone destruction, which may be unseen on MRI, for example, and can be a useful adjunct to MRI in demonstrating calcium within an undiagnosed brain lesion. Haemorrhage is easily detected on MR images, with the exception of recent subarachnoid haemorrhage (which is almost invisible), and patients suspected of having this diagnosis should have CT as their first investigation.

Risks of MRI

There are occasions when MRI may be hazardous or cannot be tolerated. Patients with cardiac pacemakers must not have MRI, and warnings should be posted to prevent them coming within range of the fringe fields. Other implanted devices, such as peripheral-nerve or spinal-cord stimulators, may malfunction or be permanently damaged. Some surgical implants are ferromagnetic and will move when the patient enters the magnetic field. The importance of this effect depends on their position, with catastrophic effects recorded following migration of an intracranial aneurysm clip. The majority of intracranial devices, however, are not ferromagnetic and MRI can be undertaken in perfect safety. The results of comprehensive testing of a range of implants for safety are published from time to time (Shellock *et al.*, 1993; Shellock & Kanal, 1994).

Incidental ferromagnetic intraocular foreign bodies pose a danger, particularly as the accident may not be remembered. Large metallic implants, such as hip replacements and spinal rods, cause some local degradation of the images by distorting the magnetic field but do not put the patient at risk.

Although not shown to be harmful to the fetus, MRI scanning is avoided in the first trimester of pregnancy.

Claustrophobia is a problem mainly with superconducting magnets, where the scanning tunnel tends to be long and narrow. Where reassurance fails, sedation may work, but occasionally general anaesthesia must be used. In either case, careful patient monitoring is required.

References

Babcock, E.E., Brateman, L., Weinreb, J.C., Horner, S.D. & Nannully, R.L. (1985) Edge artefacts in MR images: chemical shift effect. *J. Computer Assisted Tomogr.* **9**, 252–7.

Bailes, D.R., Young, I.R., Thomas, D.J., Straughan, K., Bydder, G.M. & Steiner, R.E. (1982) NMR imaging of the brain using spin–echo sequences. *Clin. Radiol.* **33**, 394–414.

Bellon, E.M., Haacke, E.M., Coleman, P.E., Sacco, D.C., Steiger, D.A. & Gangarosa, R.E. (1986) MR artefacts: a review. *Am. J. Roentgenol.* **147**, 1271–81.

Bloch, F., Hanson, W.W. & Packard, M. (1946) Nuclear induction. *Phys. Rev.* **69**, 127.

Bottomley, P.A., Foster, T.H., Argersinger, R.E. & Pfeifer, L.M. (1984) A review of normal tissue hydrogen NMR relaxation times and relaxation mechanism from 1–100 MHz: dependence on tissue type, NMR fre-quency, temperature, species, excision and age. *Med. Phys.* **11**, 425–48.

Bottomley, P.A., Hardy, C.J., Argersinger, R.E. & Allen-Moore, G. (1987) A review of 1H nuclear magnetic resonance relaxation in pathology: are T1 and T2 diagnostic? *Med. Phys.* **14**, 1–37.

Bydder, G.M. & Young, I.R. (1985) MR imaging: the clinical use of the inversion recovery sequence. *J. Computer Assisted Tomogr.* **9**, 659–75.

Bydder, G.M., Stiener, R.E., Young, I.R. *et al.* (1982) Clinical NMR imaging of the brain: 140 cases. *Am. J. Roentgenol.* **139**, 215–36.

Crooks, L., Arakawa, M., Hoenninger, J. *et al.* (1982a) Nuclear magnetic resonance whole body imager operating at 3.5 kGauss. *Radiology* **143**, 169–74.

Crooks, L.E., Mills, C.M., Davies, *et al.* (1982b) Visualisation of cerebral and vascular abnormalities by NMR imaging: the effects of imaging parameters on contrast. *Radiology* **144**, 843–52.

Edelstein, W.A., Hutchinson, J.M.S., Johnson, G. & Redpath, T.W. (1980) Spin warp NMR imaging. *Phys. Med. Biol.* **25**, 751–6.

Frahm, J., Haase, A. & Matthaei, D. (1986) Rapid three-dimensional MR imaging using the FLASH technique. *J. Computer Assisted Tomogr.* **2**, 363–8.

Haacke, E.M. & Tkach, J. (1990) Fast MR imaging: techniques and applications. *Am. J. Roentgenol.* **155**, 951–64.

Hennig, J., Nauerth, A. & Friedburg, H. (1986) RARE imaging: a fast imaging method for clinical MR. *Magnetic Resonance Med.* **3**, 823–33.

Jolesz, F.A. & Jones, K.M. (1993) Fast spin–echo imaging of the brain. *Topics Magnetic Resonance Imaging* **5**, 1–13.

Kumar, A., Welti, D. & Ernst, R.R. (1975) NMR Fourier zeugmatography. *J. Magnetic Resonance* **18**, 69–83.

Lauterbur, P.C. (1973) Image formation by induced local interactions: examples employing nuclear magnetic resonance. *Nature* **242**, 190–1.

Purcell, E.M., Torrey, H.C. & Pound, R.V. (1946) Resonance absorption by nuclear magnetic moments in a solid. *Phys. Rev.* **69**, 37–8.

Shellock, F.G. & Kanal, E. (1994) *Magnetic Resonance Bioeffects, Safety and Patient Management.* Raven Press, New York.

Shellock, F.G., Morisoli, S. & Kanal, E. (1993) MR procedures and biomedical implants, materials, and devices: 1993 update. *Radiology* **189**, 587–99.

Smith, H.J. & Ranallo, F.N. (1989) *A Non-mathematical Approach to Basic MRI.* Medical Physics Publishing Corporation, Madison, pp. 128–46.

Teresi, L.M., Lufkin, R.B. & Hanafee, W.N. (1992) In Stark, D.D. & Bradley Jr, W.G. (eds) *Magnetic Resonance Imaging,* 2nd edn. Mosby Year Book Inc., St Louis, pp. 1135–63.

Tweig, D.B. (1983) The k-trajectory formulation of the NMR imaging process with applications in analysis and synthesis of imaging methods. *Med. Phys.* **10**, 610–21.

Wood, M.L. (1992) Fourier imaging. In Stark, D.D. & Bradley Jr, W.G. (eds) *Magnetic Resonance Imaging,* 2nd edn. Mosby Year Book Inc., St Louis, pp. 21–66.

Further reading

Elster, A.D. (1994) *Questions and Answers in Magnetic Resonance Imaging.* Mosby Year Book Inc., St Louis.

Horowitz, A.L. (1991) *MRI Physics for Radiologists,* 2nd edn. Springer-Verlag, New York.

Rinck, A. (1993) *Magnetic Resonance in Medicine,* 3rd edn. Blackwell Scientific Publications, Oxford.

Smith, H.J. & Ranallo, F.N. (1989) *A Non-mathematical Approach to Basic MRI.* Medical Physics Publishing Corporation, Madison.

Stark, D.D. & Bradley Jr, W.G. (eds) (1992) *Magnetic Resonance Imaging,* 2nd edn. Mosby Year Book Inc., St Louis.

Wehrli, F.W. (1991) *Fast-scan Magnetic Resonance: Principles and Applications.* Raven Press, New York.

Appendix

Table 3.1 Mobile hydrogen ion concentration.

Tissue	H⁺ concentration
CSF/most pathology	High
Fat/grey matter	↓
White matter	Low
Cortical bone	Very low

Table 3.2 T1 values and signal intensities in soft tissue on a T1-weighted image.

Tissue	T1 constants	Signal intensity
CSF	Long	Low
Pathology (most)		
Grey matter	↓	↓
White matter		
Fat	Short	High

Table 3.3 T2 values and signal intensities in soft tissue on a T2-weighted image.

Tissue	T2 constants	Signal intensity
CSF	Long	High
Pathology (most)		↓
Grey matter	↓	Low
White matter		
Fat	Short	Moderate*

*Complete T1 relaxation, a high proton density and complex T2-relaxation processes usually give fat a moderately high signal on T2-weighted sequences.

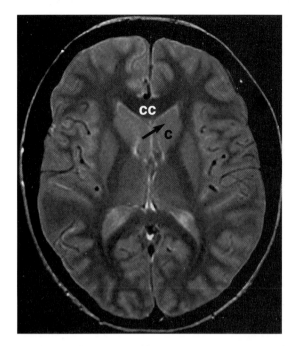

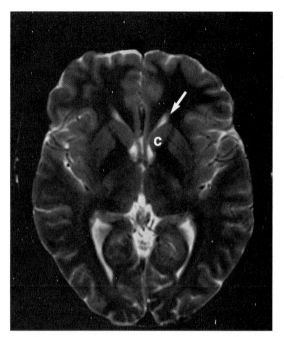

Fig. 3.A1 Proton-density scan. First echo of a double-echo sequence. Axial section (TR 2800 ms, TE 30 ms; at 1.5 T). Grey matter has a higher proton density than white matter and therefore gives a stronger signal. CSF gives a similar signal to grey matter because, even though T1 relaxation is incomplete at this TR (tending to reduce its signal intensity), T2 effects are beginning to affect image contrast at this TE (see Fig. 3.34). C, head of caudate nucleus; CC, corpus callosum; arrow, CSF in frontal horn of lateral ventricle.

Fig. 3.A2 T2-weighted scan. Second echo of a double-echo sequence. Axial section (TR 2800 ms, TE 90 ms; at 1.5 T). Grey and white matter have similar T2 constants and therefore any contrast between them must be due to a difference in their respective proton densities. T2 relaxation of CSF is prolonged and CSF now gives high signal (see Fig. 3.34). C, head of caudate nucleus; arrow, CSF in frontal horn of lateral ventricle.

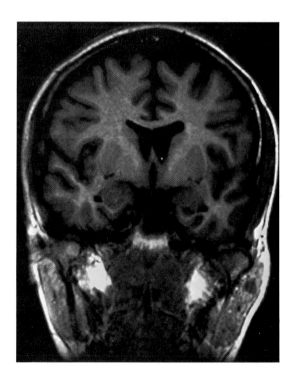

Fig. 3.A3 Inversion-recovery scan. Coronal section (TR 2000 ms, TI 700 ms, TE 16 ms; at 1.5 T). A moderately short inversion time (TI) gives strong contrast between grey and white matter (see Fig. 3.37). CSF has a low signal intensity with these sequence parameters.

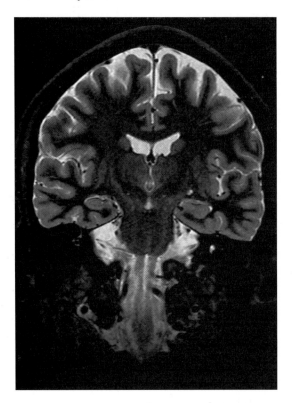

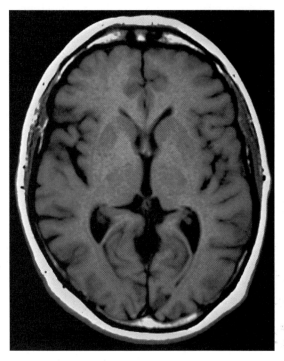

Fig. 3.A5 T1-weighted scan. Unenhanced. Axial section (TR 540 ms, TE 14 ms; at 1.5 T). A short TR accentuates T1 differences between brain and CSF (see Fig. 3.30). Grey matter has a longer T1 constant than white matter and therefore lower signal but grey/white contrast is not as strong as in the inversion-recovery image.

Fig. 3.A4 STIR sequence. Coronal section (fast spin–echo) (TR 4380 ms, TI 160 ms, effective TE 34 ms; at 1.5 T). Contrast here is largely dependent on T1 differences between tissues but signal intensities are inverted compared with normal T1-weighted scans. Fat signal is suppressed. Some T2 weighting is added at this value of TE, augmenting signal from water (see text and Fig. 3.39).

4: Normal Brain Anatomy
Imaged by CT and MRI

J. N. P. Higgins

Acknowledgement to Professor Nieuwenhuys

The author wishes to thank Professor Nieuwenhuys for kind permission to reproduce Figs 7, 8, 11–13, 21, 23, 26, 28, 29, 191, 192, 195 and 214 from Nieuwenhuys et al: The Human Central Nervous System: A Synopsis and Atlas.

Introduction

The radiological diagnosis of intracranial pathology is more frequently based on location and morphology than on density (computed tomography (CT)) or signal intensity (magnetic resonance imaging (MRI)). This may be comforting to the clinician faced with a plethora of images following a request for MRI, but it also implies that a clear understanding of anatomy is of prime importance in their interpretation.

Until recently, radiological investigation of the central nervous system relied almost entirely upon indirect methods of demonstrating pathology. On plain skull films, for example, enlargement of the pituitary fossa raised the possibility of a pituitary tumour. Special techniques such as air encephalography and cerebral arteriography allowed a more comprehensive assessment, but even here the presence and position of an abnormality could only be inferred by its effect on the ventricles or vessels (Robertson, 1957; Greitz & Lindgren, 1971; du Boulay, 1980).

Interpretation of these investigations required not only an expertise in neuroanatomy but also an understanding of the way in which the neuroanatomy was displayed by the particular technique

employed. Both air encephalography and angiography result in the formation of complex images stemming from the projection of the internal architecture of a three-dimensional object on to a two-dimensional surface (X-ray film). Structures sited widely apart in the brain may appear closely related or even contiguous when presented in this way, and mentally separating them into their correct anatomical relationships requires practice.

With the advent of CT and MRI, it has become possible to image the central nervous system directly. However, these techniques display the brain in a series of slices so that abnormalities are rarely visualised in their entirety on a single image and the internal anatomy of the brain is viewed piecemeal. Understanding the anatomical relationships between normal structures and pathological lesions presented in this way also requires practice, and experienced observers build up a mental picture of a lesion by reviewing multiple adjacent slices and by reference to imaging in different planes. Accurate interpretation of such images requires first an understanding of the complex interrelationships between the various structures that make up the normal brain and second a knowledge of how they appear in section.

It might seem appropriate to start with a description of the brain suface. However, localisation of gyral surface markings is not straightforward even in the anatomical specimen and such difficulties are reflected in the interpretation of sectional imaging. Moreover, it is the internal architecture of the brain that generally forms the most striking feature of a brain scan. CT and MRI brain anatomy is therefore best learnt from inside outwards.

For purposes of description, the internal structure of the brain has traditionally been divided into well-recognised components or systems known to interact in a more or less well-understood manner. This chapter also takes this approach but combines it with references to sectional imaging. MRI with its excellent grey/white matter contrast is ideally suited to display these anatomical features. Drawings of the gross anatomy accompany the text and axial, coronal and sagittal MRI sections are collected in 'atlas' format in the Appendix at the end of the chapter.

Anatomical knowledge is not accrued without effort. Repeated reference will have to be made both to the anatomical drawings and to the radiographic images in order to appreciate the anatomical relationships between the structures described. This can be tedious, and a much better approach would be to read the text at the same time as you have unlabelled MRI or CT scans available on an X-ray viewing box. The quality of an image on film is always better than that on paper and in this way you can easily review several brain sections at once. Work through the text and try to reconcile the appearance of the gross anatomy as described and drawn with its appearance on sectional imaging. Where necessary, use the annotated images at the end of the chapter as a crib. In unfamiliar territory, a full understanding of the anatomical drawing often follows rather than precedes an understanding of the sectional image. Each representation of anatomy complements the other in the learning process. CT sections, which are less cluttered by anatomical detail, are sometimes better studied before the MRI images.

As far as a description of brain anatomy is concerned, this chapter is necessarily incomplete. Even so, some of the anatomy described may not seem immediately relevant to psychology or psychiatry but has been included for the sake of a better understanding of neuroanatomy in general and sectional anatomy in particular. The emphasis, however, is on supratentorial structures and structures which are visible on sectional imaging. The limbic system is considered in some depth. References for more detailed description of both the radiological and macroscopic neuroanatomy are provided at the end of the chapter.

Glossary of terms used without explanation in the text

Axial plane transverse to the axis of the body
Sagittal plane perpendicular to axial plane, 'front to back'
Coronal plane perpendicular to axial plane, 'side to side'

Rostral/caudal towards the nose/'tail'
Anterior/posterior towards the face/occiput
Superior/inferior towards the top of the head/feet

Neocortex found around the central sulcus and over the major part of the cerebral hemispheres
Allocortex primitive cortex found in the hippocampus and limbic system

Telencephalon cerebral hemispheres and underlying nuclei
Diencephalon third ventricle and adjacent structures including thalamus, hypothalamus, etc.
Foramen of Munro interventricular foramen
Ambient cistern cerebrospinal fluid (CSF) space on either side of midbrain and over quadrigeminal plate

Internal structure of the cerebral hemispheres

The ventricular system

The ventricular system comprises a complex interconnecting cavity surrounded by brain and lined by a thin layer of cells called the ependyma, which forms a partial barrier between neural tissue and contained CSF. It is readily identified on sectional imaging and provides a useful reference for the identification of adjacent anatomical structures in all three imaging planes.

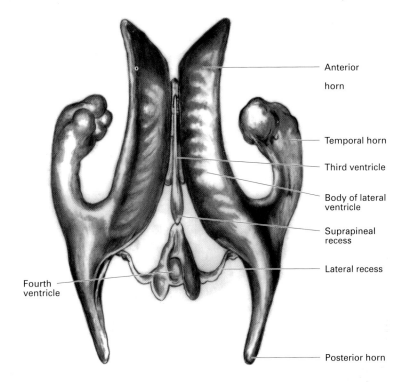

Anterior horn

Temporal horn

Third ventricle

Body of lateral ventricle

Suprapineal recess

Lateral recess

Fourth ventricle

Posterior horn

Fig. 4.1 Superior view of the ventricular system. After Retsius in *Gray's Anatomy*, 1989.

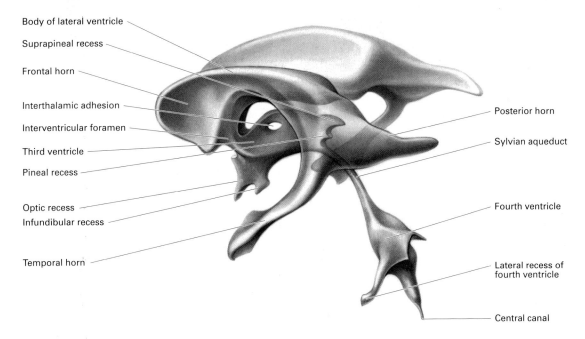

Body of lateral ventricle

Suprapineal recess

Frontal horn

Interthalamic adhesion

Interventricular foramen

Third ventricle

Pineal recess

Optic recess

Infundibular recess

Temporal horn

Posterior horn

Sylvian aqueduct

Fourth ventricle

Lateral recess of fourth ventricle

Central canal

Fig. 4.2 Oblique view of the ventricular system. After Nieuwenhuys *et al.*, 1988.

The paired lateral ventricles lie deep in the cerebral hemispheres. Each is shaped in the form of a C which is open anteriorly and which has a small tail attached to its back (Figs 4.1 & 4.2). Each is divided into a frontal horn in front of the interventricular foramen and behind into a body, trigone and posterior and temporal horns. The frontal horns and the bodies of the lateral ventricles lie in close apposition in the midline separated by the septum pellucidum, with the body of the fornix running in its inferior edge (Figs. 4.3 & 4.10). The lateral ventricles diverge from the midline posteriorly, where they are separated by the splenium of the corpus callosum, and pass down to the trigone (Fig. 4.11).

From the trigone the posterior horn projects to a variable extent into the occipital lobe and the temporal horn runs forward into the temporal lobe. The temporal horn is narrow and usually not visible on axial section except distally, where it curves medially around the head of the hippocampus. Here a thin cleft (uncal recess) usually divides the amygdala anteriorly from the hippocampal head posteriorly (Fig. 4.8).

The third ventricle forms a narrow slit which lies in the midline between and below the bodies of the lateral ventricles (Figs 4.3, 4.4, 4.5, 4.9 & 4.10). CSF formed in the lateral ventricles passes into the third ventricle through the foramen of Munro, which is situated in its anterosuperior corner and leaves through the Sylvian aqueduct, whose opening lies inferiorly in its posterior wall.

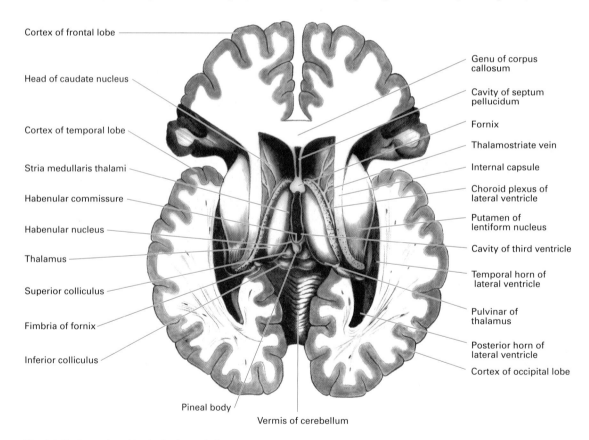

Cortex of frontal lobe
Head of caudate nucleus
Cortex of temporal lobe
Stria medullaris thalami
Habenular commissure
Habenular nucleus
Thalamus
Superior colliculus
Fimbria of fornix
Inferior colliculus
Pineal body
Vermis of cerebellum

Genu of corpus callosum
Cavity of septum pellucidum
Fornix
Thalamostriate vein
Internal capsule
Choroid plexus of lateral ventricle
Putamen of lentiform nucleus
Cavity of third ventricle
Temporal horn of lateral ventricle
Pulvinar of thalamus
Posterior horn of lateral ventricle
Cortex of occipital lobe

Fig. 4.3 Brain sectioned in the horizontal plane at two levels to show the lateral and third ventricles and related structures. After Snell, 1982.

The roof of the third ventricle lies below the body of the fornix and is formed from a double layer of pia mater called the tela choroidea evaginated forwards to the foramen of Munro from the ambient cistern. The upper layer is reflected from the posterior part (splenium) of the corpus callosum. The lower layer is continuous with pia over the back of the third ventricle. Vessels supplying the choroid plexus run between them.

The floor of the third ventricle is formed by the optic chiasma, hypothalamus and mamillary bodies (Fig. 4.4). The anterior wall is formed by the lamina terminalis, which is a thin sheet of grey matter passing between the hemispheres, orient-ated in the coronal plane. The anterior commissure crosses immediately behind the lamina terminalis, forming a prominent posterior bulge in sagittal section. The posterior wall evaginates into the suprapineal and then the pineal recesses above the opening of the Sylvian aqueduct. The lateral walls are formed by the thalamus above and the hypothalamus below. The thalami are connected in the midline across the third ventricle by the interthalamic adhesion.

The fourth ventricle is triangular in sagittal section, its floor formed by the dorsal pons and medulla and its roof projecting into the cerebellum (Fig. 4.4). It communicates with the

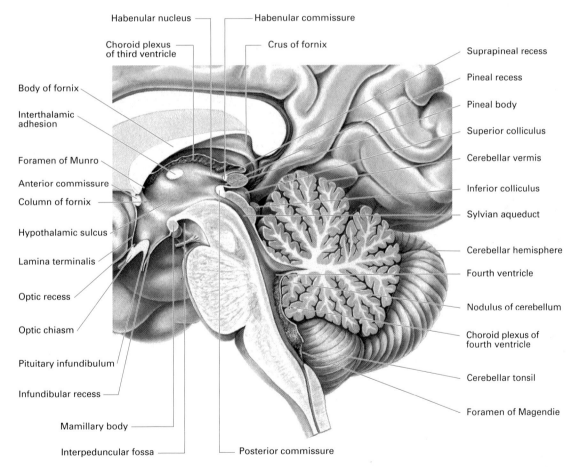

Fig. 4.4 Third and fourth ventricles in sagittal section. After Nieuwenhuys *et al.*, 1988.

third ventricle via the Sylvian aqueduct, which runs above the tegmentum of the midbrain and under the quadrigeminal plate, opening into the fourth ventricle at the level of the upper pons. Inferiorly, the fourth ventricle narrows and becomes continuous with the central canal of the spinal cord. A wide midline aperture in the posterior part of its roof allows communication with the subarachnoid space between the cerebellar tonsils (foramen of Magendie).

In axial section the cavity of the fourth ventricle is square at the level of the pons (Fig. 4.8), develops an inverted U shape at the level of the middle cerebellar peduncles (because of posterior indentation by the nodulus of the cerebellar vermis (Fig. 4.7) and becomes a coronal slit at the level of the medulla. At the pontomedullary junction, the paired lateral recesses of the fourth ventricle extend anteriorly, communicating with the subarachnoid cisterns on either side of the brainstem (foramina of Luschka).

Within the ventricular system the choroid plexus can be identified, particularly on CT if there is calcification. It forms a continuous band of tissue running through the lateral ventricles from the temporal horns to the interventricular foramen (Fig. 4.3). Here it turns down, through the foramen, and then passes posteriorly as paired

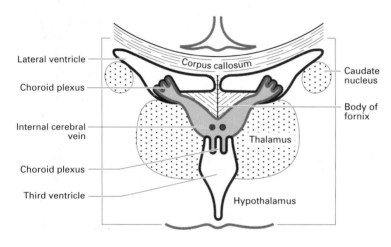

Fig. 4.5 Schematic drawing of a coronal section through the bodies of the lateral and third ventricles. The choroid plexus is formed where the ependymal lining (dark grey) and pia matter (light grey) are apposed.

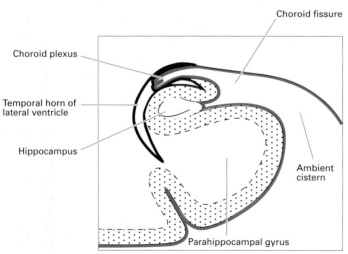

Fig. 4.6 Schematic drawing of a coronal section through the temporal horn of the right lateral ventricle to show the choroid fissure and choroid plexus. Ependyma, dark grey; pia mater, light grey.

projections in the roof of the third ventricle (Fig. 4.4). Choroid is also found on the posterior part of the roof of the fourth ventricle (Fig 4.4), with extensions into the lateral recesses bilaterally. Calcification may be seen here as well.

The choroid plexus is formed where the innermost meningeal covering (pia mater) and the ependyma are apposed (and fuse). This occurs across defects (choroidal fissure, roof of the third

ventricle) where the ventricles are not covered by neural tissue, although these defects do remain covered by ependyma (Figs 4.5 & 4.6). The choroid and its vasculature therefore lie not so much within the ventricles as outside but nevertheless deeply invaginating them from the subarachnoid space.

In the temporal horn the choroid plexus projects into the ventricle from the choroidal

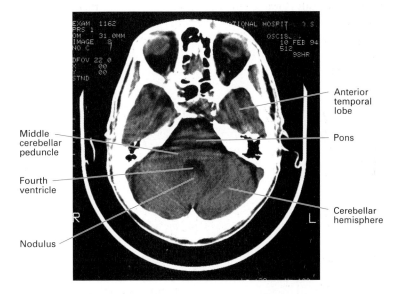

Fig. 4.7 Axial CT section through the posterior fossa showing the fourth ventricle between the middle cerebellar peduncles.

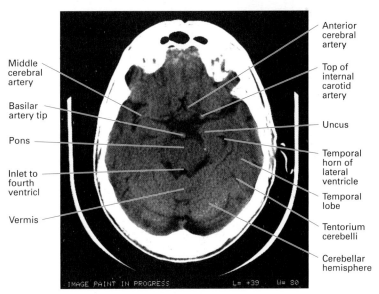

Fig.4.8 Axial CT section through the pons and base of the brain. The tentorium cerebelli separates the temporal lobe from the cerebellum at this level. The temporal horn of the lateral ventricle expands distally around the head of the hippocampus.

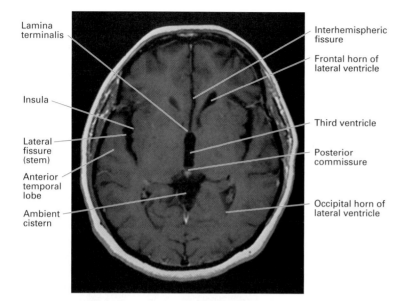

Lamina terminalis

Insula

Lateral fissure (stem)

Anterior temporal lobe

Ambient cistern

Interhemispheric fissure

Frontal horn of lateral ventricle

Third ventricle

Posterior commissure

Occipital horn of lateral ventricle

Fig. 4.9 Axial T1-weighted MRI section through the third ventricle.

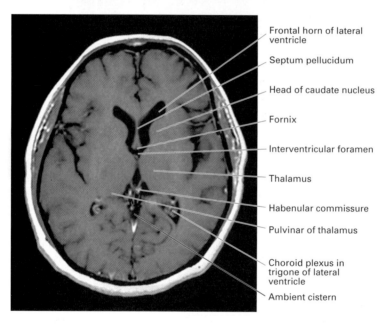

Frontal horn of lateral ventricle

Septum pellucidum

Head of caudate nucleus

Fornix

Interventricular foramen

Thalamus

Habenular commissure

Pulvinar of thalamus

Choroid plexus in trigone of lateral ventricle

Ambient cistern

Fig. 4.10 Axial T1-weighted MRI section through the foramen of Munro. The habenular commissure marks the back of the third ventricle at this level. The choroid plexus invaginates the trigone of the lateral ventricle from a lateral recess of the ambient cistern behind the pulvinar of the thalamus.

fissure, taking its arterial supply (anterior choroidal artery) with it. The choroidal fissure is easily identified on coronal MRI scans above the body of the hippocampus on the medial temporal lobe. It forms a point of reference in the identification of hippocampal anatomy. The choroid plexus then turns with the lateral ventricle, following the concavity of its C-chaped curve, into which it projects from the medial side. As the ventricle turns up through the trigone, it is invaginated by choroid from behind the posterior part of the thalamus (Fig. 4.10) and then, as it turns forward again adjacent to the midline choroid, invaginates its floor from above the third ventricle (Figs 4.5 & 4.11). Choroid in the third ventricle projects downwards from the roof.

CSF formed in the choroid plexus passes out of the ventricular system through the foramina in the fourth ventricle into the subarachnoid cisterns. Description of these complex interconnecting CSF spaces which surround the brain will not be attempted here; suffice it to say that CSF density (CT) and signal intensity (MRI) in the subarachnoid cisterns are indistinguishable from those in the ventricular system except where the MRI signal is affected by regions of high or turbulent CSF flow.

The thalamus and basal ganglia

The terminology involved in the description of the deep structures of the brain can be confusing. Names have been given to numerous different combinations of grey and white matter (usually with a functional interrelationship in mind), with the result that the use of a particular term often has to be qualified with an explanation, and there is as yet no universal agreement on nomenclature (Gray, 1989c). Here basal ganglia refers only to the caudate and lentiform nuclei and to the claustrum.

Thalamus

The thalami are paired ovoid masses of grey matter which form the lateral walls of the third ventricle and which are usually joined across it by the interthalamic adhesion (Figs 4.3, 4.4 & 4.12). On axial scans they are easily identified on either side of the third ventricle as areas of grey-matter signal (or density) posterior to the interventricular foramen and medial to the posterior limb of the internal capsule. The posterior part of the thalamus, known as the pulvinar, overhangs the quadrigeminal plate and is outlined by CSF in a lateral recess (or wing) of the ambient cistern (Fig. 4.10).

The superior and inferior relations of the thalamus are best appreciated on coronal images (Figs 4.6, 4.A16 – 4.A18). The upper surface of

the thalamus forms part of the floor of the body of the lateral ventricle. Superolaterally it is related to the body of the caudate nucleus and supero-medially across the tela choroidea of the third ventricle to the body of the fornix. Antero-inferiorly it is related to the posterior part of the hypothalamus. Inferiorly it is related to the subthalamus, red nucleus and geniculate bodies (see below).

Caudate nucleus

The caudate nuclei are elongated paired structures closely related to the lateral ventricles on either side. Each has a head, body and tail and conforms to a C shape, to some extent mirroring the concavity of the lateral ventricles (Fig. 4.12).

The expanded head of the caudate nucleus is easily seen on axial and coronal images where it indents the floor of the frontal horn of the lateral ventricle. The anterior limb of the internal capsule lies on its lateral side. Behind the head, the body of the caudate narrows considerably and is best seen on coronal sections. It lies against the floor of the lateral ventricle, with the posterior limb of the internal capsule on its lateral side. The caudate body follows the curve of the lateral ventricle into the temporal lobe. Here its tail continues along the roof of the temporal horn (Fig. 4.A19) before turning medially to fuse with the inferior part of the lentiform nucleus (and amygdala).

Anterior to the foramen of Munro the characteristic shape of the lateral ventricle results from the prominent impression on the frontal horn by the head of the caudate nucleus (Fig. 4.10). Posterior to the foramen of Munro the shape of the lateral ventricle in coronal section is partly derived from impressions on its floor by the thalamus medially and by the body of the caudate laterally. The thalamocaudate groove between them marks the site of the thalamostriate veins (Fig. 4.A18). These veins run towards the interven-tricular foramen (Figs 4.3 & 4.A6) before turning back in the tela choroidea of the third ventricle as the internal cerebral veins. The constancy of this anatomical arrangement

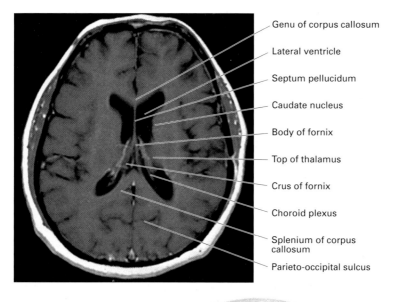

Genu of corpus callosum

Lateral ventricle

Septum pellucidum

Caudate nucleus

Body of fornix

Top of thalamus

Crus of fornix

Choroid plexus

Splenium of corpus callosum

Parieto-occipital sulcus

Fig. 4.11 Axial T1-weighted MRI section through the floor of the body of the lateral ventricle. The choroid plexus projects into the lateral ventricle through the choroid fissure (see Fig. 4.5). The top of the thalamus is just included in the plane of section.

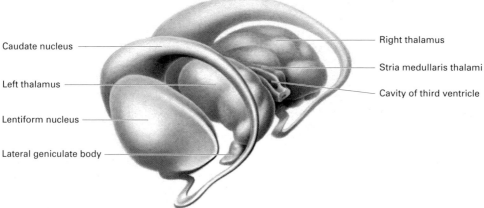

Caudate nucleus

Left thalamus

Lentiform nucleus

Lateral geniculate body

Right thalamus

Stria medullaris thalami

Cavity of third ventricle

Fig. 4.12 Oblique posterior view of the thalamus, caudate and lentiform nuclei. After Nieuwenhuys *et al.*, 1988.

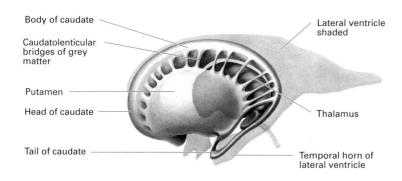

Body of caudate

Caudatolenticular bridges of grey matter

Putamen

Head of caudate

Tail of caudate

Lateral ventricle shaded

Thalamus

Temporal horn of lateral ventricle

Fig. 4.13 Lateral view of the lentiform and caudate nuclei to show the caudatolenticular bridges of gery matter through which fibres of the internal capsule pass. After Nieuwenhuys *et al.*, 1988.

previously formed an important landmark in the angiographic localisation of disease.

Lentiform nucleus and claustrum

The lentiform nucleus is a lens-shaped condensation of grey matter in each cerebral hemisphere which lies within, but slightly lateral to, the arc formed by the caudate nucleus. It is separated from the caudate nucleus by the internal capsule except where it is fused with the caudate head anteroinferiorly and with the caudate tail posteroinferiorly. Numerous radially aligned strands of grey matter bridge the gap between the caudate and the lentiform nucleus through which the fibres of the internal capsule have to pass (Figs 4.13 & 4.A12). These strands are often visible on MRI and their striking appearance in the sectioned brain gave rise to the term 'corpus striatum', encompassing the caudate and lentiform nuclei and intervening internal capsule (Gray, 1989c).

Each lentiform nucleus is divided by a sagittally orientated lamina into two main parts. The larger putamen lies laterally. The smaller and more medial globus pallidus is itself further divided into medial and lateral parts. The globus pallidus takes its name from its relative pallor in section, caused by numerous white-matter tracts which traverse it. This and a high concentration of stored iron allow the globus pallidus to be distinguished from the putamen on MRI (Figs 4.A4 & 4.A10) (Drayer *et al.*, 1986). On CT, distinction between these structures is not possible unless there is differential calcification.

The characteristic biconvex shape of the lentiform nucleus is clearly demonstrated on axial scans, bordered medially by the anterior and posterior limbs of the internal capsule and laterally by the external capsule deep to the insular cortex. The larger putamen is the dominant structure on MRI. On coronal scans the globus pallidus and putamen present a triangular configuration, the globus pallidus forming the apex of the triangle pointing downwards and medially and the putamen forming the base

against the external capsule laterally. Fusion between the inferior part of the caudate head and the putamen is seen on anterior sections. More posteriorly the internal capsule separates the lentiform nucleus, at first from the caudate head and then from the caudate body and the thalamus (Fig 4.A13–4.A19).

The claustrum is the name given to a thin sheet of grey matter orientated in the sagittal plane which is interposed between the external capsule and the insular cortex (Figs 4.A11 & 4.A14). A few fibres passing lateral to the claustrum are sometimes referred to as the extreme capsule.

Vascular territories

Arterial supply to the basal ganglia is mainly via small perforating arteries from the proximal middle cerebral artery. These vessels, known as the lenticulostriate arteries, pass up through the anterior perforated substance in the base of the brain to the lentiform nucleus, internal capsule and caudate nucleus. Wide CSF spaces often mark their position on both coronal and axial imaging (Fig. 4.A3) (Jungries *et al.*, 1988). A small recurrent branch (of Heubner) from the proximal part of the anterior cerebral artery joins the lenticulostriate arteries supplying the basal ganglia and also part of the anterior thalamus.

Arterial supply to the thalamus is mainly via thalamoperforating arteries derived from the posterior communicating, posterior cerebral and basilar arteries. The medial part of the thalamus is supplied by the medial posterior choroidal artery (itself derived from the posterior cerebral artery).

The cerebral peduncles, internal capsule and corona radiata

The majority of neuronal connections between the neocortex and the brainstem and spinal cord are condensed from the corona radiata on to the internal capsule and cerebral penduncle (Fig. 4.14).

The corona radiata describes the fan-shaped

convergence of these fibres from the cortex on to the internal capsule. The internal capsule describes their further convergence, between the lentiform nucleus laterally and the caudate and thalamus medially, on to the cerebral peduncle. The cerebral peduncle transmits these fibres to the brainstem and spinal cord.

The shape of the internal capsule is imposed on it by the lentiform nucleus, around the medial side of which fibres from the corona radiata must pass to reach the cerebral peduncle inferomedially. The result is a broad cone of white-matter tracts, split anteroinferiorly but otherwise passing the lentiform nucleus above, below, in front and behind, which converge to an apex on the cerebral peduncle (Fig. 4.15).

Axial sections at the level of the basal ganglia divide the 'cone' of the internal capsule into anterior and posterior limbs, seen as bands of white-matter signal or density. The genu describes the region where they join. MRI signal from the posterior part of the posterior limb of the internal capsule may be increased on T2-weighted sequences, owing to a relatively low concentration of iron locally (Fig. 4.A4) (Drayer *et al.*, 1986).

Frontopontine fibres run in the anterior limb. The pyramidal tracts are found in the genu and posterior limb.

The cerebral peduncles lie on the anterolateral surface of the midbrain, separated in the midline by the interpeduncular cistern. They are easily recognised in axial section, where they give a characteristic broad Y configuration to the upper midbrain (Fig. 4.24).

Coronal sections at the level of the cerebral peduncles show the posterior limb of the internal capsule continuous with the cerebral peduncles inferiorly and the corona radiata superiorly (Figs 4.A18 & 4.A19).

The hypothalamus and subthalamus

Beneath the readily identifiable mass of grey matter that forms the thalamus lie the hypothalamus and subthalamus. These areas are more difficult to recognise on imaging because for the most part they comprise neural tissue with limits defined more by the boundaries of neighbouring structures than by any distinctive morphology or imaging feature. Their superior extent is marked

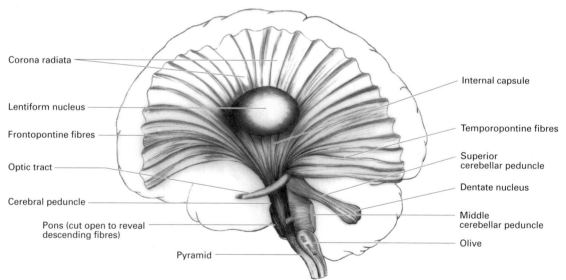

Fig. 4.14 Lateral view of left corona radiata, internal capsule and cerebral peduncle. The internal capsule lies on the medial side of the lentiform nucleus. After Snell, 1982.

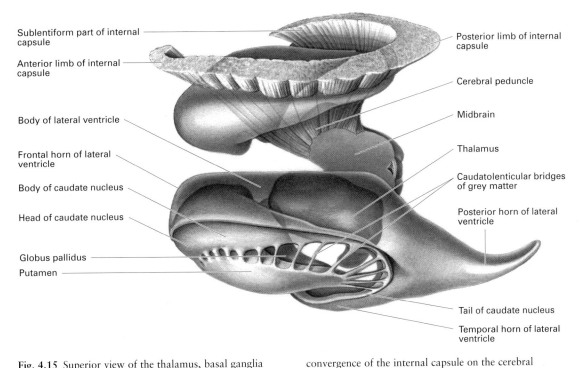

Sublentiform part of internal capsule

Anterior limb of internal capsule

Body of lateral ventricle

Frontal horn of lateral ventricle

Body of caudate nucleus

Head of caudate nucleus

Globus pallidus

Putamen

Posterior limb of internal capsule

Cerebral peduncle

Midbrain

Thalamus

Caudatolenticular bridges of grey matter

Posterior horn of lateral ventricle

Tail of caudate nucleus

Temporal horn of lateral ventricle

Fig. 4.15 Superior view of the thalamus, basal ganglia and internal capsule. The lateral ventricle and thalamus have been removed on the right side to show the convergence of the internal capsule on the cerebral peduncle. After Nieuwenhuys *et al.*, 1988.

on the lateral wall of the third ventricle by a shallow groove (the hypothalamic sulcus) running posteriorly from the foramen of Munro to the Sylvian aqueduct (Fig. 4.4). This groove may be visible on sagittal section as a thick line of pure CSF signal intensity, signifying the widest part of the third ventricle.

The hypothalamus tends to be discussed in the singular but nevertheless refers to paired regions on either side of the third ventricle and to structures forming its floor (Fig. 4.16). The lamina terminalis defines its anterior limit (including the preoptic area), and a line drawn vertically upwards from the mamillary bodies approximately defines its posterior limit. It lies below the anterior part of the hypothalamic sulcus. On each side, the hypothalamus is divided into medial and lateral nuclei, the anterior column of the fornix and mamillothalamic tract (see below) running in the paramedian plane between them. Behind the optic chiasma, hypothalamic

nuclei are found in a thickening of the floor of the third ventricle around the base of the pituitary stalk, named the tuber cinereum, and more posteriorly in the paired mamillary bodies.

On midline sagittal MRI, the hypothalamus on either side of the third ventricle is often marked by signal which is intermediate between grey matter and CSF because of partial-volume averaging, below the hypothalamic sulcus. On axial MRI the hypothalamus and anteroinferior part of the third ventricle can appear as an island of tissue in front of the cerebral peduncles, bordered laterally by the optic tracts (Fig. 4.A2).

The subthalamus refers to the region directly inferior to the thalamus and posterosuperior to the main bulk of the hypothalamus. It is bordered laterally by the cerebral peduncle as it merges with the internal capsule and medially by the posterior nuclei of the hypothalamus, which separate it from the third ventricle. The anterior parts of both the red nucleus and the substantia nigra project in the caudal part of the subthalmic area.

On axial scans the subthalamic areas are found on the section between the one containing the easily recognized cerebral peduncles below and the one containing the easily recognised thalami above. The red nuclei are often seen as circular regions of relative low signal on T2-weighted images in the same section on either side of the interpeduncular cistern (Fig. 4.A3).

Working backwards from the anterior commissure, coronal sections first show the hypothalamus on either side of the third ventricle below the hypothalamic sulcus. Next the mamillary bodies are visible in the floor of the third ventricle, with the subthalamic areas lying just above and lateral to them (and below the

thalami). The internal capsules separate these structures from the lentiform nuclei. More posteriorly still, the red nuclei are seen directly below the thalami (Figs 4.A14–4.A18).

The substantia nigra and red nuclei

The substantia nigra refers to paired bands of pigmented cells running the length of the midbrain, posteromedial to the cerebral peduncles, from the upper border of the pons into the subthalamus. Their position is best appreciated on axial sections (Fig. 4.24).

Axial scans through the upper midbrain also show the red nuclei, which are paired, nearly spherical masses situated close to the midline, medial and posterosuperior to the substantia

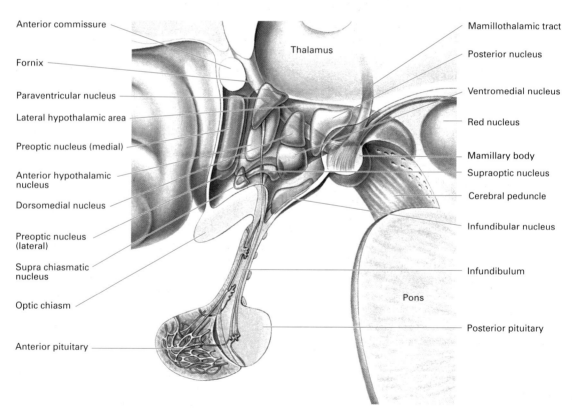

Fig. 4.16 Medial view of inferior part of right hemisphere showing the major hypothalamic nuclei in the wall and floor of the third ventricle below the hypothalamic sulcus

(see also Fig. 4.5). The red nucleus projects into the subthalamic area. After Nieuwenhuys *et al.*, 1988.

nigra. Local iron deposition means they return a reduced signal on T2-weighted MRI relative to surrounding tissue, often giving them a striking, dark appearance (Fig. 4.C). The proximity of the red nuclei to the thalami is apparent on coronal scans.

The anterior and posterior commissures and the corpus callosum

Within the brain, neuronal connections between left and right run in the commissures, which form dense transversely orientated white-matter bundles spreading out symmetrically on either side of the midline to merge with the white matter of each cerebral hemisphere.

The corpus callosum is the largest and takes fibres from the frontal, parietal, occipital and temporal lobes . It is divided into a rostrum, genu, body and splenium and is easily identified in sagittal section (Fig. 4.30). The rostrum of the corpus callosum is thin and extends anteriorly from the upper end of the lamina terminalis, under the septum pellucidum, where it forms the floor of the anterior horns of the lateral ventricles. It thickens considerably as it approaches the genu, turning upwards and then posteriorly as the body to form the roof of the lateral ventricles and enclosing the septum pellucidum. The body ends in a thickened downturned ridge – the splenium — which projects into the ambient cistern.

The forceps major describes the convergence of fibres from the occipital lobes on to the splenium and the forceps minor a similar convergence on to the genu from the anterior frontal lobes (Fig. 4.17). However, these tracts cannot be identified as separate structures on imaging, and lateral to the midline the radiations of the corpus callosum rapidly intersect and merge with the fibres of the corona radiata.

The anterior commissure crosses the midline in the anterior wall of the third ventricle, forming a prominent indentation just below the foramen of Munro, which is visible on sagittal section (Fig. 4.4). It provides a useful marker for adjacent structures (Naidich *et al.*, 1986). Looking from

above, it has the shape of bicycle handlebars with the outer ends turned back towards the temporal lobe (Fig. 4.18). This is not immediately apparent on axial scans because the lateral parts of the anterior commissure are inclined, both inferiorly and posteriorly, and therefore only parts of it can be seen on a single section.

Immediately lateral to the midline, the anterior commissure passes in front of the anterior columns of the fornix, which at this level lie on either side of the anterior part of the third ventricle (Fig. 4.A3). Running very slightly forwards, it passes just under the anterior limb of the internal capsule before turning posteriorly and inferiorly to cross the anteroinferior part of the lateral nucleus of the globus pallidus. Further laterally, it passes above the amygdala into the temporal lobe and merges with fibres of the external capsule, after which it can no longer be distinguished as a separate structure.

The site of the posterior commissure is marked on sagittal section by a thickening of the posterior wall of the third ventricle just above the origin of the Sylvian aqueduct and below the pineal recess (Fig. 4.4). It merges rapidly with tissue postero-inferior to the thalamus in the upper midbrain.

The habenular commissure and the commissure of the fornix are described below, under the limbic system.

Limbic system

The limbic system defines a complex arrangement of cortical gyri, grey-matter nuclei and inter-connecting white-matter tracts lying on the medial surfaces of the cerebral hemispheres and around the third ventricle, which are functionally so closely related that they can be considered as a single unit. In evolutionary terms these areas are older than other parts of the cerebral hemispheres (telencephalon) and histologically the limbic cortex appears primitive, generally lacking the well-defined lamination found elsewhere (Gray, 1989b).

The limbic system is concerned with emotion, instinct and memory and, through the hypo-

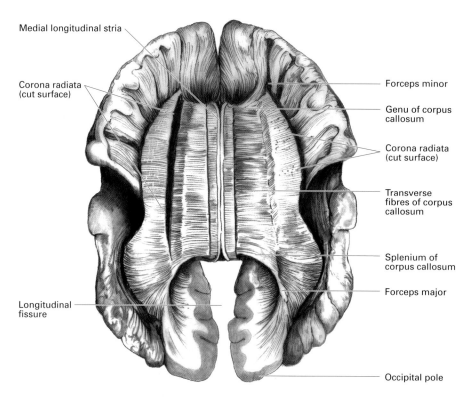

Medial longitudinal stria

Corona radiata
(cut surface)

Forceps minor

Genu of corpus
callosum

Corona radiata
(cut surface)

Transverse
fibres of corpus
callosum

Splenium of
corpus callosum

Forceps major

Longitudinal
fissure

Occipital pole

Fig. 4.17 Superior view of the brain dissected to show the
fibres of the corpus callosum and corona radiata. After
Snell, 1982.

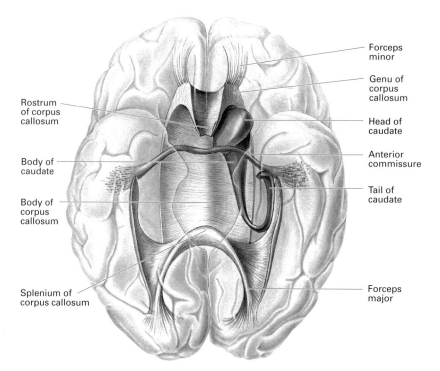

Forceps
minor

Genu of
corpus
callosum

Rostrum
of corpus
callosum

Head of
caudate

Anterior
commissure

Body of
caudate

Tail of
caudate

Body of
corpus
callosum

Splenium of
corpus callosum

Forceps
major

Fig. 4.18 Inferior view of the corpus callosum, anterior
commissure and caudate nucleus. After Nieuwenhuys *et
al.*, 1988.

thalamus, with the maintenance of homoeostasis (Isaacson, 1982a). Large parts of the limbic system are contained in distinctive structures whose morphology is easily amenable to anatomical description and which can be identified on imaging. Other areas are submerged in surrounding brain and cannot be resolved. Naming and describing the tracts and nuclei of the limbic system is relatively straightforward but, not unexpectedly, ascribing particular functions to named areas is problematic. Nevertheless, understanding the gross morphology of limbic structures, even without fully understanding their function, at least facilitates communication between workers.

Any description of the limbic system is complicated by a lack of agreement on what structures should be included under the term and furthermore by an inconsistency in the naming of its components (Gray, 1989b; Bronen, 1992). Some authors include the olfactory structures. Others do not. Some authors consider the hypothalamus to be the central component of the limbic system (Isaacson, 1982b) but often (as here) it is described separately. The term hippocampus is used here to describe a well-defined mass of tissue aligned along the medial temporal lobe. Elsewhere hippocampus/hippocampal formation often includes its continuation over the corpus callosum. The purpose of this chapter is not to contribute to this debate, but to develop an understanding of the anatomy of limbic structures and hence of how they appear on sectional imaging.

The majority of the limbic efferent, afferent and intrinsic neuronal impulses pass through the hypothalamus, and the limbic system can be considered to lie in a series of paired concentric C-shaped curves on either side of the midline with the hypothalamus at the centre (Nieuwenhuys *et al.*, 1988) (Fig. 4.19). The innermost curve is represented by the stria medullaris thalami, habenular nucleus and the habenulointerpeduncular tract. Next the amygdala and stria terminalis form a curve similar to that of the caudate nucleus already described. Around this

run the fimbria and fornix which connect each hippocampus to its ipsilateral mamillary body. More peripherally still the hippocampus and its extension runs over the corpus callosum to the septal nuclei and lastly the widest curve is formed by the parahippocampal gyrus and the cingulum. The anterior commissure has already been described but it also contains fibres related to the limbic system.

In this section the emphasis is mainly on those limbic structures which can be identified on MRI (Naidich *et al.*, 1987a,b; Tien *et al.*, 1992). The approach taken does not follow the orderly pattern outlined above but starts in the temporal lobe, where a knowledge of the anatomy has particular clinical relevance. The fimbria and fornix seem to form the primary pathway for hippocampal efferents (Nieuwenhuys *et al.* 1988), but even these structures contain hippocampal afferents and descriptions of nerve-fibre tracts as running forwards, downwards, etc. are not meant to be taken as an indication of the direction of nerve conduction.

The mesial temporal lobe—uncus, hippocampus

If a cerebral hemisphere, with brainstem, cerebral peduncles and thalamus removed, is viewed from its medial aspect, the hippocampus and parahippocampal gyrus can be seen aligned along the medial (or mesial) surface of the temporal lobe (Fig. 4.20). Anteriorly these structures turn sharply upwards to form the uncus (hook), which itself forms a prominent medial protuberance on the temporal lobe. Anterior to the uncus the medial temporal cortex, no longer a part of the limbic system, turns away laterally to the temporal pole.

The hippocampus probably derives its name from a supposed resemblance to a sea serpent when viewed through the lateral ventricle (Bronen, 1992). From this aspect a broad head is visible anteriorly, which reduces to a smaller body and tail posteriorly (Fig. 4.21). Its anterior extent is marked medially by the uncus and laterally by the uncal recess of the lateral ventricle. Where it

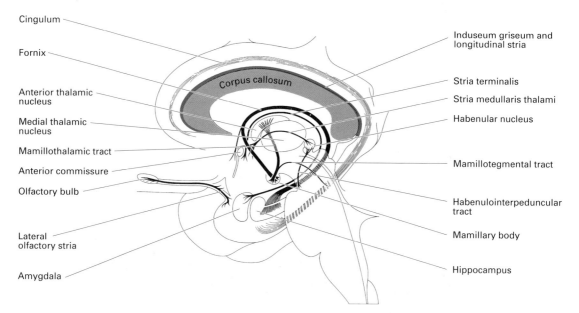

Cingulum

Fornix

Anterior thalamic nucleus

Medial thalamic nucleus

Mamillothalamic tract

Anterior commissure

Olfactory bulb

Lateral olfactory stria

Amygdala

Corpus callosum

Induseum griseum and longitudinal stria

Stria terminalis

Stria medullaris thalami

Habenular nucleus

Mamillotegmental tract

Habenulointerpeduncular tract

Mamillary body

Hippocampus

Fig. 4.19 Schematic diagram of the five limbic rings on the medial surface of the cerebral hemisphere. After Nieuwenhuys *et al.*, 1988.

projects into the ventricle, the head is folded into a number of interdigitations called the pes hippocampi. Posteriorly the hippocampus runs upwards into both the fornix and the indusium griseum (see below). Laterally its border is delineated by the temporal horn of the lateral ventricle. Medially the hippocampus and parahippocampal gyrus form the lateral margins of the ambient cistern on either side of the cerebral peduncles.

The origin of the term 'hippocampus' has become obscured because when sectioned at right angles to its long axis it can be taken to resemble a sea horse. Several distinct components are visible in this plane: the dentate gyrus, the cornu ammonis, the subiculum, the alveus and the fimbria (Figs 4.22 & 4.23).

The dentate gyrus (called after characteristic corrugations that run along its medial surface) lies in an upturned arc, into which the medial downturned margin of the cornu ammonis is invaginated. The rest of the cornu ammonis is folded around the lateral side of the dentate gyrus, merging with the subiculum and then with the

cortex of the parahippocampal gyrus. The parahippocampal gyrus is limited by the collateral sulcus. The alveus is a condensation of white matter derived from the subiculum and parahippocampal gyrus that covers the lateral and superior surface of the cornu ammonis and converges medially on the fimbria.

The dentate gyrus abuts the subiculum inferiorly across the hippocampal sulcus. The fimbriodentate sulcus is a medial groove which partly separates the fimbria from the dentate gyrus and, above this, the choroid fissure separates the fimbria from the diencephalon. Occasionally the hippocampal sulcus is not completely obliterated (Sasaki *et al.*, 1993).

An axial section tilted along the plane of the temporal lobe frequently gives an excellent overview of the hippocampus (Fig. 4.24). However, hippocampal anatomy (and pathology) is best evaluated in the coronal plane, despite the difficulties of interpretation presented by its changing orientation along the medial temporal lobe (Jack *et al.*, 1990; Watson *et al.*, 1992; Jackson *et al.*, 1993; Mieners *et al.*, 1994). These

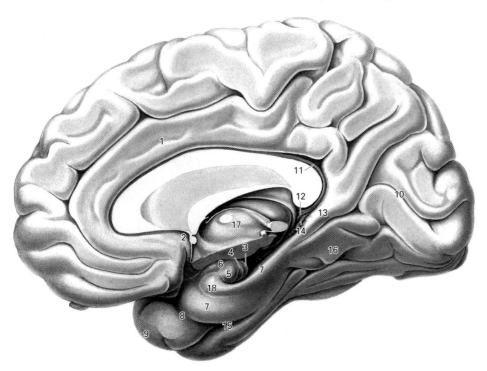

1	Cingulate gyrus	2	Paraterminal gyrus	3	Intralimbic gyrus (uncus)
4	Band of Giacomini (uncus)	5	Uncinate gyrus (uncus)	6	Semilunar gyrus
7	Parahippocampal gyrus	8	Rhinal sulcus	9	Temporal pole
10	Calcarine sulcus	11	Indusium griseum	12	Gyrus fasciolaris
13	Isthmus of the cingulate gyrus	14	Dentate gyrus	15	Collateral sulcus
16	Medial occipitotemporal gyrus	17	Thalamus	18	Gyrus ambiens

Fig. 4.20 Medial view of right cerebral hemisphere with the brainstem, cerebral peduncles, hypothalamus and subthalamus removed to reveal the medial temporal lobe. After Nieuwenhuys *et al.*, 1988.

difficulties are particularly acute anteriorly, where the medial part of the hippocampal head turns upwards and backwards to form the uncus, taking the dentate and other gyri with it. Confident labelling of the internal structure of the hippocampus is therefore difficult in this region (Duvernoy, 1988) and typical hippocampal anatomy is best appreciated on more posterior sections.

Coronal MRI sections through the body of the hippocampus have the cerebral peduncles medially and the belly of the pons inferomedially (Fig. 4.25). The choroidal fissure, containing CSF, can be traced laterally from the ambient cistern over the parahippocampal gyrus to the point where it reaches the fimbria and dentate gyrus. On anterior sections the dentate gyrus lies buried deeply under the fimbria but more posteriorly it is increasingly exposed as the fimbria moves to a more lateral position on the hippocampus. Identification of hippocampal anatomy requires extremely close inspection of the images, the various components taking up much less room than might be imagined following study of various magnified diagrammatic representations. Nevertheless, from above downwards, between structures at the base of the diencephalon and the parahippocampal gyrus, the choroidal fissure, fimbria, cornu ammonis, fimbriodentate sulcus,

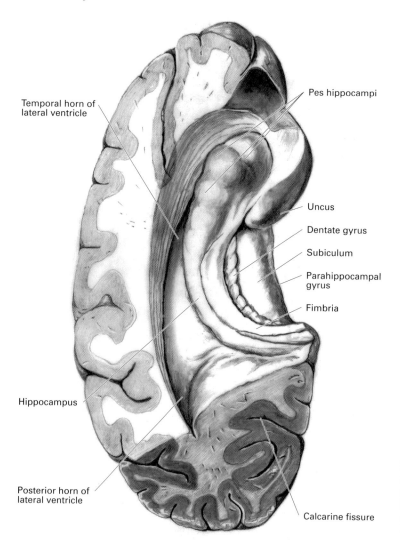

Temporal horn of
lateral ventricle

Pes hippocampi

Uncus

Dentate gyrus

Subiculum

Parahippocampal
gyrus

Fimbria

Hippocampus

Posterior horn of
lateral ventricle

Calcarine fissure

Fig. 4.21 Superior view of a dissection of left temporal and occipital lobes to reveal the hippocampus and its relations to the temporal horn of the lateral ventricle. After Sobota, 1911.

dentate gyrus, hippocampal sulcus and subiculum can often be distinguished (Fig. 4.25). The temporal horn of the lateral ventricle appears as a crescent of CSF signal laterally, outlining the cornu ammonis (covered by the alveus). The collateral sulcus is the first sulcus on the inferomedial surface of the temporal lobe.

The mesial temporal lobe—amygdala

The amygdala comprises a group of grey-matter nuclei in the medial temporal lobe, deep to the

uncus and just anterior to the hippocampal head, from which it is separated only by the uncal recess of the temporal horn of the lateral ventricle. It is named after its characteristic almond shape and is aligned with its broad anterior and posterior surfaces tilted slightly backwards from the coronal plane (Fig. 4.26).

Working backwards through coronal MRI sections the amygdala first appears as a rather amorphous thickening of grey matter on the medial temporal lobe which helps to define the uncus (Fig. 4.A15). More posteriorly, scans

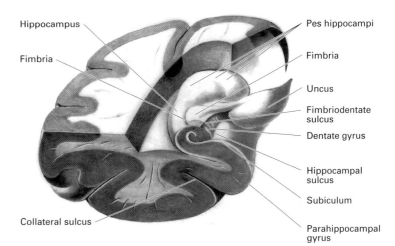

Fig. 4.22 Further dissection of the same specimen as in Fig. 4.17. A more posterior view shows the typical configuration of the hippocampus in cross-section. After Sobota, 1911.

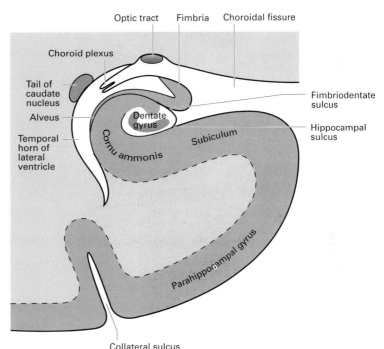

Fig. 4.23 Schematic diagram of the hippocampus in cross-section. Compare this with its appearance on coronal MRI (see Fig. 4.25).

quickly run on to the hippocampus. The inclination of the amygdala to the horizontal means that its superior (and most caudal) portion is sometimes seen just above the hippocampal head on the same section, with the uncal recess of the lateral ventricle in between them (Fig. 4.A16). This appearance is exaggerated when coronal scans are angled forwards so as to section the temporal lobe at right angles to its long axis (Watson *et al.*; 1992).

The fimbria, fornix, mamillary bodies and anterior thalamus

Hippocampal efferents are found mainly in the fimbria and fornix which describe (working

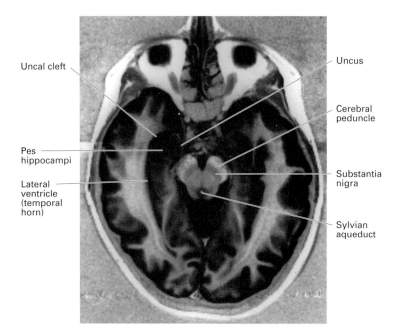

Uncal cleft

Pes
hippocampi

Lateral
ventricle
(temporal
horn)

Uncus

Cerebral
peduncle

Substantia
nigra

Sylvian
aqueduct

Fig. 4.24 Tilted axial T1-weighted
MRI scan through the body and
head of the hippocampus.

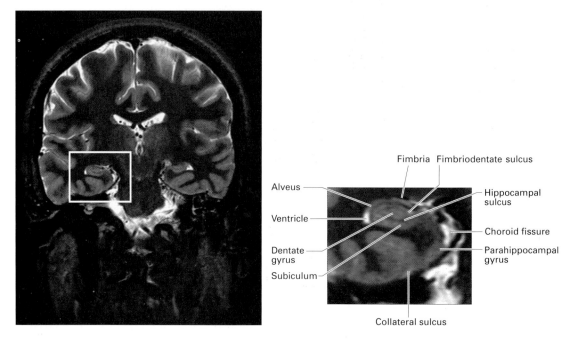

Alveus

Ventricle

Dentate
gyrus

Subiculum

Fimbria   Fimbriodentate sulcus

Hippocampal
sulcus

Choroid fissure

Parahippocampal
gyrus

Collateral sulcus

Fig. 4.25 Coronal T2-weighted (short-inversion-time
inversion-recovery (STIR) sequence) MRI scan through
the body of the hippocampus.

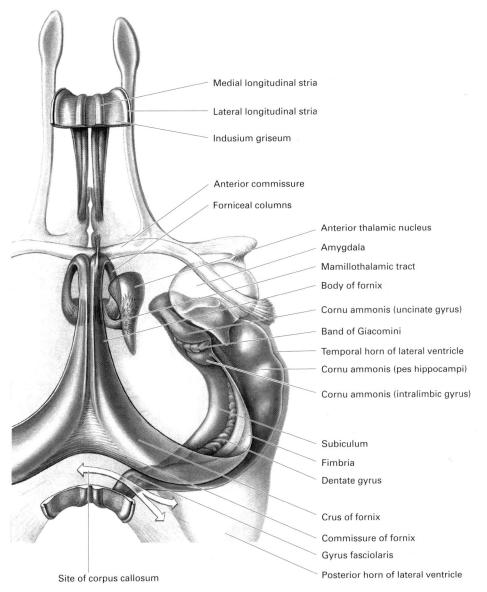

Medial longitudinal stria

Lateral longitudinal stria

Indusium griseum

Anterior commissure

Forniceal columns

Anterior thalamic nucleus

Amygdala

Mamillothalamic tract

Body of fornix

Cornu ammonis (uncinate gyrus)

Band of Giacomini

Temporal horn of lateral ventricle

Cornu ammonis (pes hippocampi)

Cornu ammonis (intralimbic gyrus)

Subiculum

Fimbria

Dentate gyrus

Crus of fornix

Commissure of fornix

Gyrus fasciolaris

Posterior horn of lateral ventricle

Site of corpus callosum

Fig. 4.26 Superior view of limbic structures including the anterior commissure. Temporal and posterior horns of the lateral ventricle are shaded. The amygdala lies tilted back from the coronal plane deep to the uncus and is separated from the hippocampus by the uncal recess of the lateral ventricle. After Nieuwenhuys *et al.*, 1988.

outwards) the third of the five pairs of C-shaped curves taken by limbic structures. From each temporal lobe the fimbria, containing fibres condensed from the alveus of the hippocampus, run upwards and posteriorly (Figs 4.21, 4.26 & 4.27). The fimbria has to diverge from the tail of the hippocampus in order to pass under the corpus callosum, and its continuation forms the

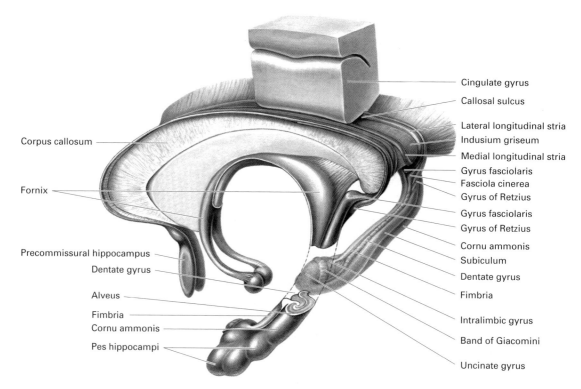

Cingulate gyrus

Callosal sulcus

Lateral longitudinal stria

Indusium griseum

Medial longitudinal stria

Gyrus fasciolaris

Fasciola cinerea

Gyrus of Retzius

Gyrus fasciolaris

Gyrus of Retzius

Cornu ammonis

Subiculum

Dentate gyrus

Fimbria

Intralimbic gyrus

Band of Giacomini

Uncinate gyrus

Corpus callosum

Fornix

Precommissural hippocampus

Dentate gyrus

Alveus

Fimbria

Cornu ammonis

Pes hippocampi

Fig. 4.27 Posterior oblique view of the hippocampus and related structures showing the continuation of the fimbria into the fornix and of the cornu ammonis and dentate gyrus into the indusium griseum and longitudinal stria. After Nieuwenhuys *et al.*, 1988.

crus of the fornix. Each crus arches upwards and anteriorly, fusing with its opposite number in the midline to form the body of the fornix, which at first lies in close proximity to the inferior surface of the corpus callosum. Further anteriorly, as the fornix curves down towards the foramen of Munro, it becomes increasingly separated from the corpus callosum, the septum pellucidum occupying the intervening space (Fig. 4.30).

The body of the fornix passes anterior to the foramen of Munro before its bilateral components begin to diverge again, forming the fornical columns. A few fibres pass in front of the anterior commissure to the septal nuclei, but the majority descend in the fornical columns behind the anterior commissure and then on either side of the third ventricle into the mamillary bodies. From here the mamillothalamic tracts pass antero-superiorly to the anterior thalamic nuclei and the

mamillotegmental tracts pass posteriorly to the midbrain (Fig. 4.16). The commissure of the fornix refers to a thin veil of transversely orientated fibres which join the crura beneath the splenium of the corpus callosum.

Midline sagittal sections show the body of the fornix posterior to the foramen of Munro running in the posterior margin of the septum pellucidum (Fig. 4.31). Axial sections show the body of the fornix where it runs perpendicular to the plane of scanning, for example anterior to the foramen of Munro (Fig. 4.10). The fornical columns can be seen at lower levels and in the same section the mamillothalamic tracts more posteriorly (Fig. 4.A3).

Coronal sections best demonstrate the crura, which, together with the fimbria, form the medial walls of the trigones of the lateral ventricles. More anteriorly the crura approximate under the body of the corpus callosum, each crus now forming the medial wall of the posterior part of the body of the lateral ventricle. Further anteriorly still, the septum pellucidum appears as a thin line separating the body of the fornix from the corpus callosum. In these anterior sections, the paired deep middle cerebral veins, running posteriorly beneath the fornix in the tela choroidea of the third ventricle, can be identified by their prominent signal flow void (Figs 4.A15–4.A20).

The indusium griseum and longitudinal stria

Where the crus of the fornix separates from the hippocampus, it leaves behind the dentate nucleus, cornu ammonis and subiculum (Figs 4.26 & 4.27). These gyri form the fourth limbic curve, passing upwards and posteriorly as narrow bands (fasciola cinerea, gyrus fasciolaris, gyrus of Retzius) around the splenium and on to the upper surface of the corpus callosum. On each side their extensions continue forwards, closely applied to the upper surface of the corpus callosum, as the medial and lateral longitudinal stria, with the indusium griseum a thin veil of grey matter between them. Anteriorly these structures turn around the genu of the corpus callosum and merge in the paraterminal gyrus, anterior to the lamina terminalis of the third ventricle (Fig. 4.27).

On coronal sections, just posterior to the crura of the fornix, the fasciola cinerea, gyrus fasciolaris and gyrus of Retzius may be visible together as a strip of grey matter on the medial surface of each cerebral hemisphere, running up to the underside of the splenium of the corpus callosum. More commonly, however, they cannot be distinguished from the grey matter of the isthmus of the cingulate gyrus (see below). The indusium griseum and longitudinal stria are too small to be resolved.

The parahippocampal gyrus and cingulum (and uncus)

The parahippocampal gyrus and cingulum form the fifth and most peripheral of the C-shaped limbic arcs. The cingulum is a band of longitudi-

nally orientated short association fibres, continuous with the septal nuclei rostrally (see below) and the parahippocampal gyrus caudally. Its site is marked by the cingulate gyrus, which is a prominent feature of the medial wall of the cerebral hemisphere (Fig. 4.20). The cingulate gyrus follows the outer margin of the arch described by the corpus callosum in the sagittal plane. Anteriorly it merges with the paraterminal gyrus under the rostrum of the corpus callosum. Posteriorly it turns under the splenium of the corpus callosum, narrowing to form the isthmus, and then merges with the parahippocampal gyrus. It is separated from the corpus callosum by the callosal sulcus.

The parahippocampal gyrus runs downwards and forwards from the isthmus of the cingulate gyrus, forming the medial border of the temporal lobe (Fig. 4.22). Its rostral tip is curved upwards to form the uncus (see above). Superiorly, the parahippocampal gyrus is continuous with the hippocampus through the subiculum. Inferiorly the parahippocampal gyrus merges with the rest of the temporal lobe, the longitudinally orientated collateral sulcus defining its inferolateral border and (approximately) the region where its primitive cortex merges with the neocortex of the rest of the temporal lobe.

The appearance of the parahippocampal gyri on coronal imaging has been described above. In the axial plane the parahippocampal gyri can be identified as they pass closely around the midbrain and cerebral peduncles. The unci appear as prominent medial protuberances on each temporal lobe just posterior to the middle cerebral arteries and anterolateral to the cerebral peduncles. On each side, the CSF space separating the uncus and parahippocampal gyrus from the brainstem is part of the ambient cistern, and the prominent signal void (MRI) which is frequently seen within it is caused by flow in the posterior cerebral artery or the basal vein, both of which pass around the brainstem in this region.

The length of the cingulate gyrus can be seen on midline sagittal sections, except for the isthmus where it diverges from the midline to pass into the temporal lobe. Coronal scans through the bodies of the lateral ventricles demonstrate the cingulate gyrus in section. The cingulum bundle within the cingulate gyrus is sometimes seen on axial T2-weighted or proton-density scans as a line of low signal, in white matter, close to the midline on sections just above the corpus callosum (Daniels *et al.*, 1987).

The stria terminalis and amygdala

The stria terminalis is a thin band of nerve fibres, for the most part not resolved as a separate structure on MRI, which forms the second of the limbic arcs on each cerebral hemisphere (Fig. 4.19). It runs posteriorly from the amygdala in the roof of the temporal horn of the lateral ventricle, just medial to the tail of the caudate nucleus. Turning forward between the body of the caudate nucleus and the thalamus, its position is sometimes marked on coronal scans by a small bump on the floor of the body of the lateral ventricle beneath the thalamostriate vein (Fig. 4.A18). Anterolateral to the foramen of Munro it divides, some fibres passing in front of the anterior commissure to the septal region, some behind to the supraoptic nuclei and some turning posteriorly to join fibres in the stria medullaris thalami (see below).

The stria medullaris thalami and habenular nucleus (and pineal gland)

The innermost limbic ring is formed by the stria medullaris thalami, habenular nucleus and the habenulointerpeduncular tract. These are also paired structures, lying on the medial surfaces of the cerebral hemispheres, which terminate in the interpeduncular nucleus in the midline (Fig. 4.19).

The stria medullaris thalami takes fibres from the septal region, preoptic nuclei and stria terminalis to the habenular nucleus. It curves posteriorly over the medial side of the thalamus, forming a small ridge along the superolateral corner of the third ventricle (Figs 4.4 & 4.12). The habenular nucleus comprises a small nidus of grey matter at the end of this ridge on the medial thalamus which indents the posterior superior

part of the lateral wall of the third ventricle in front of the habenular commissure and pineal gland. The habenular commissure connects the habenular nuclei on either side of the third ventricle. The habenulointerpeduncular tract passes anteriorly and inferiorly from the habenular nucleus to the interpeduncular nucleus, which lies between the cerebral peduncles, in the anterior part of the tegmentum of the midbrain, just below the red nuclei (Fig. 4.19).

The habenular commissure runs across the posterior wall of the third ventricle between the suprapineal and the pineal recesses, but this area is difficult to see on sagittal scans. Axial scans may show the habenular nuclei as small elevations on the medial thalami at the back of the third ventricle, with the habenular commissure arching posteriorly between them. The posterior commissure crosses just below the habenular nuclei in a slightly more anterior plane and may also be seen in the same section (Figs 4.9, 4.10 & 4.A4). The pineal gland, lying posteriorly, may be identified on CT if it is calcified and on MRI if it is cystic.

The olfactory bulb and nuclei

Included in broader definitions of the limbic system, the olfactory bulb and tract (Fig. 4.26) can be identified on each side on coronal MRI in the olfactory sulcus, lateral to the gyrus rectus. Proximally (and unseen on imaging) the lateral olfactory striae pass from the olfactory tract in front of the anterior perforated substance to merge with the amygdala. The medial olfactory striae turn on to the medial surface of the hemisphere and merge with the septal region in front of the lamina terminalis.

The septal nuclei

The septal region generally refers to the precommissural septum, which lies in the medial walls of both frontal lobes, above and anterior to the lamina terminalis and anterior commissure. As described above, it is functionally intimately related to the hypothalamus and olfactory and limbic systems. Coronal MRI sections immediately anterior to the anterior commissure show the septal regions as areas of grey-matter intensity on either side of the interhemispheric fissure, medial to the inferior parts of the frontal horns of the lateral ventricles (Fig. 4.A13). The term supracom-missural septum refers to the small part of the septal region contained in the septum pellucidum.

The surface of the cerebral hemispheres

Lobar anatomy

Each cerebral hemisphere is divided into frontal, parietal, temporal and occipital lobes (Fig. 4.28). The central sulcus separates the frontal lobe from

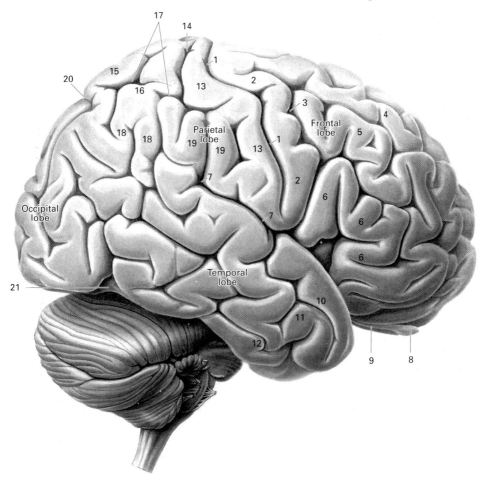

1	Central sulcus	2	Precentral gyrus	3	Precentral sulcus	4	Superior frontal gyrus
5	Middle frontal gyrus	6	Inferior frontal gyrus	7	Lateral fissure (posterior ramus)	8	Olfactory bulb
9	Olfactory tract	10	Superior temporal gyrus	11	Middle temporal gyrus	12	Inferior temporal gyrus
13	Postcentral gyrus	14	Postcentral sulcus	15	Superior parietal lobule	16	Inferior parietal lobule
17	Intraparietal sulcus	18	Angular gyrus	19	Supramarginal gyrus	20	Parieto-occipital sulcus
21	Preoccipital notch						

Fig. 4.28 Lateral view of the cerebral hemisphere. After Nieuwenhuys *et al.*, 1988.

the parietal lobe. The lateral (Sylvian) fissure transmits branches of the middle cerebral artery on to the cerebral convexity and separates the frontal lobe and anterior part of the parietal lobe from the inferiorly placed temporal lobe. The parietal lobe includes the postcentral gyrus and various gyri around the posterior part of the lateral fissure. It is separated from the occipital lobe by the parieto-occipital sulcus on the medial surface of the cerebral hemisphere and its imagined continuation over the convexity to the preoccipital notch. It is separated from the temporal lobe by the lateral fissure and its imagined posterior extension to that same line. The temporal lobe is inferior to the lateral fissure and its imagined posterior extension. It is separated from the occipital lobe, again by the line drawn from the preoccipital notch to the parieto-occipital sulcus. The insula refers to a small area of cortex buried in the lateral fissure overlying the external capsule and basal ganglia (Fig. 4.29) (Gray, 1989a).

Identifying particular gyri in the anatomical specimen is not easy; nor is it easy on sectional imaging. Nevertheless, with practice it is possible

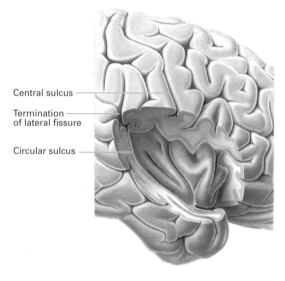

Central sulcus

Termination of lateral fissure

Circular sulcus

Fig. 4.29 Lateral view of hemisphere, dissected to show the insular cortex. After Nieuwenhuys *et al.*, 1988.

to locate some of the important surface landmarks with reasonable confidence. The following sections describe the more easily recognised surface features and conclude with a method of finding the central sulcus on axial scans.

Medial surface of the cerebrum

The orientation of the medial wall of the cerebral hemisphere (Figs 4.30 & 4.31) makes it ideally suited to imaging in the sagittal plane. The cingulate gyrus begins under the rostrum of the corpus callosum and follows its outer margin to the splenium. Here it is lost to midline sagittal scans as it narrows and passes laterally (the isthmus) around the brainstem to merge with the parahippocampal gyrus. The cingulate sulcus separates the cingulate gyrus from the superior frontal gyrus and, if traced posteriorly, turns upwards at the level of the posterior part of the body of the corpus callosum into the marginal sulcus. The marginal sulcus defines the posterior margin of the paracentral lobule and is a useful way of finding the central sulcus in this plane. The central sulcus generally does not run on to the medial hemisphere but into the superiorly placed paracentral lobule, which straddles the boundary between the frontal and parietal lobes. The postcentral gyrus runs into the back of the paracentral lobule, and the central sulcus lies approximately one gyrus width anterior to the marginal sulcus.

The anatomy of the medial temporal lobe has already been described. The parahippocampal gyrus merges with the isthmus of the cingulate gyrus posteriorly, losing the collateral sulcus but gaining the calcarine sulcus, which now separates it from the medial occipitotemporal gyrus and the rest of the temporal lobe (Fig. 4.20). The anterior part of the calcarine sulcus is found in the inferomedial part of the posterior temporal lobe, and it becomes visible on midline sagittal sections as it runs on to the medial aspect of the cerebral hemisphere, posterior to the splenium of the corpus callosum and cingulate gyrus. Here it turns down parallel to the inferomedial margin of the

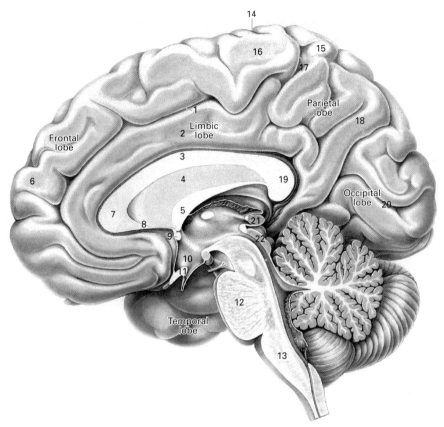

Fig. 4.30 Medial view of hemisphere. After Nieuwenhuys *et al.*, 1988.

1	Cingulate sulcus	2	Cingulate gyrus	3	Body of corpus callosum	4	Septum pellucidum
5	Fornix	6	Superior frontal gyrus	7	Genu of corpus callosum	8	Rostrum of corpus callosum
9	Anterior commissure	10	Hypothalamus	11	Optic chiasm	12	Pons
13	Medulla oblongata	14	Central sulcus	15	Superior parietal lobule	16	Paracentral lobule
17	Marginal sulcus	18	Occipitoparietal sulcus	19	Splenium of corpus callosum	20	Calcarine sulcus
21	Pineal gland	22	Quadrigeminal plate					

cerebral hemisphere (and tentorium cerebelli), terminating near the occipital pole.

The parieto-occipital sulcus runs upwards and backwards on the medial surface of the cerebral hemisphere from the point where the calcarine sulcus turns down, to gain the superomedial margin about 5 cm above the occipital pole. It separates the medial portions of the parietal lobe (precuneus) anteriorly from the occipital lobe (cuneus) posteriorly.

The cerebral convexity and central sulcus

The central sulcus runs anteriorly and inferolaterally across the cerebral hemisphere, at about 60–70° to the median plane, from the paracentral lobule, terminating just short of the lateral fissure. The precentral and postcentral gyri run on either side, in turn delineated by the precentral and postcentral sulci.

The bulk of the outer surface of the frontal lobe

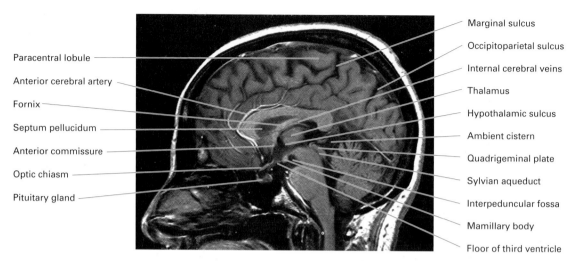

Paracentral lobule

Anterior cerebral artery

Fornix

Septum pellucidum

Anterior commissure

Optic chiasm

Pituitary gland

Marginal sulcus

Occipitoparietal sulcus

Internal cerebral veins

Thalamus

Hypothalamic sulcus

Ambient cistern

Quadrigeminal plate

Sylvian aqueduct

Interpeduncular fossa

Mamillary body

Floor of third ventricle

Fig. 4.31 Midline sagittal (T1-weighted) scan.

is divided into three convoluted, but essentially longitudinally orientated gyri: superior, middle and inferior. These gyri terminate posteriorly in the more transversely orientated precentral sulcus. The central sulcus lies behind and parallel to the precentral sulcus, with the precentral gyrus in between (Fig. 4.28).

The central sulcus can be identified on axial scans by working backwards through the frontal lobe, its relatively posterior position reflecting the frontal lobe's large size. Superior sections show the longitudinally orientated superior and middle frontal gyri, which can be traced back to the precentral sulcus running across their terminations. The central sulcus lies immediately posterior to the precentral sulcus in the same orientation, i.e. running forwards at about 60–70° to the median plane (although the observed orientation will depend on the plane of scanning) (Fig. 4.A8).

Below the topmost sections, finding the central sulcus becomes increasingly difficult. All three frontal gyri appear in the same section and the different orientation of the precentral sulcus is no longer apparent. At levels at and just above the roofs of the lateral ventricles, the central sulcus

can be located by first identifying the white-matter stems of the superior and middle frontal gyri, and then the stems of the precentral and postcentral gyri (Iwasaki *et al.*, 1991). At levels below the roofs of the lateral ventricles, the central sulcus will only be found by careful tracing downwards through serial sections.

Several subdivisions of the parietal lobe are recognised. The postcentral sulcus runs parallel to the central sulcus, delineating the back of the postcentral gyrus. The postcentral gyrus runs superiorly into the back of the paracentral lobule. The intraparietal sulcus runs posteriorly from about the middle of the postcentral gyrus, dividing the remainder of the parietal lobe into the superior and inferior parietal lobules. The inferior parietal lobule is further subdivided into the supramarginal gyrus around the upturned end of the lateral fissure and the angular gyrus more posteriorly. These features are difficult to identify on sectional imaging, but some have been used to confirm the position of the central sulcus (Iwasaki *et al.*, 1991).

The convexity boundary between the occipital and parietal lobes is difficult to define precisely on axial scans. The parieto-occipital sulcus is often visible in this plane and may be used as a guide. It is first seen as a deep sulcus on the medial border of the hemisphere, posterior to the splenium of the corpus callosum and isthmus of the cingulate gyrus, and can be followed on successively more superior scans as it runs upwards and posteriorly until it reaches the cerebral convexity (Figs 4.11, 4.A6 & 4.A7). The occipital lobe lies posterior to the parieto-occipital sulcus and (as described above) posterior to a line drawn from its appearance on the medial border of the cerebral convexity to the preoccipital notch. The preoccipital notch lies on the inferolateral border of the cerebral hemisphere, about 5 cm in front of the occipital pole (Fig. 4.28).

The stem of the lateral fissure commences under the anterior perforated substance and passes up and laterally on to the surface of the hemisphere, carrying branches of the middle cerebral artery and separating the frontal lobe from the anterior temporal lobe. This part of the lateral fissure is easily identified on axial or coronal scan (Figs 4.9 & 4.A13). At the surface, the lateral fissure divides and its largest branch (the posterior ramus) runs backwards and slightly upwards, terminating in an upwards extension into the parietal lobe. Its inclined horizontal orientation makes for easy identification on coronal scans (Fig. 4.A18), but on axial scans its location may be less obvious. In difficult cases, middle cerebral artery branches, emerging on to the surface of the cerebral hemisphere from the lateral fissure, give a clue to its position (Figs 4.A5, 4.A6, 4.A11 & 4.A12). The insula is buried within the lateral fissure and is easily found in the coronal or axial planes (Figs 4.9 & 4.A18).

The lateral aspect of the temporal lobe is divided into three longitudinally orientated gyri: superior, middle and inferior, which are fairly easily identified on coronal imaging. The superior temporal gyrus is continuous with gyri in the floor of the posterior ramus of the lateral fissure. The posterior boundary of the temporal lobe (with the occipital lobe) lies beyond the posterior limit of the lateral fissure and is a continuation of the posterior boundary of the parietal lobe. Its position on axial scans is judged by reference to surface markings described earlier.

Acknowledgement

My thanks to J.M. Stevens, FRCR, MRACR, Consultant Neuroradiologist, the National Hospital for Neurology and Neurosurgery, Queen Square, for reviewing and correcting errors in the manuscript.

References

Bronen, R.A. (1992) Hippocampal and limbic terminology. *Am. J. Neuroradiol.* 13, 943–5.

Daniels, D.L., Haughton, V.M. & Naidich, T.P. (1987) *Cranial and Spinal Magnetic Resonance Imaging: an Atlas and Guide.* Raven Press, New York, p. 66.

Drayer, B., Burger, P., Darwin, R., Reiderer, S., Herfkens, R. & Johnson, G.A. (1986) Magnetic resonance imaging of brain iron. *Am. J. Neuroradiol.* 7, 373–80.

du Boulay, G.H. (1980) *Principles of X-ray Diagnosis of the Skull,* 2nd edn. Butterworths, London.

Duvernoy, H.M. (1988) *The Human Hippocampus: an Atlas of Applied Anatomy.* J.F. Bergman Verlag, Munich.

Gray, H. (1989a) The surfaces of the cerebrum. In Williams, P.L., Warwich, R., Dyson, M. & Bannister, L.H. (eds) *Gray's Anatomy,* 37th edn. Churchill Livingstone, London, pp. 1020–8.

Gray, H. (1989b) Th e limbic system. In Williams, P.L., Warwich, R., Dyson, M. & Bannister, L.H. (eds) Gray's anatomy, 37th edn. Churchill Livingstone, London, pp. 1028–39.

Gray, H. (1989c) The basal nuclei. In Williams, P.L., Warwich, R., Dyson, M. & Bannister, L.H. (eds) *Gray's Anatomy,* 37th edn. Churchill Livingstone, London, pp. 1073–5.

Greitz, T. & Lindgren, E. (1971) The head. In Abrams, H.L. (ed.) *Abrams' Angiography,* 2nd edn, Vol. 1. Little, Brown & Co., Boston, pp. 155–269.

Isaacson, R.L. (1982a) The structure of the limbic system. In *The Limbic System,* 2nd edn. Plenum Press, New York, pp. 1–60.

Isaacson, R.L. (1982b) The graven image, Lethe and the guru. In *The Limbic System,* 2nd edn. Plenum Press, New York, pp. 239–57.

Iwasaki, S., Nakagawa, H., Fukusumi, A. *et al.* (1991) Identification of pre- and postcentral gyri on CT and MR images on the basis of the medullary pattern of cerebral white matter. *Radiology* 179, 207–13.

Jack, C.R., Sharbrough, F.W., Twomey, C.K. *et al.* (1990)

Temporal lobe seizures: lateralisation with MR volume measurements of the hippocampal formation. *Radiology* **175**, 423–9.

Jackson, G.D., Connelly, A., Duncan, J.S., Grunewald, R.A. & Gadian, D.G. (1993) Detection of hippocampal pathology in intractable partial epilepsy: increased sensitivity with quantitative magnetic resonance T2 relaxometry. *Neurology* **43**, 1793–9.

Jungries, C.A., Kanal, E., Hirsch, W.L., Martinez, A.J. & Moossy, J. (1988) Normal perivascular spaces mimicking lacunar infarction: MR imaging. *Radiology* **169**, 101–4.

Mieners, L.C., van Gils, A., Jansen, G.H. *et al.* (1994) Temporal lobe epilepsy: the various MR appearances of histologically proven mesial temporal sclerosis. *Am. J. Neuroradiol.* **15**, 1547–55.

Naidich, T.P., Daniels, D.L., Pech, P., Haughton, V.M., Williams, A. & Pojunas, K. (1986) Anterior commissure: anatomic–MR correlation and use as a landmark in three orthogonal planes. *Radiology* **158**, 421–9.

Naidich, T.P., Daniels, D.L., Haughton, V.M., Williams, A., Pojunas, K. & Palacios, E. (1987a) Hippocampal formation and related structures of the limbic lobe: anatomic–MR correlation. Part 1. Surface features and coronal sections. *Radiology* **162**, 747–54.

Naidich, T.P., Daniels, D.L., Haughton, V.M. *et al.* (1987b) Hippocampal formation and related structures of the limbic lobe: anatomic–MR correlation. Part 2. Sagittal sections. *Radiology* **162**, 755–61.

Nieuwenhuys, R., Voogd, J. & van Huijzen, C. (eds) (1988) Olfactory and limbic systems. In *The Human Central Nervous System: a Synopsis and Atlas*, 3rd edn. Springer Verlag, Berlin, pp. 293–363.

Robertson, E.G. (1957) *Pneumoencephalography*. Blackwell Scientific Publications, Oxford.

Sasaki, M., Sone, M., Ehara, S. & Tamakawa, Y. (1993) Hippocampal sulcus remnant: potential cause of change in signal intensity in the hippocampus. *Radiology* **188**, 743–6.

Snell, R.S. (1982) *Clinical Anatomy for Medical Students*, 2nd edn. Little, Brown & Co, Boston.

Sobota, J. (1911) *Atlas and Textbook of Human Anatomy*, McMurrich, J.P. (ed), Vol. 3. W.B. Saunders & Co., Philadelphia.

Tien, R.D., Felsberg, G.J. & Crain, B. (1992) Normal anatomy of the hippocampus and adjacent temporal lobe: high resolution fast spin–echo MR images in volunteers correlated with cadaveric histologic sections. *Am. J. Roentgenol.* **159**, 1309–13.

Watson, C., Andemann, F., Gloor, P. *et al.* (1992) Anatomic basis of amygdaloid and hippocampal volume measurement by magnetic resonance imaging. *Neurology* **42**, 1743–50.

Further reading

Daniels, D.L., Haughton, V.M. & Naidich, T.P. (1987) *Cranial and Spinal Magnetic Resonance Imaging: an Atlas and Guide*. Raven Press, New York.

Duvernoy, H.M. (1988) *The Human Hippocampus: an Atlas of Applied Anatomy*. J.E. Bergman Verlag, Munich.

Nieuwenhuys, R., Voogd, J. & VanHuijzer, C. (1988) *The Human Central Nervous System: a Synopsis and Atlas*, 3rd edn. Springer Verlag, Berlin.

Williams, P.L., Warwich, R., Dyson, M. & Bannister, L.H. (eds) (1989) *Gray's Anatomy*, 37th edn. Churchill Livingstone, London.

Appendix: MRI atlas

The axial images presented are the first and second echoes of a spin–echo sequence (time to repetition (TR) 2800, time to echo (TE) 30 and TR 2800, TE 90) on the same subject. The second echo is shown first because its strong T2 weighting gives CSF a high signal and allows the ventricular system to be identified without difficulty. Magnetic susceptibility effects are pronounced on these images, and structures which have a high iron content are marked by regions of relatively low signal. The first echo gives better contrast between grey and white matter but, because signal from CSF is similar to that from grey matter, it is sometimes necessary to refer back to the T2-weighted image to understand the anatomy.

T2-weighted sequence (2800/90)

CSF bright; grey matter higher intensity than white matter; flow very dark.

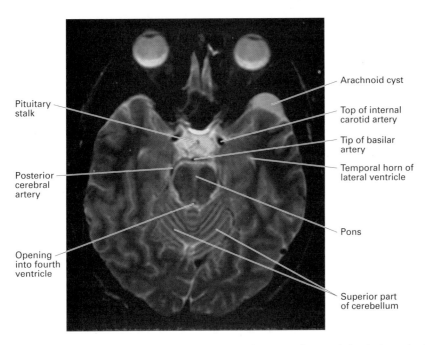

Fig. 4.A1 Level of the upper pons and chiasmatic cistern. The optic chiasma is above and the pituitary gland below this level.

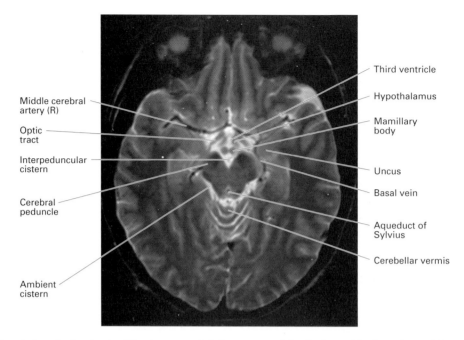

Middle cerebral artery (R)

Optic tract

Interpeduncular cistern

Cerebral peduncle

Ambient cistern

Third ventricle

Hypothalamus

Mamillary body

Uncus

Basal vein

Aqueduct of Sylvius

Cerebellar vermis

Fig. 4.A2 Level of cerebral peduncles. The deep anteroinferior recesses of the third ventricles lie in front of the mamillary bodies, with the hypothalamic nuclei in the ventricular wall on either side. The optic tracts lie just further laterally as they diverge from the optic chiasma (not seen). CSF in the Sylvian aqueduct has low signal because of flow.

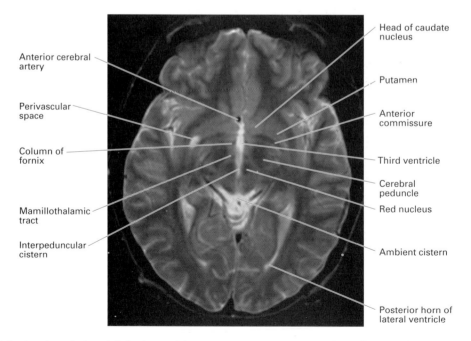

Anterior cerebral artery

Perivascular space

Column of fornix

Mamillothalamic tract

Interpeduncular cistern

Head of caudate nucleus

Putamen

Anterior commissure

Third ventricle

Cerebral peduncle

Red nucleus

Ambient cistern

Posterior horn of lateral ventricle

Fig. 4.A3 Section through the subthalamic area. The anterior commissure crosses the midline out of the plane of section but marks the site of the lamina terminalis of the third ventricle. The sloping floor of the third ventricle makes the boundary between it and the interpeduncular fossa (cistern) indistinct in the axial plane, owing to partial-volume averaging.

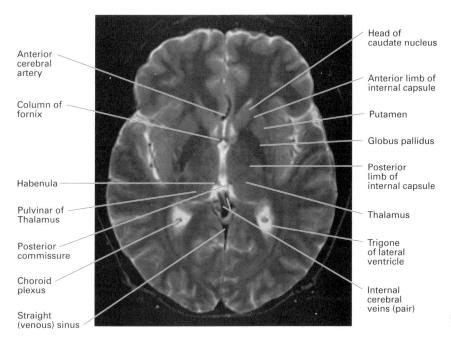

Anterior
cerebral
artery

Column of
fornix

Habenula

Pulvinar of
Thalamus

Posterior
commissure

Choroid
plexus

Straight
(venous) sinus

Head of
caudate nucleus

Anterior limb of
internal capsule

Putamen

Globus pallidus

Posterior
limb of
internal capsule

Thalamus

Trigone
of lateral
ventricle

Internal
cerebral
veins (pair)

Fig. 4.A4 Level of the thalami and internal capsule. The globus pallidus is dark on this sequence (because of contained iron) and easily distinguished from the putamen. The posterior limb of the internal capsule has moderately high signal (because of reduced iron) and is difficult to differentiate from the lateral border of the thalamus (cf. Fig. 4.A10).

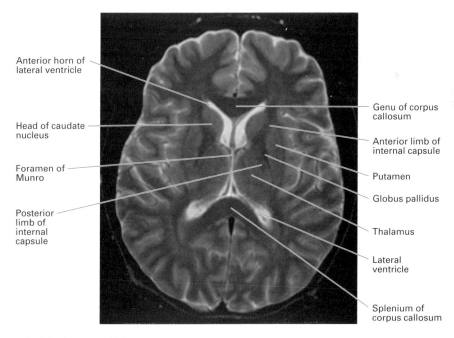

Anterior horn of
lateral ventricle

Head of caudate
nucleus

Foramen of
Munro

Posterior
limb of
internal
capsule

Genu of corpus
callosum

Anterior limb of
internal capsule

Putamen

Globus pallidus

Thalamus

Lateral
ventricle

Splenium of
corpus callosum

Fig. 4.A5 Level of the foramen of Munro.

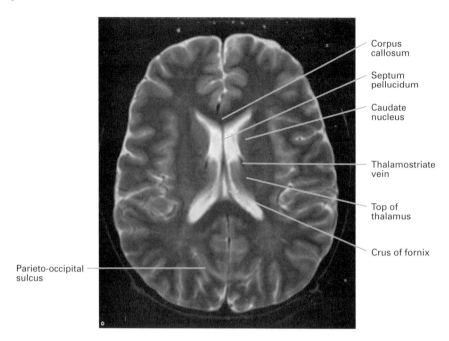

Fig. 4.A6 Section through the floor of the body of the lateral ventricle. The thalamostriate veins run anteriorly towards the interventricular foramen in the thalamocaudate groove.

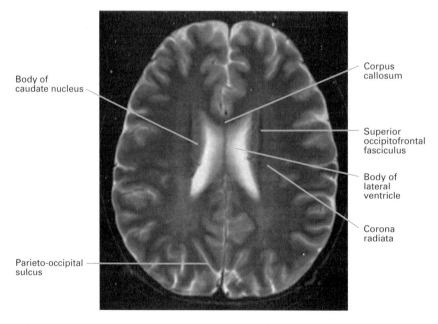

Fig. 4.A7 Section through the top of the lateral ventricles and corona radiata. The condensation of white-matter fibres in the superior longitudinal fasciculus is dark on T2-weighted sequences.

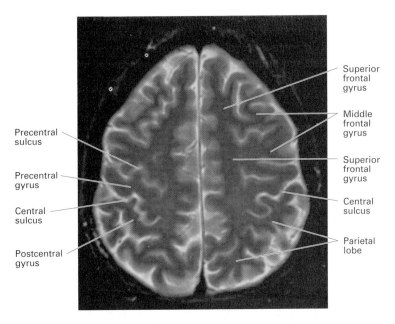

Superior
frontal
gyrus

Middle
frontal
gyrus

Superior
frontal
gyrus

Central
sulcus

Parietal
lobe

Precentral
sulcus

Precentral
gyrus

Central
sulcus

Postcentral
gyrus

Fig. 4.A8 Above the lateral ventricles the central sulcus runs across the line of the superior frontal gyrus.

The First echo–'proton-density' sequence (2800/30)

Grey matter still has higher signal than white matter
but contrast is greater than on the T2-weighted scans.
CSF has signal close to that of grey matter.

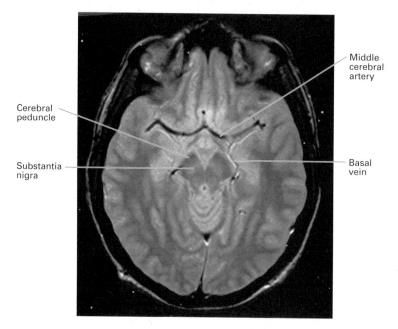

Middle
cerebral
artery

Cerebral
peduncle

Substantia
nigra

Basal
vein

Fig. 4.A9 Level of cerebral peduncles. The substantia nigra is brighter and more easily differentiated from the cerebral peduncle on the proton-density scan because its signal is less affected by contained iron (cf. Fig. 4.A2).

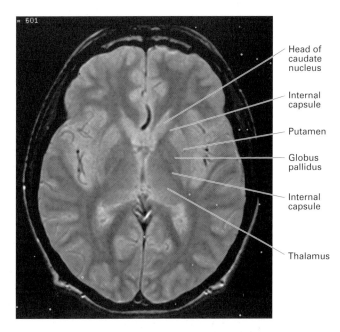

Fig. 4.A10 Level of the thalamus and internal capsule. The globus pallidus is traversed by more white-matter fibres than the putamen and has signal close to that of the internal capsule. Magnetic-susceptibility effects of iron deposition are less marked on this sequence and signal from the posterior limb of the internal capsule is similar to white matter elsewhere, allowing differentiation from the thalamus (cf. Fig. 4.A4).

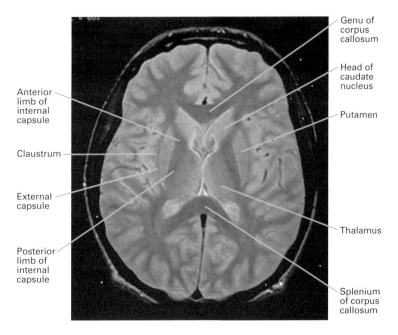

Fig. 4.A11 Level of the internal capsule, also showing the external capsule and claustrum deep to the insular cortex (cf. Fig. 4.A5).

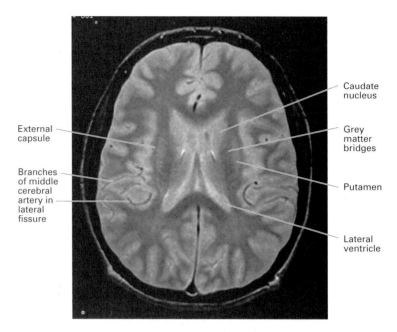

External capsule

Branches of middle cerebral artery in lateral fissure

Caudate nucleus

Grey matter bridges

Putamen

Lateral ventricle

Fig. 4.A12 Section through the floor of the body of the lateral ventricle showing the caudatolenticular bridges of grey matter. Branches of the middle cerebral artery running on to the surface define the area where the posterior ramus of the later fissure crosses the plane of section (cf. Fig. 4.A6).

Coronal STIR images

Different subject from that of the preceding dual-echo scans.
This sequence is T2-weighted, giving bright CSF.
Grey matter has high signal compared with white matter.
Signal from fat is suppressed.

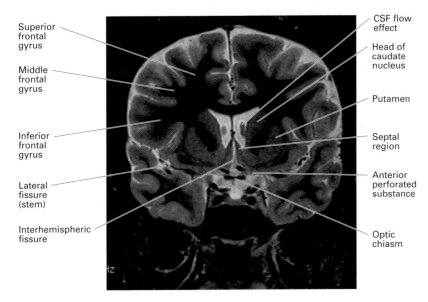

Superior frontal gyrus

Middle frontal gyrus

Inferior frontal gyrus

Lateral fissure (stem)

Interhemispheric fissure

CSF flow effect

Head of caudate nucleus

Putamen

Septal region

Anterior perforated substance

Optic chiasm

Fig. 4.A13 Section through the frontal horns of the lateral ventricles shows the head of the caudate nucleus and the putamen fusing above the anterior perforated substance. Flow artefact (dark) is present in the ventricles. Branches of the middle cerebral artery are represented by regions of flow void in the lateral fissure.

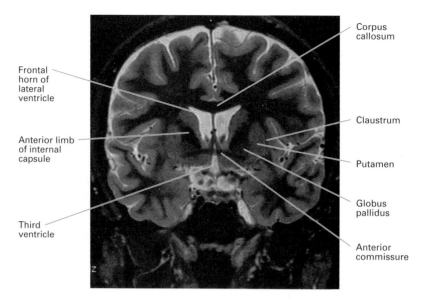

Frontal horn of lateral ventricle

Anterior limb of internal capsule

Third ventricle

Corpus callosum

Claustrum

Putamen

Globus pallidus

Anterior commissure

Fig. 4.A14 Section through the anterior commissure, which passes under the anterior limb of the internal capsule before turning posteriorly. The globus pallidus has signal similar to that of white matter.

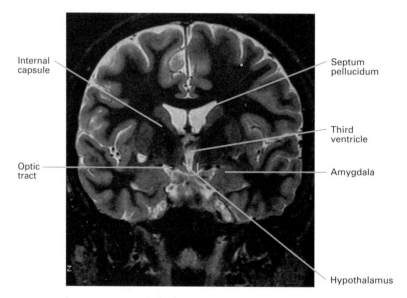

Internal capsule

Optic tract

Septum pellucidum

Third ventricle

Amygdala

Hypothalamus

Fig. 4.A15 Just posterior to the plane of the foramen of Munro. The hypothalamus lies on either side of the inferior part of the third ventricle, with the optic tracts laterally. The amygdala appears just above the most anterior part of the temporal horn of the lateral ventricle.

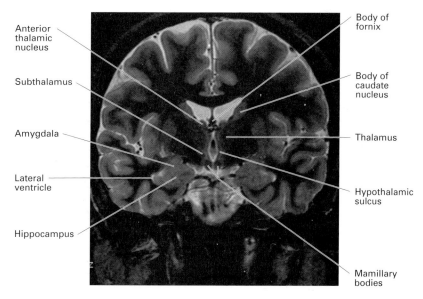

Anterior thalamic nucleus

Subthalamus

Amygdala

Lateral ventricle

Hippocampus

Body of fornix

Body of caudate nucleus

Thalamus

Hypothalamic sulcus

Mamillary bodies

Fig. 4.A16 Flow artefact produces low signal in the third ventricle. Subthalamic nuclei and the hypothalamus lie below the level of the hypothalamic sulcus. Amygdala and hippocampal head appear in the same section, one above the other.

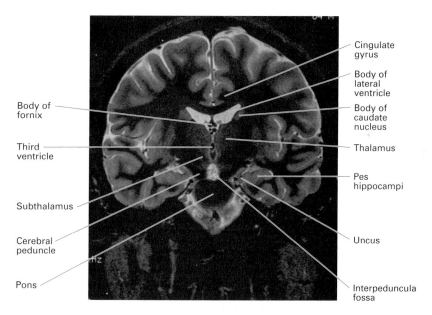

Cingulate gyrus

Body of lateral ventricle

Body of caudate nucleus

Thalamus

Pes hippocampi

Uncus

Interpeduncula fossa

Body of fornix

Third ventricle

Subthalamus

Cerebral peduncle

Pons

Fig. 4.A17 Section through the uncus, with the cerebral peduncles medially and the ambient cistern in between.

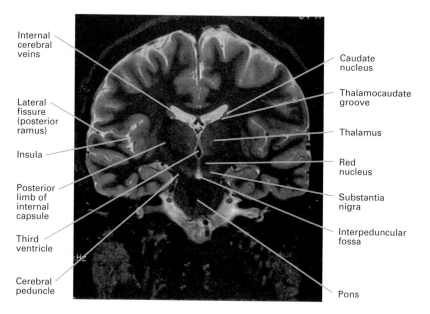

Internal
cerebral
veins

Lateral
fissure
(posterior
ramus)

Insula

Posterior
limb of
internal
capsule

Third
ventricle

Cerebral
peduncle

Caudate
nucleus

Thalamocaudate
groove

Thalamus

Red
nucleus

Substantia
nigra

Interpeduncular
fossa

Pons

Fig. 4.A18 The red nuclei (dark because of contained iron) and substantia nigra project into the subthalamic area.

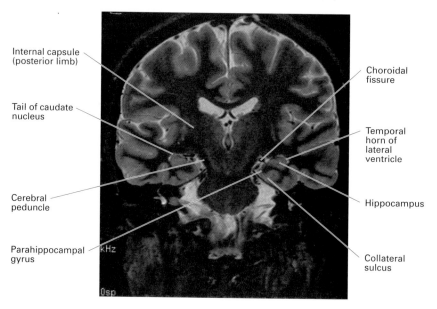

Internal capsule
(posterior limb)

Tail of caudate
nucleus

Cerebral
peduncle

Parahippocampal
gyrus

Choroidal
fissure

Temporal
horn of
lateral
ventricle

Hippocampus

Collateral
sulcus

Fig. 4.A19 Section through the body of the hippocampus. The tail of the caudate nucleus runs in the roof of the temporal horn of the lateral ventricle.

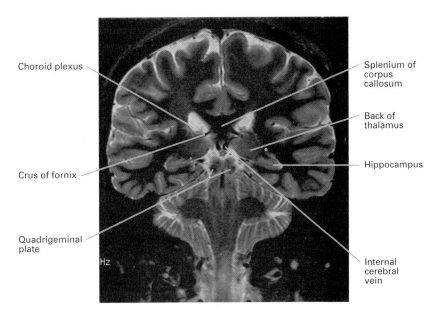

Choroid plexus

Crus of fornix

Quadrigeminal plate

Hz

Splenium of corpus callosum

Back of thalamus

Hippocampus

Internal cerebral vein

Fig. 4.A20 The splenium of the corpus callosum curves down between the lateral ventricles. The crus of the fornix merges with the fimbria round the back of the thalamus.

5: Functional Brain Imaging

S. W. Lewis

Introduction

The visualisation of brain function has become a central research paradigm in psychiatry. Unlike the measurement of brain structure, the measurement of brain function has less in the way of clinical diagnostic applications. Its main applications so far have been in research. Alterations in brain function must at some level underlie all disorders in psychiatry.

This chapter will introduce the two important and related techniques of *single-photon emission* and *positron emission tomography* (SPET and PET). The techniques and their applications in schizophrenia will be examined further in Chapter 11. Subsequent chapters will also deal with functional MR, brain electrical activity mapping and magnetoencephalography.

The functioning brain

In 1890, Roy and Sherrington proposed, in a remarkable piece of foresight, that 'the chemical products of cerebral metabolism' caused alterations in small cerebral arterial vessels so that 'its vascular supply can be varied locally in correspondence with local variations of functional activity'. This position is essentially that held currently, although Roy and Sherrington's proposal was not taken seriously until the second half of the twentieth century. Prior to that it was assumed that, unlike other tissues, brain did not require an increase in regional cerebral blood flow (rCBF) when particular local regions were doing work, in the form of perceiving, controlling movement or thinking.

The main functions of the brain include controlling motor activity, sensation and the storage, retrieval and processing of information. This activity is mediated by neurons. When activated, resting neurons undergo a very rapid change. Ion channels in the cell membrane open and allow entry of sodium ions. The resulting depolarisation continues along the axon and causes the release of a neurotransmitter when it reaches the synapse. These processes use energy. The highest energy turnover occurs in brain regions having the highest density of synapses, where glucose metabolism is highest. Glucose metabolism requires oxygen and adenosine triphosphate (ATP). Oxygen is delivered through oxyhaemoglobin in arterial and capillary blood. The very rapid and localised increases in glucose metabolism which underlie increases in brain activity occur with rapid local changes in blood flow to meet the increased demand. This change in rCBF forms the basis of much SPET and PET imaging. Rapid haemodynamic response at the capillary level is probably mediated by nitric oxide acting on precapillary vessels.

The cerebral cortex contains about 10^{12} (one trillion) neurons, and each neuron averages 10^4 (10 000) synapses. How this vast network organises itself in the execution of particular cognitive functions is still a matter for investigation. What has become more clear is that interconnecting regions or cortical and subcortical fields interact in a correlated or reciprocal way to mediate thought. The pattern of activation depends on the nature of the cognitive task being undertaken. The evidence for this has come from a variety of sources, including the study of the effects of brain lesions in animals and humans, direct electrical stimulation in animals and humans, and inferences drawn from how the cortex is organised anatomically. Classically, the cerebral cortex can be divided up into evolutionarily old parts—the palaeocortex, including the olfactory cortex, hippocampus and dentate gyrus—and the newer parts, which comprise the majority of the cortex, usually called the neocortex. Subdividing the neocortex on the grounds of cytoarchitecture or the histological appearance of individual cells started with Brodmann and Von Economo. Brodmann produced his classic maps from the detailed study of one or two individual brains (Fig. 5.1). He described about 50 different cytoarchitectonic areas in humans, although how this actually relates to cortical activity is not simple. Other more recent approaches, such as mapping of cortical receptors, can lead to other pictures of cortical subdivision on a functional basis.

The development of the first functional brain-imaging technique that was used in humans was developed by a psychiatrist, Seymour Kety. Kety and his co-worker Schmidt developed a method using inhaled nitrous oxide for quantitative determination of cerebral blood flow. In 1948 they had already applied this to normal volunteers and patients with schizophrenia, including the effects of insulin and electroconvulsive treatment (Kety *et al.*, 1948). These studies demonstrated that the global cerebral blood flow and oxygen consumption measured in schizophrenia was essentially normal, although they also pointed out that this did not preclude there being regional differences in blood flow.

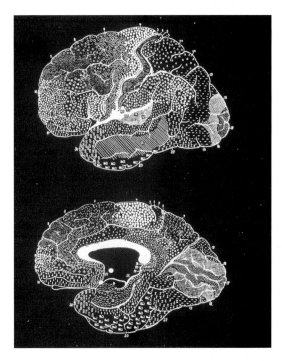

Fig. 5.1 Brodmann's maps of cytoarchitectonic fields in the human cerebral cortex.

SPET and PET compared

Both SPET (or single-photon emission computed tomography (SPECT), the same technique) and PET rely on the same underlying principle: the introduction into the working brain of radioactive isotopes which are linked to particular tracers (Table 5.1). These radiolabelled tracers cross the blood–brain barrier and emit gamma radiation whilst decaying. Depending on the property of the tracer, the concentration of this radioactivity will be related to the presence of particular

Table 5.1 PET and SPET compared for rCBF studies (see also Table 6.2).

	PET	Multidetector SPET
Absolute rCBF values possible	Yes	No
Spatial resolution	5 mm	7 mm
Biological relevant isotopes	Yes	No
Within-subject activation designs possible	Yes, especially with ^{15}O-water	Partly, with split-dose techniques
Half-life of isotopes	Minutes	Hours
Receptor imaging possible	Yes	Yes

receptors, to areas of altered glucose metabolism or to focal areas of increased blood flow. Gamma rays, or photons, are detected by gamma-ray detectors placed outside the head and a slice-by-slice image is constructed.

The crucial difference between these two techniques lies in the properties of the two different types of isotopes used. SPET uses as radioactive tracers isotopes which decay with the emission of single photons, such as iodine and technetium isotopes. PET uses a different class of isotopes, those of carbon, nitrogen, oxygen and fluorine, which decay with the emission of a positron. This travels a very small distance before producing a pair of photons simultaneously emitted in precisely opposite directions. It is this particular type of decay event which means that the source of the two photons, when they are detected simultaneously, can be pinpointed accurately. Thus, PET is a more informative imaging technique. It also uses a series of isotopes of potentially greater biological relevance, although they have relatively short half-lives.

All radioisotopes decay in an exponential way: quickly at first and then tailing off gradually towards zero activity. This property is expressed in terms of *half-life*, the half-life of a particular isotope being the time it takes for the radioactivity to decay to half of its original maximum value. The isotopes used with PET often have half-lives of minutes rather than hours. This carries a big disadvantage as well as a big advantage. The disadvantage is that these isotopes must be made within a very short period of time before being injected or inhaled; otherwise they are of little use. Most PET imaging therefore requires a cyclotron or particle accelerator on site next to the scanner. This is expensive. The scientific advantage, however, is that the short half-life enables several studies to be done with the same subject during the same scanning session. Thus, sequential studies of the same subject at rest and then during conditions of cognitive activation allow a very powerful methodology to be used with PET, subtracting one image from the next (see below). The comparatively long half-life of SPET isotopes with higher radiation exposure mean that this is more difficult to do. A further advantage of PET is that it is possible to calculate absolute (rather than relative) rCBF values.

The advantages of SPET are practical rather than scientific. SPET tracers with iodine or with technetium isotopes can be made in routine clinical nuclear medicine departments at relatively low cost. A long half-life means that administration of the tracer is not so urgent. As well as less flexibility because of the long half-life, the long half-life of SPET isotopes has another important disadvantage in terms of relative safety. Gamma radiation will continue to be emitted for a significant time after the scanning session is completed, which is wasteful in terms of a scientific risk–benefit equation. The cumulative dose of radiation is potentially biologically more harmful with SPET isotopes than with the short-lived PET isotopes.

The principles of detection of photons are the same for PET and SPET and have been used in various forms for many years. Each detector is made up of a lead septum or *collimator*, which serves to absorb any misleading photons coming in from unusual angles, which are the result of scatter. Scatter is a more important artefact for SPET than for PET, since the former uses isotopes which emit lower-energy photons. The central part of the detector is a crystal of material which has the property of scintillation. When a photon hits a crystal, a tiny flash of light is produced. This is amplified by a photomultiplier, which converts the light energy into an electrical signal. Further aspects of SPET and PET are discussed in Chapter 11, as is the less used but related dynamic cortical-probe technique.

Positron emission tomography

The nuclei of some radioactive isotopes, such as ^{11}C, ^{13}N, ^{15}O and ^{18}F, decay emitting a positively charged particle called a positron. In biological tissue this travels a few millimetres before colliding with a negatively charged electron, which leads to mutual annihilation. The result of this event is to release two high-energy photons in completely opposite directions. Each of these has an energy, expressed in kiloelectronvolts (keV), of 511 keV. This pair of photons travels in opposite directions out of the head and is detected by an opposing pair of detectors placed in a complete circle around the subject.

PET scanners typically have any number from 256 to 1024 crystals in the detector ring. Scanners also vary in the number of rings, which determines the number of slices it is possible to examine. The detectors are linked in order to detect 'coincidence events', where a pair of detectors opposite one another are both triggered simultaneously as a result of a single positron annihilation event. A coincidence circuit keeps track of all such coincidences between detector pairs.

The spatial resolution of PET depends on several factors. The smaller the size of the crystal, the thinner the slice thickness it is possible to view in the axial plain. This can also be improved further by moving the detector slightly in relation to the subject. Spatial resolution also depends on the energy of the positrons emitted by the particular isotope being used. The energy of the positron (as opposed to the resulting photon) dictates how far it is likely to travel in biological tissue before being annihilated. Low-energy positrons, such as those emitted from ^{18}F, typically travel 0.2 mm. Higher-energy positrons, such as those emitted by ^{15}O, can travel several millimetres, which introduces a lessening of the spatial resolution possible. In practice, spatial resolution of 5–6 mm in the plane of each slice is possible.

As well as the possibility of scattering (called Compton scattering), photons sometimes hit atoms in the brain and are absorbed. This leads to attenuation, in a way not dissimilar to the attenuation of X-rays (which are of lower energy than gamma rays) described in Chapter 2. The higher the density of the intervening tissue, the more likely attenuation is, and a mathematical correction has to be made for this in interpreting the levels of gamma rays arriving at gamma detectors. The data are then filtered and back-projected in a way analogous to that described in Chapter 2 to give a cross-sectional image of the distribution of radioactivity in the brain. Depending on the nature of the isotope and the tracer

used, this equates with rCBF, regional cerebral metabolic rate (rCMR), or receptor densities and characteristics.

As well as spatial resolution, an important property of functional imaging in research into cognition is the *temporal resolution* possible. This is the minimum duration between two events which is separable by repeated imaging. The better the temporal resolution a technique has, the potentially more informative it is for 'tracking' changes in brain activity over time. In PET, the temporal resolution is largely determined by the half-life of the isotope being used: 2 min for ^{15}O, 20 min for ^{11}C and 2 h for ^{18}F.

Single-photon emission tomography

Like PET, SPET brain imaging involves the detection of gamma rays (photons) emitted from the brain after inhaling or intravenous injection of a radiotracer isotope. The essential difference from PET is that the isotopes used in the tracers emit single photons. This means that the localisation of the source of each detected photon is a more complicated, less exact process. Both the energy and the trajectory of individual photons are taken into account in calculating the source.

Collimators mean that SPET can have good spatial resolution but at the expense of sensitivity. *Sensitivity* in this context is the fraction of all photon emissions which result in a recorded event. Estimates of the effect of attenuation by intervening tissues are done mathematically (attenuation correction). With PET, absolute quantitation of rCBF can be made if arterial concentrations of radiotracer are known. This is not possible with SPET, where measures are given in terms of relative rCBF, in which the region of interest is compared with some neutral reference area (perhaps the cerebellum or visual cortex) or else to the mean of the whole-brain rCBF value.

Most SPET systems available in clinical practice are of the type known as *rotating gamma cameras*. These are well suited for clinical nuclear medicine uses in the body as a whole, but their limited resolution, which also depends on the distance from the detector, precludes their wide use in brain research. So-called 'head-dedicated' systems have a circular array of detectors with focused collimators and can only be used for brain imaging. These can give high-resolution images, with spatial resolutions approaching those with PET.

SPET uses isotopes with longer half-lives than those for PET: ^{133}xenon 5 days, ^{99}technetium 6 h and ^{123}iodine 13 h. Unlike the PET isotopes of carbon, oxygen and nitrogen, these are much less biologically relevant elements. Considerable radiochemical expertise is needed to design molecules which will carry these isotopes across the blood–brain barrier. The exception is ^{133}xenon rCBF imaging, which is an inhalation technique and capable of giving 'dynamic' SPET images, due to the rapid washout of this isotope. However, resolution with the ^{133}xenon technique is poor. Radiotracer molecules designed to cross the blood–brain barrier quickly and in proportion to blood flow include ^{123}iodine-iodoamphetamine and more recently ^{99}technetium-hexamethylpropyleneaminoxime (^{99}technetium-HMPAO or Exemetazine). With the latter compound, the HMPAO carries the ^{99}technetium atom across the blood–brain barrier on first pass. It is taken up intracellularly and the change in pH makes it hydrophilic. This means it is trapped within the cells and remains in a stable distribution directly related to rCBF for several hours. This gives a 'snapshot' image of rCBF as it exists during the 3 or 4 min window after intravenous injection.

Strategies for functional image analysis

As we saw above, functional imaging, particularly PET, has the potential ability to delineate cortical and subcortical brain areas involved in individual cognitive processes. If the experimental task is properly designed, cognitive tasks can be 'dissected' such that the cerebral component which is responsible for each step is delineated. PET is better suited to this design strategy, since it is better able to give repeated scans within the same experimental session. The general principle is that the image taken while the subject is at rest or performing a simple cognitive task is subtracted from a second image taken while the subject is engaged in the particular cognitive activity being investigated. The pattern of rCBF or glucose metabolism during the initial scan is subtracted from that during the activated state in the second scan. The pattern of activity shown in the second scan over and above that shown in the first is assumed to then reflect only that cerebral activity which is involved in performing the task.

This procedure is relatively straightforward when one is subtracting a baseline image of a particular subject from an activated image of the same subject a few minutes later. So long as the cognitive task is appropriately designed, the only precautions that are important to take are to keep other variables constant: to preclude the head moving within the scanner between the first and second scans, for example. Moulded headrests are usually used for this purpose.

Image analysis becomes much more complex when between-group designs are needed, for instance comparing subjects with a particular psychiatric disorder and matched healthy volunteers. Until recently, the image-analysis approach which has been used to compare groups has been the 'region of interest' technique. In this, each subject's image would be displayed on a visual display unit and a tracker ball or pen would be used to outline regions of interest. The mean activity for each region for the experimental subjects would then be compared with that for the controls. The main drawback with this technique is that it takes no account of structural brain differences which might exist between subjects. Using a human operator to decide the boundaries of regions of interest on the functional image requires the assumption that the operator knows where to place the boundaries. On a functional image the inference that structural boundaries can be identified is obviously a circular one. There are two solutions to this problem. The first is to obtain structural imaging data as well as functional imaging data for each subject. Then, data-processing techniques can be used to 'co-register' the imaging data on a voxel-by-voxel basis, such that a superimposed map for each subject is obtained. In reality, this process is complex, although many worth while attempts at co-registration techniques have been used, usually between PET and structural magnetic resonance imaging (MRI).

The second technique has been to develop statistical methods by which normal structural differences between one subject and another can be eliminated, by transforming each functional image slightly so that it fits into a standard brain shape. This 'elastic transformation', as it is called, is usually accomplished by identifying several constant brain landmarks in each image and superimposing these. With this method, variations in levels of radioactivity between subjects must also be taken into account. Analysis of covariance is one method of doing this. The most well-known technique using these principles has been that developed by Friston, Liddle and colleagues. The set of constant landmarks used in this technique is that derived from the Talairach atlas of stereotactic coordinates (Talairach *et al.*, 1967). Liddle describes this approach further in Chapter 11. An example is given in Fig. 5.2.

The application of functional imaging, particularly PET, to the delineation of normal functional brain anatomy has been immense over the past 10 years. To illustrate this, two functional areas with particular relevance to neuropsychiatry will be reviewed briefly: movement and speech.

The functional anatomy of movement

Classically, the brain areas contributing to the control of voluntary movement have been studied from the effects of brain lesions in humans and from experimental ablation studies in animals. From considerations of the microscopic anatomy, the only neurons which are directly applied to the descending spinal neurons are those in the primary motor cortex (PMC), forming the pyramidal tract. Early functional-imaging studies demonstrated increased rCBF in the contralateral motor cortex during unilateral hand and finger movement and soon began delineating other important accessory areas (Table 5.2).

In order to produce this understanding, a series of elegant subtraction experiments has been performed with PET by many different researchers. These experiments have been constructed to address a series of questions concerning movement. How are willed ideas for action represented in the brain? How does willed action differ from action in response to sensory input?

Three main areas of cortex are involved in voluntary movement: the PMC, supplementary motor area (SMA) and premotor cortex. These form part of functional systems involving basal ganglia (corticostriatal) and corticothalamic, corticocerebellar and pyramidal (corticospinal)

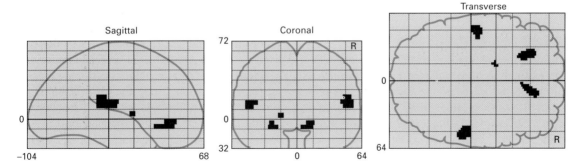

Fig. 5.2 An example of images given by the statistical parametric mapping technique of Friston and Liddle, applied in this case to SPET rCBF images. Sagittal, coronal and transverse views are given of mean differences at $P < 0.001$ level of two groups of schizophrenic subjects who perform (i) well and (ii) poorly on an eye-movement task. The poor performers as a group show statistically significantly ($P < 0.001$) reduced rCBF in the indicated areas in the anterior cirgulate and superior temporal sulcus area, bilaterally.

Table 5.2 Unilateral sequential finger movements: change in rCBF.

Contralateral only	Bilateral	Ipsilateral only
Primary motor cortex	Supplementary motor area	Anterior cerebellum
Thalamic (ventrolateral) and subthalamic nuclei	Premotor area (frontal)	
	Putamen and globus pallidus	

systems. PET studies have been crucial in understanding the functional relationships of the three cortical areas.

The PMC lies in the precentral gyrus. It is somatopically organised, that is, each body part has its own region of PMC operating it. This can be clearly shown with PET or SPET studies of rCBF or rCMR. The PMC receives afferent inputs from the SMA and premotor cortex, both of which are loosely somatopically organised, and from the cerebellum via the ventrolateral thalamus. The PMC is activated during any voluntary muscular movement (including speech), except eye movements. In absolute terms, the increase in rCBF in PMC during finger or hand movement is in the order of 10–30 ml/100 g/min, that is an increase of about 10–15%. The increase is somewhat greater for rapid or complex movements.

The SMA lies just in front of the PMC, posterior to the rear boundary of the prefrontal cortex, equivalent to Brodmann area 6. Early electrical-stimulation studies of human cortex showed that, whereas stimulation of the PMC led to simple movements, stimulation of the SMA leads to more complex movements. The SMA connects with its contralateral opposite via the corpus callosum and to cingulate cortex. The SMA is activated strongly during the learning of motor tasks and planning motor activity, but much less so during simple well-practised movements (Roland *et al.*, 1980). During motor tasks, bilateral SMA activity occurs, although it is usually stronger on the contralateral side. Dominant-hemisphere SMA activity occurs during speech.

The premotor cortex is an area in the superolateral region of the posterior prefrontal cortex. It is a higher-order organisational area. PET studies show it to be particularly active during the incorporation of sensory information into new motor programmes. Intention for motor action involves bringing on-line learned motor programmes (memories) initially, if the movement is already learned.

Deiber *et al.* (1991) used PET to investigate how different motor programmes were selected for different movement conditions, and is an elegant example of functional dissection or deconstruction. All test conditions involved the subject using a hand to move a joystick. The control condition was moving the joystick forwards repeatedly. Four test conditions were: (i) random movement; (ii) moving the joystick in a well-learned sequence of directions; (iii) moving it according to the identity of a tone; and (iv) moving it the opposite way to that dictated by the tone. Self-initiated movements compared with those secondary to a tone were characterised by increased SMA and premotor activity. It is possible to divorce motor planning from motor action by studying subjects who are internally rehearsing a motor activity rather than actually doing it. SMA and premotor areas but not primary motor cortex are activated (Fox *et al.*, 1987).

Speech

The use of functional imaging, particularly PET, to investigate mechanisms involved in speech function has been similarly fruitful. As with more general issues of movement production, much attention has been given to the different cortical areas involved in internally generating words, compared with giving verbal responses to auditory stimuli. The final common pathway of speech production involves the posterior inferior frontal area (Broca's area), the SMA and the PMC subserving the larynx and mouth.

The word-generation or word-fluency task has been studied extensively and is a further example of the use of functional deconstruction through subtraction techniques through PET. In this task, subjects are asked to speak out loud as many words starting with a particular letter as they can manage. The control task, which is subtracted from this condition, is usually the subject simply repeating a word presented to him/her. The difference between these two conditions is that, during internal generation, increases in rCBF were seen in left prefrontal and anterior cingulate cortex (Frith *et al.*, 1991). In association with these increases during word generation, a proportionate decrease in superior temporal cortex can also be seen. Using the statistical image analysis approaches to measuring connectivity between different activated brain regions, whose principles are described by Liddle (Chapter 11) and by Frith and colleagues (1991), this reciprocal relationship has been interpreted as essential to the normal self-monitoring of internally generated speech. Frith and colleagues (1991) have shown how these normal relation-ships might be disrupted in disorders such as schizophrenia,

where a failure of self-monitoring of willed action might be a central neuropsychological deficit (Friston *et al.*, 1995).

References

Deiber, M.P., Passingham, R., Colbach, J.G., Friston, K.J., Nixon, P.D. & Frackowiak, R.S.J. (1991) Cortical areas in the selection of movement: a study with PET. *Exp. Brain Res.* **84**, 393–402.

Fox, R.T., Pardo, J.V., Petersen, S.E. & Raichle, M.E. (1987) Supplementary motor and premotor response to actual and imagined hand movements with PET. *Soc. Neurosci. Abstr.* **13**, 1433.

Friston, K.J., Herald, S., Fletcher, P. *et al.* (1995) Abnormal fronto-temporal interactions in schizophrenia. In Watson, S.J. (ed.) *Biology in Schizophrenia and Affective Disorders.* Raven Press, New York, pp. 445–81.

Frith, C.D., Friston, K., Liddle, P.F. & Frackoviak, R.S. (1991) Willed action and the prefrontal cortex in man: a study with PET. *Proc. Roy. Soc. London* **244**, 241–6.

Kety, S.S., Woodford, R.B., Harmell, M.H., Freyhan, F.A., Apel, K.E. & Schmidt, C.F. (1948) Cerebral blood flow and metabolism in schizophrenia: the effects of barbiturate semi-narcosis, insulin coma and electro-shock. *Am. J. Psychiatry* **104**, 765–70.

Roland, P.E., Larsen, B., Lassen, N. & Skinhoje, A. (1980) Supplementary motor area and other cortical areas in the organisation of voluntary movements in man. *J. Neurophysiol.* **43**, 118–36.

Roy, C.S. & Sherrington, C.S. (1890) On the regulation of the blood supply of the brain. *J. Physiol.* **11**, 85–108.

Talairach, J., Szikla, G., Tournoux, P. *et al.* (1967) *Atlas d'Anatomie Stéréotaxique du Télencéphale.* Masson, Paris.

6: Magnetic Resonance Spectroscopy and Functional MRI

M. S. Keshavan and J. D. Cohen

Introduction

The understanding of the pathophysiology of major neuropsychiatric disorders has been limited by the fact that, until recently, direct access to the human brain for research studies has been mainly via post-mortem studies. The introduction of brain imaging techniques such as computerised tomography (CT), magnetic resonance imaging (MRI) and 'functional' techniques, such as positron emission tomography (PET), functional magnetic resonance imaging (fMRI) and magnetic resonance spectroscopy (MRS), have changed the scene in neuropsychiatric research. MRS and fMRI are non-invasive *in vivo* approaches to the measurement of metabolic and physiological changes in living tissues and are based on the principles of nuclear magnetic resonance (NMR), explored in Chapter 3. In this chapter, we review the history and elementary physical principles of magnetic resonance (MR), the techniques and the physiological insights potentially provided by fMRI and MRS, as well as their potential applications to psychiatry. For more extensive analyses of these rapidly expanding fields, the interested reader is referred to more elaborate reviews (Keshavan *et al.*, 1991a; Cohen *et al.*, 1993).

Magnetic resonance spectroscopy

Historical review

NMR was first demonstrated by Rabi and his colleagues at Columbia University, New York, in 1939 (Andrew, 1984). However, it was Edward Purcell and Felix Boch who, working independently, first discovered in 1946 that the magnetic dipoles of molecules in ordinary matter resonate in response to an externally applied field (nuclear magnetic resonance, or NMR). Bloch and Purcell also pioneered biological applications of NMR. Bloch obtained an NMR signal from his finger inserted into the radio frequency (RF) coil of his spectrometer, while Purcell recorded signals from his own dental fillings (Bloch *et al.*, 1946; Purcell *et al.*, 1946). Early biological applications included ^{31}P-MRS studies of erythrocytes and then of intact organs from animals. Human limbs were subsequently studied, made possible by the advent of stronger magnets with larger bore sizes. The use of *in vivo* MRS in clinical settings has been relatively recent, beginning with the first report of a ^{31}P-MRS study of a patient with McArdle's syndrome (Ross *et al.*, 1981).

Physics

Atomic nuclei are constituted by different numbers of protons and neutrons. A proton has a positive charge, but a neutron has no charge. All nuclei which have an odd number of protons or neutrons have a spin (for example, ^{1}H has a core of only one proton, and ^{7}Li has three protons and four neutrons), generating a magnetic field. However, not every atom has a spin. Helium (^{4}He), for example, has two protons and two neutrons, which cancel each other's spin; only atoms with net spins (e.g. ^{1}H, ^{13}C, ^{19}F, ^{23}Na, ^{31}P) are NMR-sensitive.

All atoms in matter are randomly aligned in the absence of an external magnetic field (Fig. 6.1a). When an external magnetic field (B_0) is imposed, the atoms line up along the direction of the magnetic field (Fig. 6.1b) and spin ('precess') about the axis of the external field. If another field (B_1) generated by a (RF) coil is now applied, at an angle of 90° to B_0, the spinning-tops can be 'tipped' in the x–y axis (Fig. 6.1c), thus being elevated to a higher state of energy; the nuclei which were initially spinning around the B_0 axis will start 'precessing' around that axis in addition, like a top or a gyroscope spinning about the spike (Fig. 6.1d). Each distinct nuclear species resonates at a unique frequency, called the Larmor frequency (W) (Table 6.1). This frequency varies with the external magnetic field (B_0) as well as the gyromagnetic constant (γ), thus:

$$W = \frac{\gamma B_0}{2\pi}.$$

If the RF field is now turned off, the nuclei return to their original axis. This 'relaxation' induces a voltage signal in a surrounding record-ing coil; the signal decays with time (free induction decay, or FID). By Fourier transformation the FID can be translated from the time to the frequency domain, resulting in the MR spectrum (Fig. 6.2).

The resonance frequency of a nucleus (fortunately for the spectroscopists) is affected by the local magnetic field of the electron 'cloud' surrounding the nucleus, an effect called the *chemical shift* and described, by convention, in units of parts per million (p.p.m.) (i.e. millionths of the Larmor frequency) in relation to a central RF (Fig. 6.3). The chemical shift varies with bond configuration of each molecule; thus, the same element in different chemical compounds resonates at slightly different frequencies. The spectrum provides information as to what biochemicals are present by the *position* of the peak on the horizontal frequency axis. The *area under each peak* can represent the quantity of the different metabolites. The *width* of the peak is affected by intermolecular interactions, but could be broadened by magnetic-field inhomogeneities as well. Thus, in order to detect minute changes in NMR frequency caused by the *chemical shift*, an extremely homogeneous external magnetic field is therefore necessary. Since the sharpness of each peak, or line width, is determined by the homogeneity of the magnetic field, increasing the homogeneity ('shimming') is needed in obtaining narrow line widths. In order to get an acceptable signal-to-noise ratio (SNR), the MR signal has to be averaged many times; thus several minutes are needed to obtain a single MR spectrum.

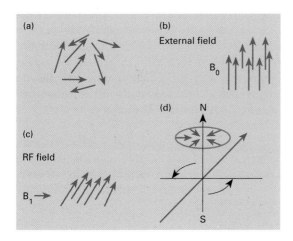

Fig. 6.1 (a) Matter as shown here is composed of nuclei which are charged and have a net spin, acting like tiny magnetic dipoles. At rest all dipoles are arranged randomly. (b) On application of an external field, B_0, the magnetic dipoles, arrange themselves along the direction of the external field. (c) On application of an additional radio-frequency (RF) field, B_1, the dipoles already aligned along B_0 are 'tipped' along the x–y axis, being elevated to a state of higher energy. (d) On removal of the radio-frequency field, the 'processing' dipole returns to alignment along axis B_0. This process, called relaxation, induces an electromotive force in the recording coil.

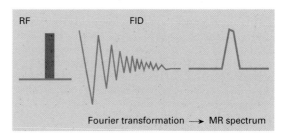

Fig. 6.2 The free induction decay (FID) induced by the radio-frequency (RF) pulse and the generation of the magnetic resonance (MR) spectrum.

Table 6.1 List of nuclei that are used in magnetic resonance spectroscopy studies.

Element	Intrinsic sensitivity (%)	Natural abundance (N%)	NMR frequency (MHz)
^1H	100.00	99.98	100.00
^{13}C	1.59	1.108	25.14
^{19}F	83.4	100.00	94.09
^{23}Na	9.24	100.00	26.45
^{39}K	5.08	93.1	4.67
^{31}P	6.64	100.00	40.48
^7Li	27.0	92.58	38.86

'Intrinsic sensitivity' reveals the relative sensitivity of a given isotope to detection by MRS.
'Natural abundance' expresses in percentage the extent to which the listed isotope constitutes the element as present in the human body under natural conditions.

To be 'visible' with MRS, the element should: (i) have a magnetic spin and thus lend itself to 'excitation' by MR; (ii) be present in a detectable concentration (Table 6.1) and produce an acceptable SNR; and (iii) be present in one or more biomolecules of interest. Further, it must be technically feasible to obtain the MR signal from the region of interest. ^{31}P, ^1H, ^{19}F, ^{13}C and ^{23}Na, which, to a varying extent, meet these conditions, have been used to study various aspects of metabolism.

Instrumentation

The instrumentation for *in vivo* MRS involves a horizontal-bore magnet (1.5–4.0 tesla (T)) for the main magnetic field (B_0), an RF transmitter and receiver coil tuned to the nucleus of interest (B_1 field), a display system and a computer. As opposed to MRI, MRS needs a higher magnetic-field strength in order to maintain chemical-shift information; a broad range of frequencies needs to be generated to study nuclei with varying resonance frequencies. Further, the source of the signal needs to be *localised* to a volume of interest. The use of a surface coil placed near the area of interest is the simplest way to acquire signals from a subject. However, volume selection is limited to a region near the surface. More recent approaches to localisation involve the use of magnetic-field gradients to select a volume of interest (VOI) and are identified by a variety of acronyms. Most involve an extension of MRI techniques, using a combination of three slice-selective RF pulses together with magnetic gradients in *x*, *y* and *z* directions that make the

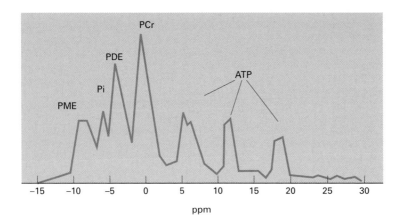

Fig. 6.3 A schematic diagram of the *in vivo* ^{31}P-NMR spectrum of the human brain. ATP, Adenosine triphosphate (α, β and γ peaks); PCr, phosphocreatine; PDE, phosphodiester; Pi, inorganic phosphate; PME, phosphomonoester.

frequency vary with the distance, thus permitting spatial encoding of the MR signal. In this way, the Larmor frequency pulse is only applied to this VOI. These include the use of chemical-shift imaging (CSI) sequences, stimulated echo-mode acquisition (STEAM), depth-resolved surface-coil spectroscopy (DRESS) and image-selected *in vivo* spectroscopy (ISIS). In CSI, one-, two- or three-dimensional spectral information can be obtained, using a series of gradient fields. In the DRESS technique, a plane parallel to the face of a surface coil is selectively excited, and this results in spectral information from a disc-shaped volume. Using ISIS, the MRS signal can be localised to an axial 'slab', a column or a cube of brain tissue at a desired anatomical location.

Because of relatively superior sensitivity, the gradient-localisation techniques are particularly well suited for ¹H-MRS (Fig. 6.4a,b). While the

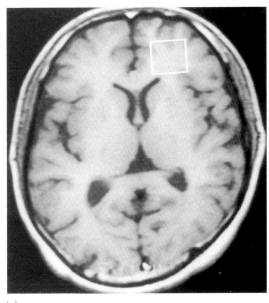

(a)

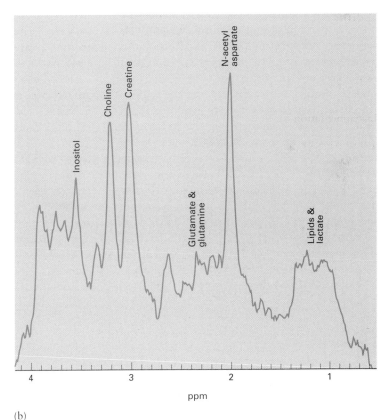

Fig. 6.4 A single voxel region of interest used for ¹H-MRS acquisition in a STEAM protocol. (b) ¹H-MR spectrum of the brain of a healthy human subject using the protocol depicted in (a).

(b)

gradient-localisation techniques offer the advantage of precise localisation of the VOI, there is a disadvantage as well. Since the gradients need to be turned off before turning on the receiver coil, there will be an acquisition delay, during which some of the signal will be lost. The differing relaxation times in different molecules could lead to varying rates of signal delay; this might lead to a disproportionate loss of signal from compounds such as phospholipids with short transverse relaxation time (T2). Approaches using 'depth-resolved pulse sequences' may therefore offer an advantage for ^{31}P-MRS studies (Pettegrew *et al.*, 1994).

Information provided by MRS

Bioenergetics

The ^{31}P-MRS resonances of α, β and γ phosphate moieties of adenosine triphosphate (ATP), phosphocreatine (PCr), adenosine diphosphate (ADP) and inorganic phosphate (Pi) provide information about energy metabolism. α and γ phosphate resonances contain a mixture of ATP and other phosphates (Fig. 6.3). ATP serves as the reservoir for energy, generated by metabolism of carbohydrates, lipids and proteins, via the Krebs cycle; any excess is saved as PCr. PCr, catalysed by creatine kinase (PCr + ADP → + ATP + creatine), serves as an 'energy shuttle' which helps brain ATP levels to be constant. Pathological states associated with hypoxia, ischaemia, anaerobic metabolism and impaired energy utilisation perturb the levels of ATP, PCr and Pi. When oxygen is lacking, a shift occurs to anaerobic metabolism, lactate is generated from pyruvate and pH is reduced. Lactate is 'visible' with ^{1}H-

MRS, and the pH can be detected by ^{31}P-MRS, as will be discussed later.

Membrane phospholipid metabolism

Cell membranes are integral to the maintenance of structure, ion conduction and signal transduction, as well as maintenance of concentration gradients, and are comprised of a phospholipid bilayer. Phosphomonoesters (PMEs) are the precursors and phosphodiesters (PDEs) are the breakdown products of membrane phospholipids (e.g. phosphatidylcholine, phosphatidylethanolamine and phosphatidylserine) (Fig. 6.5). PMEs include phosphocholine, phosphoserine, phosphoethanolamine and α-glycerophosphate; PDEs, include glycerophosphocholine and glycerophosphoethanolamine. ^{31}P-MRS *in vivo* as well as *in vitro* studies can reveal the PME and PDE resonances which reflect membrane turnover and may differ between healthy and disease states. Phospholipids themselves constitute a large part of the broad resonance underlying the PDE and PME peaks.

Carbohydrate, amino acid and fat metabolism

^{1}H-MRS can be used to measure resonances from amino acids, neurotransmitters and their derivatives; metabolites related to energy metabolism, such as glucose, phosphocreatine, creatine, lactate, acetate and *N*-acetylaspartate (NAA); metabolites related to phospholipid metabolism, such as phosphocholine and phosphoethanolamine; and metabolites related to nucleotide metabolism, such as adenine, guanine, uracil and cytosine. NAA is considered to be primarily intraneuronal, although glial cells may also contain

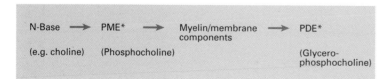

Fig. 6.5 A schematic diagram showing the major steps in membrane phospholipid metabolism. *Can be measured with ^{31}P-MRS.

some NAA (Urenjak *et al.*, 1991), and provides an index of neuronal mass and integrity. The role of brain NAA remains unclear. Its neuronal colocalisation with *N*-acetylaspartylglutamate (NAAG) suggests a possible relation to excitatory amino acids. NAAG, when cleaved by a dipeptidase, yields NAA and glutamate.

In vivo ^{13}C-MRS can be used to measure and identify triglycerides, glycogen and fats. Further definition can be obtained by enriching the diet with non-radioactive ^{13}C-labelled glucose or ^{13}C-acetate. The signal obtained from this dose of ^{13}C can be used to study the way in which ingested nutrients are incorporated, stored and metabolised.

Electrolyte and pH measurement

A largely extracellular element, such as ^{23}Na, which lends itself to MRS can be used to study electrolyte balance in health and disease states, such as injury, inflammation, oedema and tissue death, which shift the [23]Na from the extracellular to the intracellular compartment. The resonant frequencies of nuclei in relation to an acidic or basic group are also sensitive to changes in pH. For example, the chemical shift of the inorganic phosphate (Pi) varies as a function of pH. Thus, ^{31}P-MRS has been used to measure *in vivo* pH in humans. However, the sensitivity of this method is rather poor because of the imprecise definition of the Pi peak; further, in the pH range of 6.5–7.2 the Pi nucleus manifests only a 1 ppm shift. Other approaches to *in vivo* pH measurement include measuring the chemical-shift differences between γ and α peaks of ATP (Pettegrew *et al.*, 1988b).

Neuropsychiatric applications: ^{31}P-MRS

The application of MRS is relatively recent. While the clinical value of MRS appears relatively established in estimating prognosis in neonates and in detection of muscle enzyme defects, its value in the diagnosis and monitoring of neuropsychiatric disorders is far from established. However, its value in research into the subcellular

basis of neuropsychiatric disorders is clearly evident. Among the various techniques, ^{31}P-MRS has been a widely applied technique because of its 100% natural abundance, making it relatively sensitive. A variety of neuropsychiatric disorders have now been investigated using ^{31}P-MRS.

Normal development and ageing

The human brain, after birth, undergoes major maturational modifications involving substantial biochemical changes, detectable by *in vivo* MRS. Membrane phospholipid and high-energy phosphate metabolism are influenced considerably by brain development and ageing, as demonstrated by *in vitro* ^{31}P-MRS of rat brain (Pettegrew *et al.*, 1990; Hida *et al.*, 1992). *In vivo* ^{31}P-MRS studies have shown that PDEs increase and PMEs decrease during adolescence and then remain stable until senescence (Panchalingam *et al.*, 1990; van der Knapp *et al.*, 1990). Healthy elderly subjects had decreased PME and increased PDE, suggesting accelerated membrane metabolism.

Dementias

In vitro ^{31}P-MRS studies of autopsy brain from patients with Alzheimer's disease (AD) (Barany *et al.*, 1985; Pettegrew *et al.*, 1988a; Blusztajn *et al.*, 1990) have shown alterations in membrane phospholipid metabolism, with increases in PME and PDE. Early *in vitro* studies have shown increases in PME early in the disease followed by elevations in PDE as compared with non-diseased controls (Pettegrew *et al.*, 1988a; Brown *et al.*, 1989). These findings were thought to differ from the ^{31}P-MRS findings observed in association with normal ageing but are similar to the pattern seen during normal brain development (Pettegrew *et al.*, 1988a).

However, more recent studies have been conflicting; Murphy *et al.* (1993) did not find any differences between patients with AD and age-matched controls. On the other hand, Pettegrew *et al.* (1994) showed that mildly demented AD patients had increases in PME and decreases in

PCr and probably ADP, presumably related to increased oxidative metabolic rate. Methodological differences in the MRS technique may account for these variable findings in the literature. In the Murphy *et al.* (1993) study, controls were considerably younger than AD patients; the region of interest included a large inhomogeneous voxel of brain tissue. The two studies also differed in their approach to quantification of metabolites. Further studies of larger numbers of patients are needed to resolve these differences.

Similar ^{31}P-MRS findings have been observed in other dementing illnesses. Some elevations in PDE levels have been detected in deeper tissues, corresponding principally to white matter, in Binswanger's disease and in Huntington's chorea (Smith *et al.*, 1993). Brown *et al.* (1989) have shown elevations of PCr and PCr/Pi ratios in 10 patients with multi-infarct dementia (MID), as compared with patients with AD and age-matched controls. Human immunodeficiency virus (HIV)-seropositive men have been reported to have significantly decreased ATP/Pi ratios; these changes were significantly correlated with the severity of neuropsychiatric impairment (Deicken *et al.*, 1990). Bottomley *et al.* (1990) have found significant decrements in PCr in acquired immune deficiency syndrome (AIDS) dementia. Elevations in brain PME have also been seen in AIDS (Cadoux-Hudsen *et al.*, 1990).

Neurodevelopmental disorders

Studies in congenital cerebral atrophy, propionic acidaemia, arginosuccinic acidaemia and meningitis in newborn infants have revealed decreased ratios of PCr/Pi and alterations in pH. Such alterations predict poor outcome and subsequent neurological abnormalities (Hamilton *et al.*, 1986). Minshew *et al.* (1990) have shown significantly increased PCr and decreased β ATP in adult patients with Down's syndrome; PME and PDE levels were not different. In autism, Pettegrew *et al.* (1989) have demonstrated decreased levels of PCr and of α ATP, suggesting

alterations in brain high-energy phosphate metabolism. These findings are distinct from those in schizophrenia, a condition with which autism shares some clinical features.

Psychoses

Several studies suggest that schizophrenia is associated with alterations in membrane phospholipids in peripheral cells (Rotrosen & Wolkin, 1987); this has stimulated studies of brain membrane composition using ^{31}P-MRS. ^{31}P-MRS studies of the dorsal prefrontal lobe have been carried out in neuroleptic-naïve first-episode schizophrenia in comparison with age- and gender-matched controls (Keshavan *et al.*, 1989; Pettegrew *et al.*, 1991). Schizophrenic patients showed decreased PME levels, increased PDE levels, increased β-ATP levels and decreased levels of Pi. The PME and PDE results suggest decreased synthesis and increased breakdown of membrane phospholipids. A similar pattern of decreased PME and increased PDE was seen in a 'normal' control who was studied 2 years before a psychotic episode, suggesting that these alterations may represent 'trait' markers (Keshavan *et al.*, 1991b). The PDE levels correlate significantly with corpus callosal size, particularly the anterior quartile (Keshavan *et al.*, 1993).

Subsequent research has provided some support for these observations, although there are some disparities across studies. O'Callaghan *et al.* (1991) found no significant differences in the temporal lobe, except for a higher pH in schizophrenic patients. However, the normal subjects were considerably older, and the effects of neuroleptics could not be excluded. Reduction in PMEs and increases in PDEs have been replicated in drug-naïve first-episode schizophrenia (Stanley *et al.*, 1991). Williamson *et al.* (1991) reported decreased prefrontal PME, but no change in PDE, in chronic medicated schizophrenic patients compared with controls. On the other hand, Fujimoto *et al.* (1992), using ^{31}P CSI, have observed increased PDE, but no alteration in PME, in chronic schizophrenic patients in the left temporal lobes. Deicken *et al.* (1993) have observed increases in PDE in the prefrontal cortex of chronic schizophrenic patients.

Membrane phospholipid alterations, as observed by ^{31}P-MRS, may not be confined to schizophrenic illness. Decreases in PME and PDE have been noted in cocaine-dependent polysubstance abusers (MacKay *et al.*, 1993). *In vivo* ^{31}P-MRS studies of affective disorder have also been carried out. Kato *et al.* (1991) compared ^{31}P-MRS parameters in manic subjects on lithium with their euthymic state, as well as with normal controls. A significant elevation of PME was seen and was attributed to the possible accumulation of inositol-1-phosphate in brain induced by lithium. These investigations have also reported increases in PME in depressed patients (Kato *et al.*, 1992).

Pharmacological studies

The non-invasive nature of ^{31}P-MRS studies allows them to be repeated before and after administration of pharmacological agents. In a pioneering study, Renshaw *et al.* (1986) showed accumulation of PMEs following lithium administration to cats in therapeutically meaningful doses. It is possible that such effects could parallel lithium's therapeutic effects; using ^{31}P-MRS, one can non-invasively monitor second-messenger-mediated events which may mediate lithium's effects. ^{31}P-MRS has been used to detect the muscarinicagonist-induced accumulation of phosphomonoesters (such as inositol phosphate) in cats (Renshaw *et al.*, 1987). It is thus possible to carry out longitudinal and drug-related monitoring of changes in phospholipid metabolism in neuropsychiatric disorders. We have recently examined ^{31}P-MRS data in schizophrenic and schizoaffective patients before and after 1 and 2 weeks of treatment with lithium: reduced pretreatment PME and increases in nucleotide phosphates at 1 week predicted a therapeutic response (Keshavan *et al.*, in press).

^{19}F-MRS

The relatively superior sensitivity and large chemical-shift range of ^{19}F make it desirable for MRS studies. ^{19}F is the only naturally occurring fluorine isotope. There is very little mobile ^{19}F in the body, and it is biologically unimportant. Therefore, artificially introduced biocompatible fluorine-containing compounds have been used, as in ^{19}F-MRS studies with blood substitutes, chemotherapeutic drugs and fluorinated anaesthetics. Concentrations of fluorinated psychotropic agents, such as fluphenazine, trifluoperazine and fluoxetine, have been studied by ^{19}F-MRS in brains of patients receiving these drugs (Arndt *et al.*, 1988; Komorowski *et al.*, 1990; Renshaw *et al.*, 1992). Using fluorine-labelled substrates, such as 2-fluoro-2-deoxyglucose, it is possible to follow glucose metabolism. ^{19}F-MRS has also been used to measure cerebral blood flow. In the future it may also be possible to measure fluorinated neurotransmitter ligands in the human brain.

^{13}C-MRS

In naturally occurring carbon, 98.9% is ^{12}C. The 1.1% that is ^{13}C is spectroscopically 'visible' in extracts. ^{13}C-MRS has a chemical-shift range about 20 times wider than ^{1}H-MRS, although the sensitivity of this technique is rather low. Natural-abundance ^{13}C-MRS of the brain demonstrates ^{13}C chemical shifts of amino acid and neurotransmitter metabolites (glutamate, γ-aminobutyrate) and some information about phospholipid and energy metabolism. ^{13}C-labelled substrates, such as glucose, have also been used to study selected areas of metabolism *in vivo* and *in vitro*. Such studies allow metabolites of the parent compound to be simultaneously detected; successive steps in metabolism can thus be analysed in physiological states and diseases.

^{1}H-MRS

^{1}H-MRS, even though very sensitive, has limitations: (i) the dominant signal from ^{1}H in body water, being 10 000 times more abundant than any other species, 'drowns' all other signals; and (ii) ^{1}H-MRS from brain metabolites, such as lactate, can be confounded by strong signals from the extracranial lipids. However, techniques are available to 'suppress' the water and lipid resonances. Despite these disadvantages, several findings of interest have emerged from ^{1}H-MRS research.

Brain development and ageing

^{1}H-MRS has also provided valuable information about normal and abnormal brain development. During childhood and adolescence, increases in the ratios of NAA to choline and NAA to creatine have been observed; the changes are most rapid during the first 3 years of life. Since there is no increase in the number of neurons after birth, these NAA increases have been attributed to dendritic or synaptic proliferation (van der Knapp *et al.*, 1990). Elevations of choline have also been seen and have been attributed to myelination (Kreis *et al.*, 1991). Increases in the choline signal have been described with ageing in patients with Down's syndrome and have been attributed to degenerative changes in white matter (Murata *et al.*, 1993).

Dementias

Patients with AIDS dementia have been reported to have decreases in NAA (Meyerhoff *et al.*, 1993). Using *in vitro* ^{1}H-MRS, Klunk *et al.* (1992) have demonstrated decreased NAA and increased glutamate in brains of patients with AD. The decrease in NAA correlated with the number of senile plaques and neurofibrillary tangles. The decreases in NAA might reflect neuronal loss; the remaining neurons may thus be exposed to relatively high levels of glutamate, perhaps leading to neurotoxic brain damage. A recent *in vivo* study has lent some support to these findings. Miller *et al.* (1993) have found a decrease in NAA and an increase in myoinositol in patients with AD compared with age-matched healthy controls. These findings, if confirmed, suggest abnormalities in the inositol polyphosphate messenger pathway in AD.

Psychoses

Sharma *et al.* (1992) have obtained ^{1}H spectra from the frontal and occipital regions of nine psychiatric patients and nine healthy controls. The patients, notably lithium-treated bipolar disorders, showed an increased NAA/PCr ratio compared with controls. Charles *et al.* (1994) have recently observed a trend for increased choline among elderly depressives; these levels subsided following treatment. Stanley *et al.*, (1992) have compared ^{1}H-MRS data from never-treated schizophrenic patients with controls and have found significantly reduced glutamate concentration in the dorsolateral prefrontal cortex. Nasrallah *et al.* (1991) have conducted ^{1}H-MRS studies of the hippocampus in schizophrenia. They showed a decrement in NAA in the right hippocampus; they interpreted this deficit as reflecting possible neuronal loss. Further studies are needed to explore these interesting observations.

Preliminary reports of ^{1}H-MRS in major depression have appeared in the literature (Renshaw *et al.*, 1993; Charles *et al.*, 1994), showing increases in choline resonances. ^{1}H-MRS studies have been carried out recently in lithium-treated patients with bipolar disorder and lithium-free controls (Stoll *et al.*, 1992). Contrary to erythrocyte data showing accumulations of choline with lithium treatment, no changes were seen in the brain content of choline or related compounds.

Localised ^{1}H spectroscopy has been used to monitor brain metabolism following electroconvulsive therapy (ECT) (Woods & Chiu, 1990). An increase was seen in the lipid resonance; the authors speculated that this may be related to maximal activation of the phosphoinositide system. Contrary to expectations that cerebral lactate would be increased with seizures, no changes were seen in ^{1}H-MRS following ECT in one study (Felber *et al.*, 1993).

Anxiety disorders

Proton spectroscopy is likely to be of value in research into anxiety disorders. Lactate infusion, known to induce panic attacks in humans, produces a consistent and detectable elevation in brain lactate (Dager & Steen, 1992). However, lactate infusion also elevates blood lactate; the relative proportions of the total spectral signal derived from the brain and vascular compartments remain unclear.

Alcoholism

In vivo proton MRS has also been applied to alcoholism research. The methylproton signal of alcohol can be observed in the human brain using ^{1}H-MRS at levels of legal intoxication (0.1%) (Hanstock *et al.*, 1990). A significant concordance has been observed between blood and brain alcohol levels as measured by ^{1}H-MRS (Mendelson *et al.*, 1990). This approch can be used to study regional distribution and kinetics of ethanol. However, it has been suggested that ^{1}H-MRS measurements may actually underestimate actual brain alcohol levels, and that a significant portion of alcohol may be 'invisible' to MRS (Moxon *et al.*, 1991).

^{23}Na-MRS

^{23}Na is 100% naturally abundant, making it attractive for MRS studies. However, its disadvantages are that: (i) it gives rise to very broad peaks due to its rapid T2 relaxation, making it a poor choice for MRS; and (ii) Na$^+$ does not form covalent bonds with other atoms, and therefore chemical-shift information is not obtainable. Sodium exists within aqueous macromolecular complexes both inside and outside the cell; only 40% of the intracellular sodium is 'visible' with MR spectroscopy when the cell membranes are intact (Cope, 1967). Membrane-impermeable paramagnetic agents, such as dysprosium polyphosphate, by selectively changing the extracellular ^{23}Na chemical shift, can allow the resolution of the extra- and intracellular pools into distinct resonances. However, dysprosium is too toxic for human use.

^{23}Na-MRS has been applied to the study of disorders involving sodium transport and membrane disruption. ^{23}Na-MRS without shift reagents in human studies shows dramatically elevated ^{23}Na in stroke, haemorrhage and brain tumours (Hilal *et al.*, 1985).

^{7}Li-MRS

^{7}Li-MRS is a valuable approach to the study of the intracellular chemistry of lithium. Evidence from an *in vitro* ^{7}Li-MRS study suggests that lithium increases molecular motion by interaction with the membrane-associated cytoskeleton in human erythrocytes (Pettegrew *et al.*, 1987). *In vivo* ^{7}Li-NMR studies have been carried out in humans (Renshaw *et al.*, 1985; Gyulai *et al.*, 1991). In the latter two studies, the brain lithium levels, as measured by ^{7}Li-MRS, correlated well with serum levels. Kato *et al.* (1993) have reported that differences between brain lithium concentrations and serum concentrations may be related to differences in cation transport mechanisms between neurons and erythrocytes. It has been suggested that the minimum effective brain concentration of lithium for maintenance therapy in bipolar disorder is around 0.2–0.3 meq/l (Gyulai *et al.*, 1991).

Advantages and limitations of MRS

The unique advantages of MRS are its non-invasiveness and suitability for longitudinal studies. Although concerns have been raised regarding possible long-term risks, there is no established evidence that magnetic fields cause harm. A large number of chemicals, including metabolites and drugs, are potentially amenable to quantification. Nevertheless, several disadvantages, both technical and patient-related, have delayed progress in the application of MRS in clinical medicine. In addition, a variety of studies using MRS have reached varying conclusions, such that reproducible, clinically useful facts emerging from this technique are still scarce.

Poor sensitivity

MRS requires relatively strong and homogeneous magnetic fields; 'shimming' is then needed for each measurement, making it more expensive in time and cost. Since MRS signals are much weaker than the proton signals used for MRI, signal acquisition needs more time; thus the VOI has to be much larger than that for MRI, limiting spatial resolution. Another problem is that the SNR and magnetic field strength are not strictly linear. The SNR is proportional to the square root of acquisition time. Thus, the SNR will only be doubled with the signal acquisition time four times as long.

Only a select few elements can be studied by MRS

The 'overall sensitivity' of a given nucleus is its intrinsic sensitivity multiplied by its concentration in the tissue. The low intrinsic sensitivity of elements such as ^{39}K make them inaccessible to MRS. Further, the low concentrations of some elements with high sensitivity, such as ^{19}F, limit their suitability to be used in MRS studies in their natural state.

Only a few selected aspects of metabolism can be studied by MRS

Only highly mobile nuclei which are in solution are MRS-'visible'. Nuclei whose mobility is restricted because of binding to membranes or macromolecules (e.g. lipids) result in broad resonance signals with poor SNR.

Poor temporal resolution

The prolonged acquisition time limits detection of transient biochemical changes. This lack of temporal resolution limits the applicability of

MRS in cognitive or neurophysiological challenge paradigms.

Difficulties in quantification of the MR signal

One approach is relative quantification (i.e. expression of the quantity of a given compound as mole%). 'Absolute' quantification has also been attempted, using an external standard (Bottomley *et al.*, 1992). However, the use of external standards introduces several sources of random error (Pettegrew *et al.*, 1994). In particular, excitation and acquisition of an MR signal will be affected by the local environment, which will differ between an external standard and a metabolite in tissue. For these reasons, at this time relative quantification may be unavoidable. A recent study, comparing the relative quantification, using mole%, with an internal standard in an *in vitro* experiment, has supported the validity of the former approach (Klunk *et al.*, 1994).

Cost

NMR machines are quite expensive. In addition, the need for additional equipment for RF production and reception (for nuclei other than protons) adds to the cost. This raises the important question of whether MRS is cost-effective and whether the information provided is clinically useful.

Subject cooperation

Subject cooperation is a key factor and is often limited in psychiatric patients. Claustrophobia can be a particularly difficult problem, often resulting from the loud noise inside the magnet; in about 1% of subjects, NMR studies fail because of this problem. However, this can be dealt with by using benzodiazepine anxiolytics before scanning; a recent study showed no significant effects of diazepam on ^{31}P-MRS parameters (Deicken *et al.*, 1992).

Motion artefacts

Random patient motion, as well as involuntary motion caused by blood or cerebrospinal fluid (CSF) flow, respiration and peristalsis, can affect the quality of spectra in MRS. Using complex gradients, it is possible to suppress motion artefacts.

Partial-volume effects

Biochemical information provided by MRS usually conforms to geometrically shaped volumes (e.g. spherical), and not to the shapes of anatomical structures of interest to the psychiatrist. Further, signal 'bleed' from one voxel to another, leading to blurring of voxel edges, as well as regional differences in brain structure (e.g. superficial vs. deeper structures), could affect the interpretability of MRS data. Another limitation refers to the inherent heterogeneity of brain tissue; unless homogeneous regions of brain (e.g. gray or white matter; brain or CSF) are chosen, erroneous conclusions may be drawn. This is because of variations in metabolite quantities in diverse brain regions (Frahm *et al.*, 1989).

In addition to the above limitations, the field of MRS is plagued by problems in interpreting data generated by research studies and by frequent non-replications of findings. These difficulties arise from failure to address methodological problems at various levels, such as appropriate choice and matching of controls, varying MRS signal-acquisition protocols, differing approaches to quantification of peaks and metabolite concentrations and the lack of 'gold standards' to compare with (Bottomley, 1991). However, these are the 'growing pains' of any young field of enquiry and are likely to improve as the field matures.

MRS and other functional imaging techniques

PET and single-photon emission tomography (SPET) scans provide alternative, promising approaches to functional brain imaging (Table 6.2). The advantages of PET scanning include relatively high sensitivity, high spatial resolution and the feasibility of investigating a wide range of biochemical processes, including glucose and oxygen consumption, neurotransmitter turnover and neuroreceptor binding. The disadvantages include the use of radioactive tracers with its attendant risks and the need for an expensive cyclotron nearby to make such isotopes. SPET scanning offers the advantage of not requiring such an expensive facility and can potentially provide information about a wide range of biochemical processes, but it has a relatively low resolution. Thus it can be seen that PET and SPET scanning have advantages not seen with MRS: MRS likewise has unique advantages. These techniques may therefore be complementary among the developing brain-imaging technologies.

Future directions

Clinical research applications of MRS are still in their infancy. Future clinical and research

Table 6.2 Relative merits of functional imaging techniques.

	PET	SPET	MRS	fMRI
Spatial resolution	+++	++	+	++
Temporal resolution	+++	++	+	+++
Low cost	+	+++	++	++
Safety	+	++	+++	+++
Sensitivity	+++	++	+	++
Biochemical information	++	++	++	−

applications will benefit from: (i) the use of instruments with higher field magnets (up to 4 T); (ii) spectroscopy contrast agents which enhance chemical shift; (iii) the use of spectroscopic imaging, which may include three-dimensional phase encoding, allowing mapping of proton metabolites in all three spatial dimensions of the human brain (Duyn *et al.*, 1991); and (iv) simultaneous use of multinuclear spectroscopic techniques *in vivo*, e.g. using ^{31}P nuclei for ATP and ^1H for lactate. The technologies of MRI and MRS are increasingly converging to yield spatial chemical images providing novel opportunities for clinical research; recent attempts (Hennig *et al.*, 1994) to marry the techniques of fMRI and MRS (functional spectroscopy) hold considerable promise in imaging research.

Nevertheless, despite the promising prospects, potential clinical applications of MRS in the psychiatric setting are still far away. Future research in neuropsychiatric MRS will need to address: (i) specificity of MRS findings in carefully selected patients with major neuropsychiatric disorders and appropriate controls; (ii) validation of *in vivo* information from patients in the light of modern neurochemistry, (iii) anatomical–biochemical relationships by careful spatial localisation; and (iv) the potential value of biochemical parameters in predicting treatment effects and the course of illness and to develop novel treatment strategies.

Much of the research thus far in neuropsychiatric MRS has involved exploratory 'fishing expeditions'. It is only recently that clinical needs are driving experimental research and vice versa in an effort to exploit the wealth of information that MRS can yield. Focused, hypothesis-driven research is likely to help address some of these vexing questions.

Functional MRI

As discussed above (and shown in Table 6.2), one of the great strengths of using MRI for functional neuroimaging is its safety and non-invasive nature, relative to radionucleotide-based techniques such as PET and SPET. MRS, in particular, offers the opportunity to measure metabolic activity directly. However, we have also noted that MRS currently has relatively limited spatial and temporal resolution.

A new MRI-based method, commonly referred to as functional MRI (fMRI), offers all of the advantages of an MRI-based neuroimaging technique, with additional advantages that complement those of MRS. In this section, we briefly review the principles underlying this technique, its relative advantages and disadvantages, recent applications of this new method and directions in which it is likely to evolve.

The principles of fMRI

As described earlier, MRI relies on the energy released by protons in atomic nuclei, as they return to their resting state after having been temporarily perturbed. Protons precess (wobble) as they return to rest, producing a characteristic energy signal. The production of a signal strong enough to be recorded requires that a large number of protons return to their resting state in a coherent fashion—that is, that they precess in unison. When this occurs, the individual signals sum and produce an aggregate signal that can be detected by the MR scanning device. The large magnet used in MR scanners produces a strong ambient magnetic field, which ensures that a sufficiently large number of protons within the field are in a similar resting state (i.e. sitting upright). To generate an image, the scanner produces a brief RF energy pulse within the plane to be imaged, which momentarily perturbs (tilts) the protons within that plane. It then records the energy that is released as those protons precess back to their original state.

T1, T2 and T2* decay

The two time constants associated with the decay in the MR signal, as protons return to their resting state following an RF pulse, are the T1 and T2 relaxation times. T1 corresponds to the decay in the signal that results from the protons gradually returning to their initial state (which can be thought of as the longitudinal component, since the protons are 'tilting' back up to their 'upright' state). T2 corresponds to the decay in the MR signal that occurs as the protons gradually fall out of phase in their precession (this can be thought of as a transverse component, since it is in this plane that the motion of the protons is becoming non-uniform). T2 decay results from inherent, random variations in the precession frequency of individual protons, or local interactions between nearby nuclei. However, larger-scale inhomogeneities in the magnetic field can also produce differences in precession frequency, resulting in dephasing and signal reduction. When T2 dephasing is attributable to one or more localisable sources, it is referred to as T2*. This provides the basis for fMRI techniques (Young, 1988).

There have been two basic approaches to fMRI, both of which take advantage of two basic phenomena: (i) the ability of paramagnetic agents to produce contrast in the MR signal; and (ii) the fact that regional changes in brain activity are associated with local haemodynamic changes. An elementary understanding of each of these is necessary for understanding how fMRI is used to record regional changes in brain activity.

Paramagnetism and T2*-weighted imaging

Paramagnetism is the ability of an otherwise non-magnetic material to exhibit magnetic properties in the presence of a magnetic field (e.g. the ability of a paper clip to attract others when it is in the presence of a magnet). The initial efforts to record physiological activity with MRI used paramagnetic contrast agents (such as gadolinium-diethylenetriaminepenta-acetic acid (DTPA)), injected into the blood, to measure regional blood flow (Rosen *et al.*, 1990). In the presence of the MR magnet, the molecules in these agents produce local magnetic fields. Recall that MRI requires that large numbers of protons recover their initial state in phase, so that their effects sum to produce a signal that is detectable by the

imaging apparatus. The larger the number of protons that are in phase, the larger the signal. The molecules in the contrast agent introduce local inhomogeneities in the magnetic field, which reduce the coherence of, or 'dephase', the signal generated by the protons at that location. This dephasing reduces the size of the signal detected by the scanner. As a result, brain regions that are receiving greater blood flow produce a weaker MR signal than other regions. The difference in signal due to local dephasing effects can be detected in images acquired using MR parameters that are sensitive to T2* decay. Therefore, blood-borne contrast agents, in conjunction with T2*-weighted imaging, can be used to produce an image of brain perfusion. By comparing perfusion in activated and non-activated states, areas of relative brain activity can be identified (Belliveau *et al.*, 1991). One obvious limitation of this approach, however, is the need to use exogenous contrast agents to produce the image. In this respect, this method shares some of the limitations of PET, in terms of the practicality and cost of conducting studies and the number and extent of studies that can be performed in single individuals.

However, several groups have developed methods that do not require the use of injected contrast agents (Ogawa *et al.*, 1990; Turner *et al.*, 1991; Kwong *et al.*, 1992). These are based on the observation that haemoglobin (Hb) becomes highly paramagnetic in its deoxygenated state (Thulborn *et al.*, 1982). In other words, it appears that deoxygenated Hb can be used as a naturally occurring contrast agent: Highly oxygenated areas should produce a larger MR signal than less well-oxygenated regions. These changes in signal intensity related to the oxygenation of Hb should therefore be detectable in T2*-weighted images. This method is often referred to as the BOLD (*blood oxygen-level-dependent*) technique (Ogawa *et al.*, 1992), and it offers great promise because of its lack of invasiveness.

Exploiting the oxygen sensitivity of the MR signal for functional brain imaging relies on another physiological phenomenon. A number of studies (e.g. Fox *et al.*, 1988; Raichle, 1988) have demonstrated that, in a number of brain areas, blood flow increases disproportionately to metabolic need when those areas become active. This results in a net *increase* in tissue oxygenation. As a result, the T2*-weighted component of the MR signal is increased in those areas relative to others, and this contrast can be used to produce MR images of the activated region.

This method has already begun to see wide application. In particular, Kwong *et al.* (1992), Bandettini *et al.* (1992) and Ogawa *et al.* (1992) have all shown activity-related changes in occipital cortex in response to visual stimuli comparable to those that have been demonstrated using paramagnetic contrast media (Belliveau *et al.*, 1991). We shall review other applications of this technique below.

Types of scanning equipment

Most of the initial efforts to image oxygen-related changes directly (without the use of contrast agents) have used specialised MRI equipment. For example, the original studies by Kwong *et al.* (1992) and Bandettini *et al.* (1992) used *echo planar imaging* (EPI) techniques, which provide a means of acquiring MRI images much faster than with ordinary equipment. Ogawa *et al.* (1992) and Turner *et al.* (1992) have reported success using high-field (4T) magnets. Unfortunately, high-field magnets and the equipment necessary for EPI are costly and still limited in availability. Other laboratories have begun to report similar results using conventional MRI equipment (Gore *et al.*, 1992; Frahm *et al.*, 1993; Schneider *et al.*, 1993). In particular, the use of specialised pulse sequences (e.g. spiral scanning—Ahn *et al.*, 1986; Noll *et al.*, 1993) permit image acquisition at high resolution, with rates approximating those possible with specialised equipment. Some of the considerations associated with these different approaches, and likely directions in which fMRI will develop, will be discussed below following a brief review of recent applications.

We should note that, as with other functional neuroimaging methods, design of the behavioural tasks used to produce activation and the statistical procedures used to generate activation maps are critical features of any study, influencing both the results and their interpretation. Unfortunately, a discussion of these factors is beyond the scope of this chapter. Readers interested in these and other issues related to the application of fMRI to psychology and psychiatry are referred to Cohen *et al.* (1993) and David *et al.* (1994) for a detailed discussion.

Recent applications of fMRI

Studies of sensory and motor cortex

Most of the initial studies using fMRI have been directed, justifiably, at validating this technique by replicating the results of studies using more established neuroimaging techniques. Thus, Kwong *et al.* (1992), Frahm *et al.* (1993) and Schneider *et al.* (1993) have all conducted studies of activation in occipital cortex in response to visual stimuli. The latter demonstrated the high spatial resolution of which fMRI is capable: distinct areas of activity were observed for stimuli presented in different regions of the visual field, with borders between regions observed over distances as short as 1 mm. Furthermore, this study provided direct evidence for the existence of topographically distinct areas of visual cortex, similar to those that have been observed in animal electrophysiology studies. This work was conducted on a standard clinical-grade scanner. A more recent study has succeeded in distinguishing receptive field locations less than 1.4 mm apart within primary visual cortex (Engel *et al.*, 1994).

At the same time, several groups have demonstrated expected patterns of activation in primary motor cortex. For example, both Bandettini *et al.* (1992) and Kim *et al.* (1993) have distinguished between areas within the primary motor strip associated with separate fingers. In a recent case study, S.B. Baumann and D.C. Noll (unpublished study, 1993) demonstrated the clinical utility of these techniques. They conducted a study in a patient with a prediagnosed arteriovenous malformation (AVM) in a posterior frontal cortex. A functional study was performed to determine the relationship of the AVM to primary motor cortex. Based on the findings, which showed the lesion to be adjacent to the primary motor strip, a decision was made to pursue a non-surgical intervention. The results of these initial studies have helped to validate the BOLD technique as a functional neuroimaging method and to demonstrate some of its capabilities, including its potential use as a clinical instrument. More recently, this method has begun to receive amplification in the study of higher cognitive functions, which are more likely to be relevant to psychiatric illness.

Cognitive studies

The greatest number of studies using fMRI to study cognitive function have been on language function. Again, the goal of most of these has been to replicate established findings using other methods, such as PET. Most of these have used versions of a word-generation task (Hinke *et al.*, 1993; McCarthy *et al.*, 1993a; Rueckert *et al.*, 1993). replicating PET findings of activation in Brodmann's areas 45 and 10 (e.g. Petersen *et al.*, 1989).

More recently, fMRI has begun to see application to the study of other cognitive functions. Our group recently completed a study of non-spatial working-memory function, in which bilateral activation of the inferior and middle frontal gyri (corresponding roughly to Brodmann's areas 45 and 46) was reliably observed in single subjects (Plate 6.1, facing p. 230). Preliminary results have also been reported from another study of working memory, this time using spatial stimuli, in which activation in regions corresponding to Brodmann's areas 46 and 9 was observed (McCarthy *et al.*, 1993b). Just as fMRI has been used to study the topographic organisation of sensory and motor regions and so will also lend itself to similar studies of the organisation of

association cortex. Thus, for example, it should be possible to test whether, as in the monkey (Wilson *et al.*, 1993), working-memory representations are located more dorsally and object representations more ventrally within prefrontal cortex.

Clinical studies

Because fMRI is such a recent development, there have not yet been many clinical applications. In one study, conducted by Breiter *et al.* (1993), symptoms were prevoked in patients with obsessive-compulsive disorder while being scanned. Activation was observed in the orbital gyri and dorsolateral prefrontal cortex in these patients, but not in normal subjects, in whom disgust reactions were elicited. However, a number of other studies are currently in progress, including studies of schizophrenia and depression, and the results will no doubt soon be appearing in the literature.

A comparison of fMRI with other techniques

The body of work using fMRI that has already reached the literature indicates that fMRI is capable of producing functional images that are close, if not equal, to the resolution that standard MRI provides for structural anatomy. Furthermore, the technique is non-invasive, and is not associated with any known physical risks. Given these factors and the wide availability of the basic equipment, fMRI promises rapidly to become an important new functional neuroimaging tool, for both research and clinical assessment.

As exciting and important as this new technique is, however, like any other it is also associated with limitations. These have been reviewed extensively elsewhere (Cohen *et al.*, 1993). The reader is referred to this source for a detailed discussion of both technical and methodological issues surrounding the use of fMRI, and how this method compares with other functional neuroimaging methods. Here, we shall focus our discussion on issues that are relevant to clinically related applications of fMRI. We conclude by discussing some of the directions that are being pursued for its continued development.

Safety and cost

One of the primary advantages of fMRI is its safety. As discussed above, the fact that the procedure is non-invasive and non-toxic means that multiple scans can be obtained from a single subject. This, in turn, means that sufficient data can be acquired from a single subject in order to obtain reliable results. This has obvious relevance for clinical applications, where the ability to obtain useful information about a single subject is necessary for assessment and perhaps, eventually, diagnosis. Although PET technology is rapidly advancing and single-subject designs are becoming possible, it is still the case that fMRI is both less costly and less invasive than PET, which will make it a method of choice for many applications.

Physiological and anatomical limitations

Ultimately, fMRI is limited by the physiological processes it is used to measure. Current methods appear to be detecting changes in blood oxygenation that result from the brain's local regulation of its blood supply in response to local neural activity (comparable to ^{15}O studies in PET). This limits both its temporal and spatial resolution, and may have important consequences for its application under pathophysiological conditions. Thus, animal studies suggest that the haemodynamic response can begin as rapidly as 500 ms following the onset of neural firing. However, even using high-speed MRI equipment (with temporal resolutions of 250 ms), researchers have not seen changes in the MR signal until about 2–4 s after stimulation, with peak changes taking 4–6 s (Bandettini *et al.*, 1992; Blamire *et al.*, 1992; DeYoe *et al.*, 1992). It may be possible to improve on this with more sophisticated methods (such as gated acquisition of images and

signal averaging); however, these have yet to be explored.

Although the temporal resolution of fMRI (seconds) is significantly better than that of PET (minutes), it still precludes the study of many cognitive processes which are known to occur in times of the order of 100 ms and which may be relevant to many forms of psychiatric illness. Furthermore, little is known about changes in the haemodynamic response characteristics of the brain under conditions of damage or in response to psychiatric medications. These limitations suggest two important points. First, fMRI and PET will clearly benefit by efforts to better our understanding of the basic physiological processes that regulate cerebral blood flow, its relationship to blood oxygenation and metabolism and how these processes are affected by pathophysiological changes and medications. Second, neuroimaging methods such as fMRI and PET will be put to most effective use when combined with complementary electrophysiological approaches (such as event-related potentials (ERP) and magnetoencephalography (MEG)—see Chapter 9).

Finally, there are anatomical constraints on the use of fMRI. Some brain areas lend themselves better to MR imaging than others. In particular, it is difficult to obtain good images from areas that lie near large cavities, such as the frontal sinuses. The differences in magnetic susceptibility that occur along the boundaries of these areas produce a distortion of the ambient magnetic field, which degrades the MR signal (the effect is analogous to the optical distortions produced by a glass bottle submerged in a pool of water). It is possible to compensate for these distortions by introducing appropriate additional fields. This is the process of 'shimming', and is analogous to placing a set of prisms around the bottle, to 'smooth' out the image. However, this process is time-consuming and not always reliable or fully successful. This limitation may have important consequences for the study of illnesses that are believed to involve these brain regions, such as schizophrenia.

Current and future directions

The technology behind fMRI is rapidly evolving, and represents a moving target for a review such as this. Below, we touch on some of the directions for development that seem, at the present, to hold the greatest promise for improvements in this method.

High-field magnets. The strength of the MR signal is directly related to the strength of the ambient field used to align the protons in their resting state. Most scanners that are available in clinical settings are 1.5 T. However, commercial scanners are now available at 3 T, and there are a number of 4 T research scanners that are in use. One of the primary benefits of increased field strength is an increase in the SNR. Clearly, improvements in SNR will provide improved spatial, and possibly improved temporal, resolution. However, as field strength increases, so too does the energy of the RF pulse needed to generate a signal. At present, this energy is well below levels that are considered to be safe for human subjects. However, the safety limit, together with the technical problems associated with building larger magnets, is likely to significantly constrain developments in this direction.

High-speed imaging. In addition to larger magnets, faster imaging techniques are also becoming available. There have been a number of recent developments in MR technology aimed at reducing image acquisition time. These include EPI (e.g. Bandettini *et al.*, 1992; Kwong *et al.*, 1992), spiral-scan pulse sequences (Noll *et al.*, 1993) and others. Some of these require additional apparatus and all rely on special software. The technical details of these developments are beyond the scope of this discussion. What they offer, however, is much more rapid imaging times: Images can be acquired as quickly as four per second, rather than once every 7 s or longer using conventional techniques. One or more of these techniques are likely to become widely available within the next few years. These will open up a number of ways for improving functional studies. A given number of images can be acquired over a much shorter period of time, reducing subject fatigue, minimising motion artefact, etc.; this may be especially important for clinical studies, in which subjects may find it more difficult to remain still or engaged in the behavioural paradigm. Alternatively, a greater number of images can be acquired for the same amount of time, permitting better signal averaging, more detailed time-course data or larger areas that can be scanned.

Use of multiple imaging modalities. As noted above, one of the greatest promises for fMRI, as for all of the other approaches to neuroimaging, may be its use in conjunction with complementary techniques. Each method has its own strengths and potentials and its areas of weakness. fMRI offers tremendous spatial resolution. However, it does not have the temporal resolution of ERP or MEG (see Chapters 8 and 9). Conversely, it has proved very difficult to localise activity identified using ERP and MEG. By applying these techniques together, however, it may be possible to identify an area of activity with fMRI, and then trace the details of its time course using ERP and/or MEG. PET and SPET, in turn, can provide neurochemical specificity not currently possible with other techniques. These can be used to trace the underlying neurotransmitter systems involved in functions whose anatomic location and time course have been identified using a combination of MRI, ERP and MEG. One of the major directions of growth in neuroimaging research over the next several years, no doubt, will be the development of techniques for coordinating the use of multiple modalities.

Acknowledgements

This work was supported in part by Scottish Rite Schizophrenia Foundation Grant No. 5-37100 (M.S.K.), the University of Pittsburgh (M.S.K. and J.D.C.) and the Pittsburgh NMR Institute and Carnegie Mellon University (J.D.C.).

References

Ahn, C.B., Kim, J.H. & Cho, Z.H. (1986) High-speed spiral-scan echo planar NMR imaging – I. *IEEE Trans. Med. Imaging* **MI-5**, 2–7.

Andrew, E.R. (1984) A historical review of NMR and its clinical applications. *Br. Med. Bull.* **40** (2), 115–19.

Arndt, B.C., Ratner, A.W., Faull, K.S. *et al.* (1988) ^{19}F magnetic resonance imaging spectroscopy of a fluorinated neuroleptic ligand: *in vitro* and *in vivo* studies. *Psychiatry Res.* **25**, 73–9.

Bandettini, P.A., Wong, E.C., Hinks, R.S. *et al.* (1992) Time course of EPI of human brain function during task activation. *Magnetic Resonance Med.* **25**, 390–7.

Barany, M., Chang, Y.-C., Arus, C. *et al.* (1985) Increased glycerol-3-phosphorylcholine in postmortem Alzheimer's brain (letter). *Lancet* **i**, 517.

Belliveau, J.W., Kennedy, J.N., McKinstry, R.C. *et al.* (1991) Functional mapping of the human visual cortex by magnetic resonance imaging. *Science* **254**, 716–18.

Blamire, A.M., Ogawa, S., Ugurbil, K. *et al.* (1992) Echo-planar imaging of the activated human visual cortex shows a time delay between stimulus and activation. In *11th Annual Scientific Meeting*. Society of Magnetic Resonance in Medicine, Berlin, p. 1823.

Bloch, R., Hansen, W.W. & Packard, M.E. (1946) Nuclear induction. *Phys. Rev.* **69**, 127.

Blusztajn, J.K., Gonzalez-Coviella, I.L., Logue, M. *et al.* (1990) Levels of phospholipid catabolic intermediates, glycerophosphocholine and glycerophosphoethanolamine, are elevated in Alzheimer's disease but not in Down's syndrome patients. *Brain Res.* **536**, 240–4.

Bottomley, P.A. (1991) The trouble with spectroscopy papers. *Radiology* **181**, 344–50.

Bottomley, P.A., Hardy, C.J., Cousins, J.P. *et al.* (1990) HIV dementia complex: brain high energy phosphate metabolism. *Neuroradiology* **176**, 407–41.

Bottomley, P.A., Cousins, J.P., Pendrey, D.L. *et al.* (1992) Alzheimer dementia: quantification of energy metabolism and mobile phosphoesters with ^{31}P NMR spectroscopy. *Radiology* **183**, 695–9.

Breiter, H.C., Kwong, K.J.B. *et al.* (1993) Functional magnetic resonance imaging of symptom provocation in obsessive-compulsive disorder. In *12th Annual Meeting*. Society of Magnetic Resonance in Medicine, New York.

Brown, G.G., Levin, S.R., Gorrell, J.M. *et al.* (1989) *In vivo* ^{31}P NMR profiles of Alzheimer's disease and multiple subcortical infarct dementia. *Neurology* **39**, 1423–7.

Cadoux-Hudsen, J., Rajagopalan, B., Radda, G.K. *et al.* (1990) Metabolic changes due to HIV infection in human brain *in vivo*. *Magnetic Resonance Med.* **2**, 991.

Charles, H.C., Lazeyras, F., Krishnan, R. *et al.* (1994) Brain choline in depression: *in vivo* detection of potential pharmacodynamic effects of antidepressant therapy using hydrogen localized spectroscopy. *Biol. Psychiatry* **18**, 1121-7.

Cohen, J.D., Noll, D.C. & Schneider, W. (1993) Functional magnetic resonance imaging: overview and methods for psychological research. *Behav. Res. Meth. Instruments Computers* **25** (2), 101–13.

Cope, F.W. (1967) NMR evidence for complexing of Na[+] in muscle, kidney and brain, and by actomyosin: the relation of cellular complexing of Na[+] to water structure and to transport kinetics. *J. Gen. Physiol.* **50**, 1353–75.

Dager, S.R. & Steen, R.G. (1992) Applications of magnetic resonance spectroscopy to the investigation of neuropsychiatric disorders. *Neuropsychopharmacology* **7**, 249–66.

David, A.S., Blamire, A. & Breiter, H. (1994) Functional magnetic resonance imaging. *Br. J. Psychiatry* **164**, 2–8.

Deicken, R., Hubesch, B., Jensen, P. *et al.* (1990) Alterations brain phosphate metabolite concentrations in patients with HIV infection. *Arch. Neurol.* **48**, 203–9.

Deicken, R.F., Calabrese, G., Raz, J. *et al.* (1992) A [31]Phosphorous magnetic resonance spectroscopy study of diazepam does not affect brain phosphorous metabolism. *Biol. Psychiatry* **32** (7), 628–31.

Deicken, R.F., Merrin, E., Calabrese, G. *et al.* (1993) [31]Phosphorus MRSI of the frontal and parietal lobes in schizophrenia. *Biol. Psychiatry* **33**, 46A (abstract).

DeYoe, E.A., Neitz, J., Bandettini, P.A. *et al.* (1992) Time course of event-related MR signal enhancement in visual and motor cortex. In *11th Annual Scientific Meeting*. Society of Magnetic Resonance in Medicine, Berlin, p. 1824.

Duyn, J.H., Matson, G.B. & Weiner, M.W. (1991) 3D phase encoding methods for ^{1}H spectroscopic imaging of human brain. In *Works in Progress, 10th Annual Scientific Meeting*. Society of Magnetic Resonance in Medicine, San Francisco, p. 1005.

Engel, S.A., Rumelhart, D.E., Wandell, B.A. *et al.* (1994) Receptive field localization in human primary visual cortex using functional magnetic resonance imaging. *Nature* **369**, 525.

Felber, S.R., Pycha, R., Hummer, M. *et al.* (1993) Localized proton and phosphorus magnetic resonance spectroscopy following electroconvulsive therapy. *Biol. Psychiatry* **33**, 651–4.

Fox, P.T., Raichle, M.E., Mintun, M.A. & Dence, C. (1988) Non-oxidative glucose consumption during focal physiologic neural activity. *Science* **241**, 1445–8.

Frahm, J., Bruhn, H., Gyngell, M.I. *et al.* (1989) Localized high resolution proton NMR spectroscopy using stimulated echoes: initial applications to human brain *in vivo*. *Magnetic Resonance Med.* **9**, 79–93.

Frahm, J., Merboldt, K.D. & Hanicke, W. (1993) Functional MRI of human brain activation at high spatial resolution. *Magnetic Resonance Med.* **29** (1), 139–44.

Fujimoto, T., Nakano, R., Takano, T. *et al.* (1992) Study of chronic schizophrenics using ^{31}P magnetic resonance chemical shift imaging. *Acta Psychiatr. Scand.* **86**, 455–62.

Gore, J.C., McCarthy, G., Constable, R.T. *et al.* (1992) Imaging regional brain activation at 1.5 T using conventional imaging techniques. In *11th Annual Scientific Meeting*. Society of Magnetic Resonance in Medicine, Berlin, p. 1826.

Gyulai, L., Wicklund, S.W., Greenstein, R. *et al.* (1991) Measurement of tissue lithium concentration by lithium magnetic resonance spectroscopy in patients with disorder. *Biol. Psychiatry* **29**, 1161–70.

Hamilton, P.A., Hope, P.L., Cady, E.B. *et al.* (1986) Impaired energy metabolism in brains of newborn infants with increased cerebral echodensities. *Lancet* **i**, 1242–6.

Hanstock, C.C., Rothman, D.L., Shulman, R.G. *et al.* (1990) Measurement of ethanol in the human brain using NMR spectroscopy. *J. Studies Alcohol* **51**, 104–7.

Hennig, J., Ernst, T., Speek, O. *et al.* (1994) Detection of brain activation using oxygenation sensitive functional spectroscopy. *Magnetic Resonance Med.* **31**, 85–90.

Hida, K., Kwee, I.L. & Nakada, T. (1992) *In vivo* ^{1}H and ^{31}P NMR spectroscopy of the developing rat brain. *Magnetic Resonance Med.* **23**, 31–6.

Hilal, S.K., Maudsley, A.A., Raj, B. *et al.* (1985) *In vivo* NMR imaging of sodium-23 in the human head. *J. Computer Assisted Tomogr.* **9**, 1–7.

Hinke, R.M., Hu, X., Stillman, A.E. & Ugurbil, K. (1993) The use for multi-slice functional MRI during internal speech to demonstrate the lateralization of language function. In *12th Annual Scientific Meeting*, Vol. 1. Society for Magnetic Resonance in Medicine, New York, p. 63.

Kato, T., Shioiri, T., Takahashi, S. & Inubushi, T. (1991) Measurement of brain phosphoinositide metabolism in bipolar patients using *in vivo* ^{31}P MRS. *J. Affective Disorders* **22**, 185–90.

Kato, T, Takahashi, S., Shioiri, T. & Inubushi, T. (1992) Brain phosphorous metabolism in depressive disorders detected by phosphorus-31 magnetic resonance spectroscopy. *J. Affective Disorders* **26**, 223–30.

Kato, T., Takahashi, S., Shioiri, T. & Inubushi, T. (1993) Alterations in brain phosphorous metabolism in bipolar disorder detected by *in vivo* ^{31}P and ^{7}Li magnetic resonance spectroscopy. *J. Affective Disorders* **27**, 53–60.

Keshavan, M.S., Pettegrew, J.W., Panchalingam, K. *et al.* (1989) *in vivo* ^{31}P MRS of the frontal lobe in neuroleptic-naive first-episode psychosis: preliminary observations. *Schizophrenia Res.* **2**, 123

Keshavan, M.S., Kapur, S. & Pettegrew, J.W. (1991a) Magentic resonance spectroscopy: potential, pitfalls and promise. *Am. J. Psychiatry* **148**, 976–85.

Keshavan, M.S., Pettegrew, J.W., Panchalingam, K. *et al.* (1991b) ^{31}P Magnetic resonance spectroscopy detects altered membrane metabolism before onset of schizophrenia. *Arch. Gen. Psychiatry* **48**, 1112–13.

Keshavan, M.S., Sanders, R.D., Pettegrew, J.W. *et al.* (1993)

Frontal lobe metabolism and cerebral morphology in schizophrenia. *Schizophrenia Res.* **10**, 241–6.

Keshavan, M.S., Pettegrew, J.W. & Panchalingam, K. (in press) Magnetic resonance spectroscopic studies in psychosis: psychopharmacological studies. In Nasrallah, H.A. & Pettegrew, J.W. (eds) *MRS in Psychiatric Brain Disorder*. American Psychiatric Press, Washington, DC.

Kim, S.G., Ashe, J., Hendrich, K. *et al.* (1993) Functional magnetic resonance imaging of motor cortex: hemispheric asymmetry and handedness. *Science* **261**, 615–17.

Klunk, W.E., Panchalingam, K., Moossy, J. *et al.* (1994) N-acetyl-L-aspartate and other amino acid metabolites in Alzheimer's disease brain: a preliminary proton magnetic resonance study. *Neurology* **42**, 1578–85.

Klunk, W.E., Xu, C.J., Panchalingam, K. *et al.* (1994) Analysis of magnetic resonance spectroscopic data by the mole percent method. comparison to results expressed in absolute units. *Neurobiol. Aging* **155**, 133–40.

Komorowski, R.A., Newton, J.E.D., Karson, C. *et al.* (1990) Detection of psychoactive drugs in *in vivo* humans using ^{19}F NMR spectroscopy. *Biol. Psychiatry* **29**, 711–14.

Kreis, R., Ernst, T., Arcinue, E. *et al.* (1991) Myoinositol in short TE ^{1}H-MRS: a new indicator of neonatal brain development and pathology. In *Works in Progress 10th Annual Scientific Meeting*. Society of Magnetic Resonance in Medicine, san Francisco, p. 1007.

Kwong, K.K., Belliveau, J.W., Chesler, D.A. *et al.* (1992) Dynamic magnetic resonance imaging of human brain activity during primary sensory stimulation. *Proc. Nat. Acad. Sci. USA* **89**, 5675.

McCarthy, G., Blamire, A.M., Rothman, D.L. *et al.* (1993a) Echo-planar magnetic resonance imaging studies of frontal cortex activation during word generation in humans. *Proc. Nat. Acad. Sci. USA* **90**, 4952–6.

McCarthy, G., Puce, A., Hyder, F. *et al.* (1993b) Functional magnetic resonance imaging during a spatial working memory task in humans. *Soc. Neurosci. Abstr.* **19** (1), 790.

MacKay, S., Meyerhoff, D.J., Dillon, W.P. *et al.* (1993) Alteration of brain phospholipid metabolites in cocaine-dependent polysubstance abusers. *Biol. Psychiatry* **34** (4), 261–4.

Mendelson, J.H., Woods, B.T., Chiu, T.M. *et al.* (1990) *in vivo* proton magnetic resonance spectroscopy of alcohol in human brain. *Alcohol* **7** (5), 443–7.

Meyerhoff, D.J. MacKay, S., Bachman, D.L. *et al.* (1993) Reduced brain N-acetylaspartate suggests neuronal loss in cognitively-impaired human immunodeficiency virus-seropositive individuals: *in vivo* ^{1}H magnetic resonance spectroscopic imaging. *Neurology* **43** (3, Pt 1), 509–15.

Miller, B.L., Moats, R.A., Shonk, T. *et al.* (1993) Alzheimer's disease: depiction of increased cerebral myo-inositol with proton MR spectroscopy. *Radiology* **187**, 433–7.

Minshew, N.J., Pettegrew, J.W. & Panchalingam, K. (1990)

Membrane phospholipid alterations in Alzheimer's disease are not present in Down's syndrome. *Biol. Psychiatry* **27** (9A), 41–2.

Moxon, L.N., Rose, S.E., Haseler, L.J. *et al.* (1991) The visibility of the ^{1}H NMR signal of ethanol in the dog brain. *Magnetic Resonance Med.* **19**, 340–8.

Murata, T., Koshino, Y., Omori, M. *et al.* (1993) *in vivo* proton magnetic resonance spectroscopy study on premature aging in adult Down's syndrome. *Biol. Psychiatry* **34** (5), 290–7.

Murphy, D.G.M., Bottomley, P.A., Salerno, J.A. *et al.* (1993) An *in vivo* study of phosphorus and glucose metabolism in Alzheimer's disease using magnetic resonance spectroscopy and PET. *Arch. Gen. Psychiatry* **50**, 341–9.

Nasrallah, H.A., Skinner, T.E., Schmaibrook, P.E. *et al.*, (1991) *In vivo* ^{1}H NMR spectroscopy of the hippocampus in schizophrenia. In *ACNP 30th meeting.* Puerto Rico, p. 19 (abstract).

Noll, D.C., Meyer, H.C., Cohen, J.D. & Schneider, W. (1993) Spiral scan imaging of cortical activation. *J. Magnetic Resonance Imaging* **3**, 44.

O'Callaghan, E., Redmond, O., Ennis, R. *et al.* (1991) Initial investigation of the left temporoparietal region in schizophrenia by ^{31}P magnetic resonance spectroscopy. *Biol. Psychiatry* **29**, 1149–52.

Ogawa, S., Lee, T.S., Nayak, A.S. & Glynn, P. (1990) Oxygenation sensitive contrast in magnetic resonance image of rodent brain at high magnetic fields. *Magnetic Resonance Med.* **14**, 68–78.

Ogawa, S., Tank, D.W., Menon, D.W. *et al.* (1992) Intrinsic signal changes accompanying sensory stimulation: functional brain mapping using MRI. *Proc. Nat. Acad. Sci. USA* **89**, 5951–5.

Panchalingam, K., Pettegrew, J.W., Strychor, S. & Tretta, M. (1990) Effect of normal aging on membrane phospholipid metabolism by ^{31}P *in vivo* NMR spectroscopy. *Soc. Neurosci* **16**, 843 (abstract).

Petersen, S.E., Fox, P.T., Posner, M.I. *et al.* (1989) Positron emission tomographic studies of the processing of single words. *J. Cognitive Neurosci.* **2** (1), 153–70.

Pettegrew, J.W., Short, J.W., Woessner, R.D. *et al.* (1987) The effect of lithium on the membrane molecular dynamics of normal human erythrocytes. *Biol. Psychiatry* **22**, 857–71.

Pettegrew, J.W., Panchalingam, K. Moossy, J. *et al.* (1988a) Correlation of ^{31}P magnetic resonance spectroscopy and morphological findings in Alzheimer's disease. *Arch. Neuro.* **45** (10), 1093–6.

Pettegrew, J.W., Withers, G., Panchalingam, K. *et al.* (1988b) Considerations for brain pH assessment by ^{31}P NMR. *Magnetic Resonance Imaging* **6**, 135–42.

Pettegrew, J.W., Minshew, N.J. & Payton, J.B. (1989) ^{31}P NMR in normal IQ adult autistics. *Biol. Psychiatry* **25** (July Suppl.), 182–3.

Pettegrew, J.W., Panchalingam, K., Withers, G. *et al.* (1990)

Changes in brain energy and phospholipid metabolism during development and aging in the Fischer 344 rat. *J. Neuropathol. Exp. Neurol.* **49**, 237–49.

Pettegrew, J.W., Keshavan, M.S., Panchalingam, K. *et al.* (1991) Alterations in brain high energy phosphate and membrane phospholipid metabolism in first-episode, drug-naive schizophrenics. *Arch. Gen. Psychiatry* **48**, 563–8.

Pettegrew, J.W., Panchalingam, K., Klunk, W.M. *et al.* (1994) Alterations of cerebral metabolism in probable Alzheimer's disease: a preliminary study. *Neurobiol. Aging* **15**, 117–32.

Purcell, E.M., Torrey, H.C. & Pound, R.V. (1946) Resonance absorption by nuclear magnetic movements in a solid. *Phys. Rev.* **69**, 37–8.

Raichle, M.E. (1988) Circulatory and metabolic correlates of brain function in normal humans. In Mountcastle, V.B., Plum, F. & Geiger, S.R. (eds) *Handbook of Physiology—The Nervous System V.* American Physiological Society, Bethesda, MD.

Renshaw, P.F., Haselgrove, J.C., Leigh, J.S. *et al.* (1985) *In vivo* nuclear magnetic resonance imaging of lithium. *Magnetic Resonance Med.* **2**, 512–16.

Renshaw, P.F., Summer, J.J., Renshaw, C.E. *et al.* (1986) Changes in the ^{31}P NMR spectra of cats receiving lithium chloride systemically. *Biol. Psychiatry* **21**, 691–4.

Renshaw, P.F., Schnall, M.D. & Leigh, J.S. (1987) *In vivo* ^{31}P NMR spectroscopy of agonist stimulated phosphatidylinositol metabolism in cat brain. *Magnetic Resonance Med.* **4**, 221–6.

Renshaw, P.F., Guimaraes, A.R., Fava, M. *et al.* (1992) Accumulation of fluoxetine and norfluoxetine in human brain during therapeutic administration. *Am. J. Psychiatry* **149** (11), 1592–4.

Renshaw, P.F., Stoll, A.L., Rothschild, A. *et al.* (1993) Multiple brain ^{1}H MRS abnormalities in depressed patients suggest impaired second messenger cycling. *Biol. Psychiatry* **33**, 441 (abstract).

Rosen, B.R., Belliveau, J.W., Vivea, J.M. & Brady, T.J. (1990) Perfusion imaging with NMR contrast agents. *Magnetic Resonance Med.* **14**, 249–65.

Ross, B.D., Radda, G.K., Gadian, D.G. *et al.* (1981) Examination of a case of suspected McArdle's syndrome by ^{31}P nuclear magnetic resonance. *N. Engl. J. Med.* **304**, 1338–42.

Rotrosen, J. & Wolkin, A. (1987) Phospholipid and prostaglandin hypothesis of schizophrenia. In Meltzer, H.Y. (ed.) *Psychopharmacology: the Third Generation of Progress.* Raven Press, New York, pp. 759–65.

Rueckert, L., Appollonio, I., Grafman, J. *et al.* (1993) Functional activation of left frontal cortex during covert word production. In *12th Annual Scientific Meeting*, Vol. 1. Society for Magnetic Resonance in Medicine, New York, p. 60.

Schneider, W., Noll, D.C. & Cohen, J.D. (1993) Functional

topographic mapping of the cortical ribbon in human vision with conventional MRI scanners. *Nature* 365, 150–3.

Sharma, R.P., Venkatasubramanian, P.N., Bárány, M. & Davis, J.M. (1992) Proton magnetic resonance spectroscopy of the brain in schizophrenic and affective patients. *Schizophrenia Res.* 8, 43–9.

Smith, C.D., Gallenstein, L.G., Layton, W.J. *et al.* (1993) ^{31}P magnetic resonance spectroscopy in Alzheimer's and Pick's disease. *Neurobiol. Aging* 14, 85–92.

Stanley, J.A., Williamson, P., Drost, D.J. *et al.* (1991) Membrane phospholipid metabolism abnormalities in the left prefrontal cortex in drug-naive and chronic schizophrenics via ^{31}P NMR spectroscopy. In *Works in Progress, 10th Annual Scientific Meeting.* Society of Magnetic Resonance in Medicine, San Francisco, p. 1062.

Stanley, J.A., Williamson, P.C., Drost, D.J. *et al.* (1992) *In vivo* proton magnetic resonance spectroscopy in never-treated schizophrenics. In *New Research Abstract,* # NR10. American Psychiatric Association, Washington.

Stoll, A.L., Renshaw, P.F., Sachs, G.S. *et al.* (1992) The human brain resonance of choline-containing compounds is similar in patients receiving lithium treatment and controls: an *in vivo* proton magnetic resonance spectroscopy study. *Biol. Psychiatry* 32, 944–9.

Thulborn, K.R., Waterton, J.C., Matthews, P.M. *et al.* (1982) Oxygenation dependence of the transverse relaxation time of water protons in whole blood at high field. *Biochim. Biophys. Acta* 714, 265–70.

Turner, R., Le Bihan, D., Moonen, C.T.W. *et al.* (1991) Echo-planar time course MRI of cat brain oxygenation changes. *Magnetic Resonance Med.* 22, 159–66.

Turner, R., Jezzard, P., Wen, H. *et al.* (1992) Functional mapping of the human visual cortex at 4 tesla using deoxygenation contrast EPI. In *11th Annual Scientific Meeting and Exhibition.* Society of Magnetic Resonance, Berlin, p. 304.

Urenjak, J., Noble, M., Williams, S.R. & Gadian, D.G. (1991) N-Acetyl aspartate: re-evaluation of its specificity as a neuronal marker in ^{1}H NMR spectroscopy. *Soc. Magnetic Resonance Med. Abstr.* 1, 420.

van der Knapp, M.S., van der Grond, J., van Rijen, P.C. *et al.* (1990) Age-dependent changes in localized proton and phosphorus MR spectroscopy of the brain. *Radiology* 176, 509–15.

Williamson, P., Drost, D., Stanley, J. *et al.* (1991) Localized phosphorus-31 magnetic resonance spectroscopy in chronic schizophrenic patients and normal controls. *Arch. Gen. Psychiatry* 48, 578.

Wilson, F.A.W., Scalaidhe, S.P.O. & Goldman-Rakic, P.S. (1993) Dissociation of object and spatial processing domains in primate prefrontal cortex. *Science* 260, 1955–7.

Woods, B.T. & Chiu, T.M. (1990) *In vivo* [1]H spectroscopy of the human brain following electroconvulsive therapy. *Ann. Neurol* 28, 745–9.

Young, S.W. (1988) *Magnetic Resonance Imaging: Basic Principles.* Raven Press, New York.

7: Imaging Receptors in Psychiatry

L. S. Pilowsky

Introduction

Psychotropic drugs act on cellular receptors. Understanding this interaction is critical for rationalising available treatments, and developing better, more selective pharmacotherapies for psychiatric disorders. It is now possible to visualise and measure neurotransmitter receptors in the living human brain through application of the nuclear medicine tomographic techniques, positron emission tomography (PET) and single-photon emission tomography (SPET), discussed in Chapters 6 and 11. These tools permit neuropharmacological investigation, assisting drug development *in vivo*.

This chapter will review the principles of ligand imaging and the ligands available for PET and SPET research, discuss applications of the technology to psychiatric disorders and psychopharmacology and present the findings of recent work in the field.

Principles of ligand imaging

A brief history of receptors

Present-day methods of *in vivo* receptor estimation are firmly grounded in theoretical and technical achievements in pharmacology which began around the turn of the century. A short overview will be provided here. For further detail, the reader is referred to Taylor and Insel (1990) and Dean (1989).

The concept of 'receptive substances' in tissues, involved in pharmacological response to drugs, was first formulated by Langley (1878). Erlich (1900) was to extend the proposition, suggesting that particular surface groups on cells could interact with toxin molecules showing specific binding properties. These surface groups were named receptors, and the basis of drug-receptor theory was laid. The term 'receptor' strictly implies that the macromolecule confers a response or transduces a signal (as opposed to acceptors, for example, albumin, which transport or seqester ligands) (Dean, 1989). Receptors have the ability to bind, by weak non-covalent binding, specific compounds known as *ligands*. There have developed a number of criteria defining a neuroreceptor.

In the classical pharmacological approach, distinct receptor classes are defined in terms of their pharmacological specificity. Antagonists block the responses elicited by particular agonists. *Agonists* are ligands which promote a response by receptor occupancy, and the response may be proportional to the number of occupied receptors. The potency of agonists is partly determined by their affinity for the receptor and partly by their capacity to elicit a response (efficacy). *Antagonists* are those ligands which block the response elicited by an agonist. The blockade may be functional, irreversible, competitive, non-competitive or mixed (Taylor & Insel, 1990).

The usefulness of pharmacological methods for defining receptor types remains indisputable (see Young *et al.*, 1986, for examples of representative receptors and their pharmacology). However, advances in biochemistry and molecular biology have produced continual refinements in receptor classification over the decades since the drug-receptor theory was first put forward.

Pharmacological classification, critical to structure/activity considerations, as discussed above, discriminates receptors according to the mediator to which they respond (*chemical specificity*): for example, the particular effects of acetylcholine at nicotinic and muscarinic receptors (Dale, 1914), and the division of adrenergic receptors into α and β subtypes (Alquist, 1948), based on their differing pharmacological profiles.

Receptors may also be characterised by their anatomical location, for example, muscarinic receptors on smooth muscle. Receptors may be intra- or extracellular, or located on pre- or post-synaptic cell membranes.

Following the definition of receptor type by pharmacological responsivity, evaluation of receptor density and function at the cellular level was permitted by advances in molecular pharmacology beginning in the 1950s and continuing throughout the 1970s. Neurotransmitter receptors in membrane homogenates could be measured using high specific-activity (curies/mmol) tritiated radioactive ligands (Maziere & Maziere, 1993). In the most common approach, receptor-containing tissue is incubated with radioactively tagged drug molecules, and bound and unbound radioactive material is subsequently separated and quantified. Minute amounts of receptors are now measured and, in some cases, classified according to cellular responses elicited (e.g. changes in cyclic adenosine monophosphate (AMP) concentration, glucose production or electrical/mechanical responses). Thus receptors may be biochemically characterised (with binding techniques) and visualised (by autoradiographic techniques) *in vitro*. The principles of *in vitro* receptor measurement will be discussed below.

Finally, the primary amino acid sequence of receptors can now be deduced from the sequence of the gene encoding the protein. This approach has resulted in the discovery and cloning of new receptor subtypes. Examples are the dopamine D_3 and D_4 receptor populations (Sokoloff *et al.*, 1990; Van Tol *et al.*, 1991). The previously accepted strategies of receptor typing by classical pharmacological and molecular methods are then combined with molecular genetic developments to determine the physiological significance of these novel receptors.

The molecular structure of receptors can be related to their cellular, biochemical/physical responses and pharmacological specificity in the test-tube. Extrapolation from these data into the living organism is clearly imperative for drug development. Until recently, experimental animal models were the main conduit linking ligand–receptor chemistry to behavioural drug effects. This has been a particularly difficult obstacle for psychopharmacology, as inferences made from animal behavioural paradigms to complex human psychology are obviously limited (for example, there are no satisfactory animal models of schizophrenia).

Receptor measurement *in vitro*

Understanding the methodology of receptor measurement by the use of high specific-activity tritiated ligands in the test-tube is useful in order to appreciate the procedures in PET and SPET, which borrow heavily from these concepts. Detailed reviews of this subject are available in basic pharmacology texts.

For *in vitro* studies, *specific binding* is defined as ligand binding associated with the presumed receptor and *non-specific binding* as that binding remaining in the presence of a high concentration of a specific receptor antagonist (Taylor & Insel, 1990). In the test-tube, tissue receptors (R) are incubated with various concentrations of labelled radioligand (L), and bound radioligand (LR) is determined after equilibrium is achieved. The concentration of [LR] increases in proportion to [L], until all available receptors are bound (or occupied) by the ligand. When these values are plotted graphically, a curvilinear relationship is seen between [LR] and [L], with the plateau representing saturable binding of receptors, such that increasing concentrations of [L] will not increase [LR] further. The concentration of [L] halfway to this plateau is termed the *affinity* (K_d) of the ligand for the receptor.

In the absence of a cold-competitive ligand, both specific and non-specific binding is what is measured, i.e. *total binding*. In the presence of a cold-competitive ligand, which prevents any specific binding of the radioligand (L) to receptors (R), non-specific binding is measured. Subtraction of the non-specific from the total binding curve yields the specific binding curve, which at the plateau (LR_{max}) reflects receptor density. This is graphically represented in Fig. 7.1. By algebraic manipulation and replotting of these data (through graphical methods including the Scatchard and Hill plots), receptor density (B_{max}) at saturation is obtained (Taylor & Insel, 1990).

Demonstrating and quantifying specific binding of a tracer to receptors in the living animal or human brain is necessarily more involved. The ligand must pass through the blood–brain barrier, and is metabolised locally and in the periphery. Receptor–ligand behaviour in the test-tube is highly temperature- and pH-dependent, both factors which may be impossible to predict, measure or control *in vivo*.

The configuration of receptors in isolated membrane homogenates is altered in the natural environment of the pre- or postsynaptic neuronal cell membrane, where they are subject to intra- and extracellular regulatory mechanisms. Multiple binding sites/receptor subtypes may be indistinguishable, influenced by upregulatory/downregulatory neuromodulators and linked to enzyme second messengers (Young *et al.*, 1986). Thus assumptions taken from drug or ligand–receptor behaviour in the test-tube, or even in another species, when applied to receptor estimation in humans *in vivo*, are necessarily cautious, and must take account of these structural and functional complexities.

Ligand characteristics for PET and SPET

Molecular pharmacology, physics and radiochemistry combine to produce radioligands suitable for PET and SPET studies. A useful ligand should generally be highly selective in its binding profile (and bind with high affinity), get rapidly to the target organ (in the case of the brain, pass easily through the blood–brain barrier), be metabolised efficiently away from the area of interest (without labelled active metabolites) and be reasonably easily and economically synthesised. The path from radiochemical development to use in humans is lengthy and poses a constant challenge in the field, both to generate non-toxic relevant probes and to creatively employ those which are available. Many radioligands have been prepared and evaluated. Stocklin (1992) and Maziere and Maziere (1993) have comprehensively reviewed the topic and listed and discussed currently available neuroligands for PET and SPET.

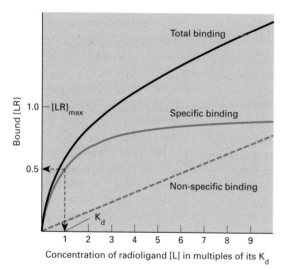

Fig. 7.1 Linear plot of saturation binding isotherm for ligand–receptor binding. Tissue receptors are incubated with various concentrations of radioligand and bound radioligand (LR) is determined after equilibrium is achieved. Subtracting values for non–specific binding from total binding yields specific binding. At [L] = K_d, the receptors are half-saturated relative to $[LR]_{max}$.

Tracer synthesis

The ideal strategy for ligand production entails labelling of an original atom on a pharmacologically active molecule with its own gamma-emitting isotope. If this is not possible, analogues of the molecule are synthesised, with replacement of an atom and attachment of a radiohalogen isotope at a suitable position.

Tracer design is rendered more complicated by analogue molecule synthesis. Steric and electronic effects alter the physiological properties of the ligand under preparation. Substitution with a halogen, for example ^{123}I, enhances lipophilicity, maximising non-specific binding or producing a flow tracer (Stocklin, 1992). Some molecules cannot be labelled with positron- or photon-emitting isotopes, excluding many interesting probes from *in vivo* studies. Exogenous antagonists are often chosen for labelling over agonists, as they are less likely to produce receptor–drug responses that may interfere with binding estimation, are not diluted by endogenous agonists and usually have higher affinity for receptor systems under investigation (Dolan *et al.*, 1990; Stocklin, 1992).

Ligand specificity

It is useful, but not essential, for a single receptor population to be under investigation during a PET or SPET scan to simplify interpretation of binding parameters. Occasionally, where anatomical localisation of receptor populations is sufficiently distinct, mixed receptor ligands may be employed. ^{11}C-*N*-methylspiperone (NMS), for example, binds to both 5-hydroxytryptamine (5-HT) receptors (localised mainly in the neocortex) and dopamine receptors (found mainly in the basal ganglia) and, as these are clearly separated anatomically, has been used to evaluate both systems (Wong *et al.*, 1984; Nordstrom *et al.*, 1993a).

Pharmacological research to determine ligand specificity *in vivo* is initially performed in animals as part of essential tracer evaluation, by similar methods to those of the *in vitro* displacement studies described above. Isomers of the ligand are given to test stereospecificity of ligand binding (Kung *et al.*, 1989). Receptor sites are blocked prior to ligand administration by predosing with a known 'cold' competitor—for example, lorazepam given prior to ^{11}C-flunitrazepam (Comar *et al.*, 1979). In a *chaser study*, a cold competitor for the receptor is administered following the radioligand. Competitive drugs or ligands that do not specifically bind to the receptor of interest will not displace the ligand from the receptor. Figure 7.2 demonstrates a typical chaser study, showing a rapid decline (so-called increased washout) in striatal activity of the D_2 ligand ^{123}I-iodobenzamide (IBZM) following an intravenous injection of the specific D_2 antagonist haloperidol (Seibyl *et al.*, 1992). The ligand distribution (which follows known patterns of receptor distribution found post-mortem) and time : activity kinetics 'on' and 'off' the receptor are observed and modelled mathematically.

In general, for PET and SPET receptor studies, areas with *high* receptor density (i.e. high specific binding to the receptor populations of interest) show a relatively longer time to peak activity but rapid clearance (displacement) following injection of a specific cold-competitive drug or ligand. Areas devoid of receptors or with negligible receptor density (i.e. mainly non-specific binding to blood proteins, capillary walls, fat, connective tissue) show a short time to peak activity and no effect of displacer on natural washout rate. A common approach (the *reference region* approach), is used to estimate receptor availability for ligand binding and generate an operational index of specific binding. The difference or ratio between high- and low-activity areas is obtained. Values over the plateau portion of the resulting 'specific' binding curve (pseudoequilibrium) reflect the saturable component of ligand binding. The choice of regions of interest (ROIs) is often guided by known receptor distribution from post-mortem studies, but the methodology of image analysis for receptor studies is under constant review.

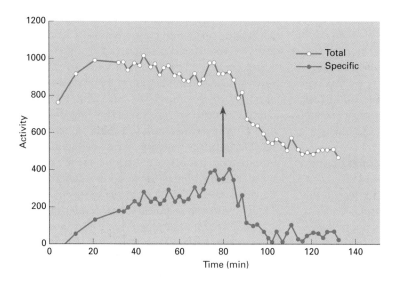

Fig. 7.2 Time–activity curve for a subject shows the effect of haloperidol on striatal and 'specific' activity washout rate. (Permission from Seibyl, *et al.*, 1992.)

Blood–brain barrier permeability

For neuroreceptor PET and SPET research, the ligand must be lipophilic enough to enter the brain (a reasonable level of uptake is >1% dose/g), but not so lipid-soluble that the blood–brain equilibrium is retarded by increased tracer binding to albumin, plasma proteins or blood cells (i.e. non-specific binding) (Young *et al.*, 1986). An optimal range of octanol:saline partition coefficient (between 0.5 and 10) has been suggested to maximise brain uptake and limit non-specific binding.

Metabolic stability

Useful tracers are metabolically stable within the time course of a scan, as tracer metabolism *in vivo* may result in labelled or unlabelled metabolites interfering with binding. To minimise this risk, suitable neuroreceptor radioligands are those which are metabolised in the periphery, with polar metabolites that do not redistribute to the brain (Young *et al.*, 1986; Stocklin, 1992). By measuring plasma metabolites of the ligand during scanning, the degree to which they are contributing to the detected activity may be incorporated when mathematically representing tracer delivery to the brain.

In vivo receptor measurement: modelling tracer behaviour

Mathematical modelling of radioligand uptake and clearance rate during a scanning experiment attempts to precisely quantify receptor binding in terms of traditional binding parameters, affinity and density (K_d/B_{max}), influx constants, volumes of distribution or specific rate constants (Dolan *et al.*, 1990). The attempt to quantify binding in these terms is not always desirable or necessary. In some instances, including clinical studies, absolute quantification may not confer additional benefits. Models requiring many estimated parameters may increase variability in the final measurement of interest. If the modelling demands repeated scans, radiation exposure to the subject is inevitably increased (Verhoeff, 1993). Thus far, the attempt to quantify ligand binding *in vivo* has been restricted to PET.

Limitations for quantification in SPET lie in the difficulty of correctly assuming that all the photons detected emerge from the region under investigation, i.e. that the activity detected in a given volume or area correctly reflects the true activity within this volume/area. Problems such as attenuation correction, scatter and correction for volume-averaging or partial-volume effects (Woods *et al.*, 1991) preclude full quantification with SPET at the present time, although solutions are under rapid development (with the use of reference phantoms to generate attenuation correction factors) and SPET quantification of both receptor and blood-flow studies is proceeding in some centres (Abi-Dargham *et al.*, 1993; Dobbeleir & Dierckx, 1993; Innis *et al.*, 1993; Laruelle *et al.*, 1993; Nikkinen *et al.*, 1993).

Nevertheless, dynamic SPET can evaluate regional binding kinetics, and provide valid *semiquantitative* indices of receptor binding by normalisation to areas of non-specific binding (Costa *et al.*, 1990; Brucke *et al.*, 1991; Pilowsky *et al.*, 1992) using a reference region approach during 'pseudoequilibrium'. This is expressed, for example, for ^{123}I-IBZM binding to dopamine D_2 receptors, as the ratio or difference between the basal ganglia region of interest (ROI) activity, representing total activity ((specific + nonspecific binding) + free ligand), and the frontal-cortex ROI activity representing background activity (non-specific binding + free ligand), at equilibrium between tracer uptake and washout (Pilowsky *et al.*, 1992). Figure 7.3 shows time : activity curves in the basal ganglia and frontal cortex following injection of ^{123}I-IBZM. Specific binding can be

seen to plateau approximately 40 min after radioligand injection, reaching a maximum stable plateau between 60 and 80 min postinjection.

Methods of *quantitative* analysis utilise the concept of brain *compartments*. Compartments represent anatomical volumes (not necessarily physically measurable) into which the tracer can distribute (Young *et al.*, 1986; Dolan *et al.*, 1990). Following tracer injection, the radioligand exists in two compartments—*intravascular* or *extravascular*. In the vascular space ligands are distributed as free or non-specifically bound. Unbound tracer can cross the blood–brain barrier, entering the extravascular compartment. Within this space the ligand is free, non-specifically bound (both states show rapid uptake and clearance) or specifically bound to receptor populations (reversibly or irreversibly). The conceptualisation of the ligand in three separate spaces (plasma, free or non-specifically bound, and specifically bound) is referred to as the three-compartment model.

Regional brain activity detected by the PET or SPET camera encompasses the radioligand in all these compartments over the time of a scanning experiment. Tracer distribution between these compartments is time-dependent, and rate con-

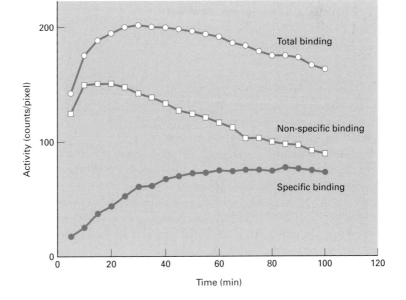

Fig. 7.3 Typical time–activity curves from a healthy volunteer. Scanning commences immediately after injection of 185 MBq of ^{123}I-IBZM. Total binding represents activity within the striatal region of interest. Non-specific binding is represented by activity in the frontal cortex region of interest and specific binding is derived by striatal – frontal cortex activity.

stants are used to describe fractional transfer of tracer across compartments.

Several different models are currently employed to quantify receptor binding (discussed by Dolan *et al.*, 1990; Verhoeff, 1993).

The equilibrium model

This applies to reversibly bound ligands; it is assumed that a steady state between the free tracer in the tissue and binding to receptors occurs in the time of the scanning experiment. Relatively few assumptions are made with regard to the mechanisms of tracer distribution in tissues. The existence of a *reference region* in the brain, devoid of receptors, but with the same non-specific volume of distribution as the receptor-containing ROI is also assumed. At equilibrium (plateau of tracer uptake and washout), ligand distribution is proportional to receptor density. To produce an absolute index of B_{max} and K_d, multiple studies are necessary at high and low specific activities of the tracer (i.e. in the presence or absence of a cold competitor—see above). Two such studies are the irreducible minimum (Lassen, 1992). A set of saturation/displacement curves are obtained transformed to linear functions and then plotted on Scatchard and Hill plots to provide the parameters B_{max} and K_d. An example is the modelling of ^{11}C-raclopride binding to dopamine D_2 receptors (Farde *et al.*, 1990).

The kinetic model

Tracers with very high affinity bind too firmly to permit quantitation in terms of B_{max} and K_d, invalidating equilibrium analysis. In these situations, *kinetic* models are used to describe exchange rates of tracer between compartments. The rate constants k_1 and k_2 are first-order rate constants, in that they represent simple diffusion forward (k_1) and back (k_2) through tissues and non-specific binding. Transfer coefficients k_3 (association constant) and k_4 (dissociation constant) describe the interaction of free tissue ligand with specifically bound ligand. The forward rate constant k_3 describes the interaction of free tissue ligand with receptor and is proportional to receptor number (B_{max}). The kinetic strategy is used when the dissociation rate (k_4) off the receptor is very slow. As an example, for modelling of ^{11}C-NMS to D_2 dopamine receptors (Wong *et al.*, 1986), two scans are required at the same specific activity of the ligand with and without haloperidol. The ratio of k_3 in the blocked and unblocked state is a measure of saturation (Andreasen *et al.*, 1988).

Multiple time-graphic analysis

The *multiple time-graphic* approach does not attempt to generate the binding parameters B_{max} and K_d, but does generate an influx constant K_i (a function of receptor availability) and volume of distribution (Patlak *et al.*, 1983). This form of analysis is used where a unidirectional transfer process is presumed. The model assumes linear transfer kinetics and consists of a blood-plasma compartment, a reversible tissue region and one or more irreversible tissue regions. When the tracer reaches equilibrium between all blood and brain compartments, constant flux into a specific compartment (from which there is no backflux) is indicated by a linear increase in the plotted data, with a slope reflecting its magnitude (Leenders *et al.*, 1990). The influx constant K_i is calculated from the slope of the tissue time : activity / plasma activity curve plotted against normalised time (integrated plasma activity/plasma activity). An example is the analysis of ^{18}F-dioxyphenylalanine (DOPA) PET data (Leenders *et al.*, 1990).

Spectral analysis

A simple spectrum of the kinetic components relating tissue response to the blood activity curve is produced. No a priori assumptions are made with respect to the number or compartments required to describe the time course of the label in the tissue (Cunningham & Jones, 1993).

These methods are under constant development.

Recent studies have focused on simplifying parameters necessary for models in order to minimise invasive and complex acquisition protocols (Lammertsma *et al.*, 1993; Patlak *et al.*, 1993) but retain accuracy. Pixel-by-pixel parametric comparisons of neuroreceptor scanning data, similar to those employed in blood-flow and metabolism studies, are enhancing the power of the above methods to detect subtle physiological and pathophysiological alterations in neuroreceptor systems (Cunningham *et al.*, 1993; Yokoyama *et al.*, 1993).

PET and SPET receptor studies and psychopharmacology

PET and SPET receptor estimation *in vivo* offers powerful new research strategies for neuropsychopharmacology. Hypotheses generated by postmortem investigations and indirect animal and human pharmacology studies can be tested in representative target populations. The main research areas in psychopharmacology are evaluation of specific receptor systems implicated in the aetiology of neuropsychiatric disorders; dynamic studies of drug and neurotransmitter: receptor interactions in animals and humans; and correlation of receptor measures with other indices of brain function, behaviour and clinical responsivity.

The enormous potential for clinical and research applications in neuroreceptor imaging is becoming clearer. However, there are still limiting factors. These include: the variety and type of probes available (for example, there are no selective ligands for D_3 and D_4 receptors, of enormous interest to schizophrenia research); the degree of radiation exposure associated with the study, as ethical restrictions increase; and the level of cooperation required for the scan (including the number of scans, the duration of the scan, and relative invasiveness of other procedures such as arterial blood monitoring), precluding examination of some patient groups.

Receptor studies in normal controls

Before evaluation of drug effects on ligand binding to receptors and comparison of healthy and ill populations can take place, normal patterns of receptor binding must be understood. The impact of demographic and physical factors, such as sex, age, weight, height, intelligence quotient (IQ) and educational level, and handedness, on the variability of binding measures is still uncertain. In the case of postsynaptic D_2 receptors, for example, the consensus from PET and SPET studies in large control samples is that receptor binding declines with age (Wong *et al.*, 1984; Martinot *et al.*, 1990, 1991; Brucke *et al.*, 1991; Rinne *et al.*, 1993; Pilowsky *et al.*, 1994). The decline is related specifically to density rather than affinity (Rinne *et al.*, 1993). Preliminary evidence suggests a sex difference, with males showing an exponential, rather than linear decline (Wong *et al.*, 1984). Other receptor systems which show age-related decreases in binding include benzodiazepine (BZ) receptors (Prevett *et al.*, 1993), 5-HT_2 receptors (Blin *et al.*, 1993; Iyo & Yamasaki, 1993) and muscarinic receptors (Suhara *et al.*, 1993). These data underline the absolute necessity for accurate age and sex matching of control and patient groups in receptor-binding studies.

Antipsychotic drugs

The clinical potency of antipsychotic drugs is linearly related to their affinity for D_2 receptors *in vitro* (Peroutka & Snyder, 1980). No similar relationship has been shown between clinical antipsychotic effect and affinity for α-adrenergic, histaminergic, cholinergic or serotonergic receptors *in vitro*. In one PET study, the degree of D_2 receptor occupancy by antipsychotic drugs correlated with clinical improvement (Nordstrom *et al.*, 1993b). For future rational antipsychotic drug development, the relationship between D_2 occupancy by antipsychotics and their clinical efficacy must be determined *in vivo*. PET and SPET have been applied to study antipsychotic drug occupancy of D_2 receptors *in vivo*, determine dose:receptor occupancy relationships and examine the relationship between D_2 receptor occupancy, extrapyramidal side-effects and clinical response.

Smith *et al.* (1988) and others (Cambon *et al.*, 1987; Lundberg *et al.*, 1989) demonstrated blockade of central D_2 receptors by typical antipsychotics in humans. A linear relationship between plasma haloperidol level and degree of D_2 occupancy (i.e. decline in striatocerebellar ratios) was shown (Smith *et al.*, 1988). After withdrawal of typical antipsychotic drugs, striatocerebellar ratios returned to high levels. Farde *et al.* (1989) showed that occupancy of D_2 receptors by 10 chemically distinct classes of typical antipsychotics was in the range 65–85% with ^{11}C-raclopride PET. Clozapine, an atypical antipsychotic, had only a 45% occupancy of D_2 receptors and a high level of occupancy of D_1 receptors (42%) compared with five other classic antipsychotics. Clozapine also had a decreased propensity to produce extrapyramidal side-effects (Farde *et al.*, 1992). This was confirmed by Brucke *et al.* (1992), who found a curvilinear dose–occupancy relationship for typical antipsychotics, but no similar relationship for clozapine. Pilowsky *et al.* (1992) showed that marked clinical improvement on clozapine (in patients previously unresponsive to typical antipsychotics) was associated with *increased* availability for D_2-receptor binding to ^{123}I-IBZM (i.e. decreased occupancy) and this was qualitatively obvious (Plate 7.1, facing p. 230). Thus neuroreceptor PET and SPET provided the first evidence for a highly effective antipsychotic whose mechanism of action did not appear to lie primarily in blockade of D_2 receptors.

Plate 7.1 (facing p. 230) shows ^{123}I-IBZM SPET scans from schizophrenic patients on typical and atypical antipsychotics. When D_2 receptors in the basal ganglia are occupied by antipsychotic drugs, fewer are available for specific binding to ^{123}I-IBZM. Thus washout of activity from this region occurs rapidly, which is seen qualitatively on the SPET image as a decrease in basal ganglia activity relative to neocortical areas at equilibrium (approximately 60 min after injection).

In vivo techniques are helpful in determining rational drug treatment and optimum dosage to achieve D_2 blockade without side-effects. Extrapyramidal symptoms, such as akathisia and dystonia, are unpleasant side-effects of antipsychotic treatment. These side-effects have been correlated with high *in vivo* occupancy of striatal D_2 receptors (Farde *et al.*, 1992). Nordstrom *et al.* (1993), from studies with ^{11}C-raclopride PET, suggest a quantitative relationship between D_2 receptor occupancy and extrapyramidal side-effects, in that patients with high levels of D_2 blockade are extremely likely to experience dystonic side-effects. This proposed relationship apparently does not hold for some of the newer antipsychotics. A recent ^{123}I-IBZM SPET study of risperidone and remoxipride (Busatto *et al.*, 1995) in schizophrenic patients showed that these drugs produced few or no extrapyramidal symptoms despite levels of D_2 blockade comparable to other, typical antipsychotic drugs. This intriguing finding suggests either that atypical antipsychotics act on distinct D_2-like receptors not associated with extrapyramidal side-effects (i.e. D_3 and D_4 receptors) or that a particular mixture of neurochemical blockade (for example at cholinergic or serotonergic receptors) attenuates these unwanted effects *in vivo*.

Although antipsychotics are clinically useful in treating psychosis, a third of schizophrenic patients are poorly responsive to neuroleptic medication, and this group may experience side-effects without therapeutic benefit. PET and SPET studies have conclusively shown that lack of response to these drugs is not due to insufficient central D_2 blockade (Wolkin *et al.*, 1989; Pilowsky *et al.*, 1993). Therefore these patients do not require the massive doses of typical antipsychotics used in the past, and may benefit from atypical drugs such as clozapine or sulpiride, which are less likely to produce extrapyramidal symptoms. It is not yet possible for PET and SPET to predict unresponsive patients prior to commencing therapy, although this is under investigation.

Other receptor systems may also be involved in antipsychotic drug action. Nordstrom *et al.* (1993a) and Nyberg *et al.* (1993) showed that clozapine and risperidone have very high occupancy of 5-HT$_2$ receptors (84–90% and 60% respectively) with ^{11}C-NMS PET, and suggest that this may account for clozapine's unique treatment profile. Comparison of 5-HT binding with other, typical antipsychotics is necessary.

In vivo probes for the recently cloned D$_2$-receptor subtypes D$_3$ and D$_4$ (Sokoloff *et al.*, 1990; Van Tol *et al.*, 1991) are not yet available. These receptors are of particular interest to antipsychotic drug development, given their distribution in mesolimbic regions. One difficulty in synthesizing a competitive antagonist radioligand for D$_3$ receptors lies in the high affinity of endogenous dopamine for this receptor subtype, which is typically saturated in normal states. A probe for the D$_3$ receptor is currently under development (Kung *et al.*, 1993). Recently, ligands with the ability to measure extrastriatal, D$_2$-like receptor (possibly related to D$_3$ and D$_4$) have been evaluated in humans (Kessler *et al.*, 1992; Wang *et al.*, 1993).

Other psychotropic drugs

PET and SPET evaluation of drug behaviour has been most applied to antipsychotic drugs. With the development of radioligands for receptors other than the dopamine D$_2$ type, the activity of many other psychotropic drugs is being assessed. A few examples are provided below.

Benzodiazepines

^{123}I-iomazenil has been used as a SPET probe of the BZ receptor to measure occupancy by agonists and antagonists. The potency of these drugs (in terms of the degree of receptor occupancy required to produce a clinical effect) may be evaluated and compared. Seibyl *et al.* (1993) assessed receptor occupancy by a clinically relevant dose of the highly potent BZ agonist lorazepam and showed that, at doses which produce sedation in humans, lorazepam occupies less than 4% of BZ receptors. This is an extremely interesting finding, suggesting that these drugs exert their effects at very low levels of receptor occupancy and raising the notion of a functional BZ/GABA 'receptor reserve' in the brain. Innis *et al.* (1992) calculated the ED$_{50}$ (median effective dose, i.e. the dose of drug required to displace 50% of brain ^{123}I-iomazenil activity) of benzodiazepine agonists and antagonists, and found the following rank order of potency: iomazenil > flumazenil > clonazepam ≈ alprazolam > diazepam.

Monoamine oxidase inhibitors

Monoamine oxidase B (MAO-B) inhibitors putatively retard the development of Parkinson's disease. As such, new drugs are under development and clinical investigation, an example being RO 19 6327, a reversible MAO-B inhibitor. Fowler *et al.* (1993) employed the MAO-B tracer ^{11}C-L-deprenyl to determine the degree and reversibility of human-brain MAO-B inhibition. The study found that this drug given at doses of 0.55 mg/kg every 12 h produces 95% inhibition of brain MAO-B activity, and that this returns to baseline values within 36 h of drug discontinuation. This information is critically relevant to dose ranging and development of new MAO-B inhibitors.

Dynamic pharmacological studies

Agonist/antagonist–receptor challenges

The capacity for endogenous neurotransmitters to compete with radioligand binding has been exploited to evaluate the functional responsivity of receptor systems. A drug agonist or antagonist is administered and the effect on ligand binding to the receptor observed. Thus interactions between pre- and postsynaptic systems and between different neurochemical pathways are deduced. It is assumed in these studies that the chosen agonist or antagonist exerts an effect only by acting on receptor systems, and not through global peripheral actions on metabolism or blood flow. Due to the limited availability of probes for other neurotransmitter systems, much of this research has focused on the consequences of a variety of drug challenges on dopaminergic pathways by observation of alterations in D_2-receptor binding.

Cholinergic challenge. Dewey *et al.* (1988) showed that a single dose of the anticholinergic drug benztropine reduced striatal binding of the D_2-receptor ligand ^{18}F-*N*-methylspiroperidol (NMS). They took this as evidence for the hypothesis that central cholinergic blockade increases synaptic dopamine levels by a poly-synaptic feedback loop. To exclude an intrinsic effect of benztropine at D_2 receptors causing the reduction, a further study with amphetamine (a dopamine-releasing agent) was performed (Dewey *et al.*, 1991). Diminished receptor availability following amphetamine challenge was also found; thus the investigators felt the decrease in binding seen after benztropine was indeed related to endogenous dopamine release, competing with ^{18}F-NMS for D_2-receptor binding. The effect has been demonstrated with other D_2-receptor ligands and anticholinergic drugs, for example, D_2-receptor binding by ^{11}C-raclopride was reduced after anticholinergic challenges by benztropine and scopolamine (Dewey *et al.*, 1988, 1993).

Amphetamine challenge. Amphetamine challenges during scans with other D_2-receptor ligands, including ^{11}C-raclopride PET (Dewey *et al.*, 1993), ^{123}I-IBZM SPET (Innis *et al.*, 1992) and ^{123}I-IBF SPET (Laruelle *et al.*, 1993), give results concordant with the above study. Validating the amphetamine-challenge paradigm in primates, Innis *et al.* (1992) used a chaser-study approach and showed that pretreatment with reserpine (a dopamine-depleting agent) abolished the increased washout of ^{123}I-IBZM usually seen after an amphetamine bolus given during tracer equilibrium. Thus amphetamine reduces D_2 binding through release of stored dopamine from presynaptic neurons. Agents such as GBR-12909

(a dopamine reuptake inhibitor) and tetrabena-zine (a biogenic amine-depleting drug), which indirectly increase the amount of endogenous dopamine in the synapse, similarly compete for D_2-receptor binding with ^{11}C-raclopride and decrease D_2-receptor availability for binding with the ligand (Dewey *et al.*, 1993).

The sensitivity of D_2 radioligands to altered synaptic dopamine levels permits study of the impact of other neurotransmitter pathways on dopaminergic function.

GABAergic challenge. Following challenge with γ-vinyl-GABA, and lorazepam (both GABA agonists), ^{11}C-raclopride binding increases, possibly as a result of GABAergic stimulation and resultant inhibition of endogenous dopamine release (Dewey *et al.*, 1992). Similar results were obtained by ethanol challenges during ^{11}C-raclopride PET imaging, suggesting a complex mode of action for ethanol in the brain (Wong *et al.*, 1993) and lending support for the putative role of dopaminergic pathways in the mainten-ance of addictive behaviours.

Receptor studies in neuropsychiatric conditions

A further highly relevant area for investigation by neuroreceptor PET and SPET attempts to define biochemical lesions underlying neuropsychiatric disorders. By evaluating receptor binding in these conditions, existing drugs may be targeted to avoid side-effects and more selective treatments developed.

Schizophrenia

Schizophrenia is one of the most common and serious psychoses, with a prevalence of 1% in the community. The mechanism of action of antipsy-chotic drugs in blocking D_2 receptors (Johnstone *et al.*, 1978; Peroutka & Snyder, 1980) suggests that overactivity or hyperdensity of these receptors may be a neurochemical substrate for the disorder (Crow, 1980). Post-mortem studies find elevations of D_2 receptors in the brains of never-antipsychotic-treated and previously treated patients (Mackay *et al.*, 1982). As neuroleptics themselves may affect D_2-receptor regulation, PET and SPET studies in never-treated (so-called drug-naïve) patient groups eliminate this potential artefact.

Crawley *et al.* (1986) first described an 11% elevation of D_2-receptor density in 12 antipsychotic-free schizophrenia patients with ^{77}Br-bromospiperone SPET, using a single fixed gamma camera. Similarly, the Johns Hopkins PET group have shown unequivocal two- to threefold increases in striatal D_2-receptor binding in up to 23 never-medicated patients by ^{11}C-NMS (Wong *et al.*, 1986, 1989; Tune *et al.*, 1992). A sex difference in D_2 binding was also noted in a preliminary report from this group, with male patients showing significantly higher striatal D_2 density than female patients and healthy controls (Tune *et al.*, 1992). Contradictory data have emerged from other studies. Farde *et al.* (1990) could not find an elevation of D_2-receptor binding in an ^{11}C-raclopride PET study of 18 never-medicated patients and 20 healthy controls. This was also the case in two PET studies of 9 and 10 never-medicated patients, respectively (Martinot *et al.*, 1990, 1991).

Subtle disturbances of D_2-receptor density in patients were shown in the Karolinska (Farde *et al.*, 1990) and Caen studies (Martinot *et al.*, 1990, 1991). Schizophrenic patients had greater asymmetry of binding than controls (Farde *et al.*, 1990). Of the 18 patients, 14 studied had higher receptor density in the left compared with the right putamen (analysis of variance for case by side-interaction, $F = 5.3$, $P = 0.027$; paired t-test, $P < 0.01$). Patients in the Caen series did not show an age-related decline in D_2-receptor binding, consistent with data mentioned above from a large post-mortem study of neuroleptic-treated patients (Mackay *et al.*, 1982). Recently, investigators from the Caen group have begun to relate D_2-binding indices to symptom patterns (in particular, psychomotor poverty (Liddle *et al.*, 1992)) in groups of highly selected patients

(Martinot *et al.*, 1994).

Pilowsky *et al.* (1994) have recently substantiated the PET data by ^{123}I-IBZM SPET in 20 antipsychotic-free schizophrenic patients (17 never medicated), finding a sex-specific relative increase in left striatal D_2 binding confined to male patients (compared with the same-sex healthy counterparts) and a failure of patients to show the expected age-related decrement in D_2-receptor binding seen in controls. No overall elevation in D_2-receptor binding was observed.

In view of these conflicting findings, the hypothesis that an *in vivo* elevation of D_2-receptor binding is a fundamental abnormality in schizophrenia remains unproved. Clarification of these issues is vital in providing markers for the disorder, understanding its pathogenesis and helping to design more selective, novel antipsychotics.

Epilepsy

Evidence for GABA/BZ receptor-complex involvement in epilepsy stems from the known efficacy of GABA/BZ agonists in the treatment of epilepsy and the reverse tendency of GABA antagonists to induce seizures. Reduced BZ-receptor binding (measured by ^{11}C-RO-15 1788 PET) has been demonstrated in the seizure foci of patients with partial epilepsy (Savic *et al.*, 1988). As the severity of focal reduction corresponds to increased seizure frequency, PET and SPET BZ-receptor imaging can give a predictive index of treatment resistance (Savic & Thorell, 1993). The diagnosis of foci prior to surgery is also greatly enhanced. Van Isselt *et al.* (1993) used ^{123}I-iomazenil SPET combined with electroencephalogram (EEG) and magnetic resonance imaging (MRI) to identify seizure foci prior to surgery, which provided the final confirmation. A true positive was found in all 80 cases examined by these methods. The impact of partial epilepsy on wider neurophysiological functioning may also be assessed. In one study, diminished BZ-receptor binding in partial epilepsy was localised to the seizure focus and did not extend to other parts of the brain (Minoshima *et al.*, 1993). A preliminary study of primary generalised epilepsy (Prevett *et al.*, 1993) found increased cerebral cortical binding and decreased cerebellar binding in patients not taking sodium valproate. The increase was interpreted as due to receptor upregulation. The pattern was reversed in patients on sodium valproate. Preliminary assessments of BZ-receptor binding *in vivo* are proving extremely useful in clarifying the aetiology, diagnosis and management of epilepsy. Future ligand development, particularly with regard to excitatory glutamatergic receptors, will extend this enterprise.

Dementia

Several biochemical alterations have been proposed as underlying Alzheimer's disease, including cholinergic, monoamin-ergic and serotonergic. Wyper *et al.* (1993) found specific deficits in muscarinic-receptor binding (measured by ^{123}I-quinuclidinylbenzylate (QNB) SPET) in the superior frontal and parietal regions of two very severely affected patients. The remainder of the sample (six cases) showed a global decrease in functional activity (by both ^{99m}Tc-hexam-ethylpropyleneaminoxime (HMPAO) and ^{123}I-QNB). This study reinforces the importance of distinguishing alterations in receptor binding from global deficits in blood flow and metabolism. Bench *et al.* (1993) showed raised cortical activity of MAO-B in Alzheimer's patients compared with controls and Parkinson's disease (PD) cases, and suggested this was due to glial/astrocytic proliferation. Blin *et al.* (1993) compared 5-HT$_2$-receptor binding in nine presumed Alzheimer's patients with 37 controls by ^{18}F-setoperone PET. A decrease in binding was noted throughout the cortex in patients. Clearly much more work is necessary to identify specific receptor systems involved in aetiology and symptomatology in dementia, and to define whether receptor alterations are simply markers for generalised neuronal loss or provide clues for the aetiology and specific opportunities for pharmacological intervention similar to those found in PD. Chapter 14 reviews this area.

Cocaine addiction

Cocaine is a potent inhibitor of the dopamine-reuptake transporter. It is thought that its action on dopamine systems is crucial to its reinforcing properties. PET studies have been applied to understand the site of action of cocaine (and thus the mechanism for addictive behaviours in other contexts). The distribution and kinetics of cocaine have been examined by ^{11}C-cocaine PET (Volkow *et al.*, 1991). The tracer showed maximal accumulation in the brain 4–8 min after injection, with a heterogeneous distribution, mainly to the basal ganglia. Rapid clearance followed (50% decrease after 20 min). The cold-competitor approach was used to demonstrate specificity of cocaine binding to the dopamine transporter. Pretreatment with nomifensine (a dopamine-transporter inhibitor) decreased ^{11}C-cocaine binding, which was unaffected by the serotonergic and noradrenergic blocker, desipramine. The timing of cocaine's euphorigenic effects corresponded to binding and release of cocaine from the transporter (Cook *et al.*, 1985).

The chronic effects of cocaine on cerebral physiology have also been studied. Baxter *et al.* (1988) found an overall decrease in uptake of ^{18}F-DOPA shortly after detoxification, consistent with decreased dopamine synthesis. Binding of ^{18}F-NMS to the postsynaptic D$_2$ receptor was decreased in the week after detoxification in chronic abusers (Volkow *et al.*, 1990), and the decrease was maintained for up to 3–4 months (Volkow *et al.*, 1993). The persistent decline in dopamine D$_2$-receptor availability was directly associated with a specific decrease in frontal cortex metabolism (Volkow *et al.*, 1993), suggesting more serious dysregulation of brain dopamine systems than previously thought and providing vital insights into the mechanisms of cocaine addiction.

Pain

The neurochemical mechanisms of pain responses are being evaluated with the opiate receptor ligand ^{11}C-diprenorphine and PET. Jones *et al.* (1993) scanned rheumatoid-arthritic patients during a flare-up of their disease and in the pain-free state. Global increases in ^{11}C-diprenorphine binding were found in relation to pain reduction. Specific regional increases, over the global increase, were noted in prefrontal, orbital, cingulate and temporal cortices. The hypothesis that inflammatory pain results in production of endogenous opiate peptides is reinforced by these data, which enlighten research into the functional anatomy of pain and could monitor the progress of medical and psychological analgesic strategies.

Movement disorders

PET ^{18}F-DOPA uptake reflects the functional integrity of nigrostriatal dopamine projections and correlates with nigral cell counts at necropsy (Snow *et al.*, 1993). In sporadic L-DOPA-responsive PD, a characteristic pattern of striatal ^{18}F-DOPA is seen. Putamen uptake is decreased by 40% and caudate by 80% of normal (Brooks *et al.*, 1990; Leenders *et al.*, 1990). This pattern is consistent with the disruption of ventrolateral nigral projections to the putamen found in PD tissue post-mortem. In progressive supranuclear palsy, where nigrostriatal projections are uniformly affected, ^{18}F-DOPA PET shows equally severe loss of uptake in anterior and posterior putamen and caudate nuclei (Brooks *et al.*, 1990). Close correlations are found between movement asymmetries, ^{18}F-DOPA and ^{11}C-nomifensine uptake asymmetries in the putamen, but not the caudate (Leenders *et al.*, 1990).

Both SPET and PET presynaptic dopamine-transporter ligands are sensitive markers for dopaminergic nerve terminals in the striatum. PD patients show loss of presynaptic dopamine-transporter sites in the caudate and putamen to 20–39% of control values (Innis *et al.*, 1993), and 48% and 55% decreases in dopamine-transporter binding in the anterior and posterior putamen respectively, measured by ^{11}C-WIN 35428 PET (Frost *et al.*, 1993). Dopamine-transporter ligands

may therefore be useful both in diagnosis and in screening populations of at-risk individuals, particularly by SPET, which is less costly and more widely available.

The beneficial effects of dopamine-agonist treatment for PD are mediated through postsynaptic D_2 receptors. In untreated PD, patients have similar D_2-binding values to controls as measured by ^{11}C-raclopride PET and ^{123}I-IBZM SPET (Brooks, 1991; Brucke *et al.*, 1991; Tatsch *et al.*, 1992). Relative upregulation of putamen D_2 receptors in PD has been found contralateral to more affected limbs, although this was not necessarily consistent (Rinne *et al.*, 1990; Sawle *et al.*, 1990). L-DOPA treatment results in a decrease in D_2-receptor availability for binding to ^{123}I-IBZM SPET (Brucke *et al.*, 1991). Patients with Parkinsonism due to other causes (multiple-system atrophy (MSA)) show marked reduction in postsynaptic D_2 receptors measured by ^{123}I-IBZM SPET, with no overlap compared with controls (Van Royen *et al.*, 1993). This group are also distinguishable from idiopathic PD by the pattern of opioid-receptor binding measured by ^{11}C-diprenorphine PET. PD patients show similar values to controls, but MSA patients, in whom loss of encephalinergic neurons is found post-mortem, show a significant decrease in binding (Brooks, 1991). Huntington's disease, associated with severe degeneration of the caudate nuclei, shows bilaterally decreased D_2 binding (Brucke *et al.*, 1991) and loss of GABAergic-binding sites compared with controls (Holthoff *et al.*, 1993). Sawle *et al.* (1993) combined ^{18}F-DOPA and ^{11}C-raclopride PET measures in nine patients diagnosed as having PD, and demonstrated postsynaptic D_2-receptor upregulation consequent on diminished presynaptic DOPA uptake. One patient did not have this pattern, showing a decrease in both pre- and postsynaptic markers, and later developed MSA.

Therapeutic responsivity can be predicted by assessing the functional status of D_2 receptors *in vivo*. This is usually done by examining response to the apomorphine challenge test. In two studies, patients with positive responses to apomorphine challenge showed significantly higher striatal D_2 binding by PET and SPET than those with a negative outcome (Schwarz *et al.*, 1992; Hierholzer *et al.*, 1993). PET ^{11}C-raclopride studies find chronically treated PD patients, with fluctuating resistance to L-DOPA, have a uniform reduction in D_2-binding sites in caudate and putamen (Brooks, 1991). These findings have now been substantiated by ^{123}I-IBZM SPET (Pizzolata *et al.*, 1993).

Neuroligand PET and SPET can help to monitor and develop therapeutic interventions. Peripheral decarboxylation of DOPA is a problem in the drug treatment of PD. Ruottinen *et al.* (1993) found that peripheral catecholamine-*o*-methyl-transferase (COMT) inhibition by drugs such as nitecapone and entacapone increases the bioavailability of ^{18}F-DOPA into the brain. The progress of neural-cell transplantation has been monitored by ^{18}F-DOPA PET, and increased uptake of the ligand at the transplant site correlated with clinical improvement (Sawle *et al.*, 1993).

PET and SPET clearly have a place in the differential diagnosis of movement disorders, screening at-risk individuals, predicting and monitoring response to dopamine agonist treatment and elucidating neurochemical mechanisms underlying these conditions.

Conclusion

This chapter has provided an overview of current uses of neuroreceptor PET and SPET in the study of the neurochemical basis of psychiatric disorders and in aiding drug development. The capacity of these techniques to image the targets of drug action continues to open fascinating new avenues for clinical and research studies. The field broadens constantly, and a review is likely to be outdated from the time it is written. It is hoped that this chapter will both act as a reference source and stimulate interest in this most exciting and challenging area.

References

Abi-Dargham, A., Seibyl, J.P., Zohgbi, S. *et al.* (1993) SPECT imaging of the benzodiazepine receptor in humans using ^{123}I iomazenil. *Schizophrenia Res.* **9**, 191.

Alquist, R. (1948) A study of adrenotropic receptors. *Am. J. Physiol.* **153**, 586–600.

Andreasen, N.C., Carson, R., Diksic, M. *et al.* (1988) Workshop on schizophrenia: PET and dopamine D2 receptors in the human neostriatum. *Schizophrenia Bull.* **14**, 471–85.

Baxter, L.R., Schwartz, J.M., Phelps, M. *et al.* (1988) Localisation of neurochemical effects of cocaine and other stimulants in the human brain. *J. Clin. Psychiatry* **49**, 23–6.

Bench, C., Lammertsma, A.A., Dolan, R.J., Brooks, D.J. & Frackowiack, R.S.J. (1993) Cerebral monoamine oxidase (MAO-B) activity in normal subjects, Alzheimer's disease and Parkinson's disease, *J. Cerebr. Blood Flow Metab.* **13** (Suppl. 1), S246.

Blin, J., Baron, J.-C., Dubois, B. *et al.* (1993) Loss of brain 5-HT2 receptors in Alzheimer's disease. *Brain* **116**, 497–510.

Brooks, D. (1991) PET: its clinical role in neurology. *J. Neurol. Neurosurg. Psychiatry* **54**, 1–5.

Brooks, D.J., Ibanez, V., Sawle, G.V. *et al.* (1990) Differing patterns of striatal ^{18}F DOPA uptake in Parkinson's disease, multiple system atrophy and progressive supranuclear palsy. *Ann. Neurol.* **28**, 547–55.

Brucke, T., Podrecka, I., Angelberger, P. *et al.* (1991) Dopamine D_2 receptor imaging with SPECT: studies in different neuropsychiatric disorders. *J Cerebr. Blood Flow Metab.* **11**, 220–8.

Brucke, T., Roth, J., Podrecka, I., Strobi, R., Wenger, S. & Asenbaum, S. (1992) Striatal dopamine D_2 blockade by typical and atypical neuroleptics. *Lancet* **339**, 497.

Busatto, G.F., Pilowsky, L.S., Costa, D.C., Ell, P.J., Verhoeff, N.P. & Kerwin, R.W. (1995) Dopamine D2 receptor blockade *in vivo* with the novel antipsychotics risperidone and remoxipride – a ^{123}I IBZM single photon emission tomography (SPET) study. *Psychopharmacology* **117**, 55-61.

Cambon, H., Baron, J.C., Boulenger, J.P., Loc, C., Zarifian, E. & Maziere, B. (1987) *In vivo* assay for neuroleptic receptor binding in the striatum. *Br. J. Psychiatry* **151**, 824–30.

Comar, D., Maziere, M., Godot, J.M. *et al.* (1979) Visualisation of ^{11}C flunitrazepam displacement in the brain of the live baboon. *Nature* **280**, 329–31.

Cook, C.E., Jeffcoat, R. & Perez-Reyes, M. (1985) Pharmacokinetic studies of cocaine and phencyclidine in man. In: Barnett, J. & Chiang, C. (eds) *Pharmacokinetics and Pharmacodynamics of Psychoactive Drugs*. Biomedical Publications, Foster City, CA, pp. 49–72.

Costa, D.C., Verhoeff, N.P.L.G., Cullum, I.D. *et al.* (1990) *In vivo* characterisation of 3-iodo-6-methoxybenzamide ^{123}I in humans. *Eur. J. Nucl. Med.* **16**, 813–16.

Crawley, J.C.W., Crow, T.J., Jonhstone, E.C. *et al.* (1986) Uptake of Br-spiperone in the striata of schizophrenic patients and controls. *Nucl. Med. Comm.* **7**, 599–607.

Crow, T.J. (1980) Molecular pathology of schizophrenia: more than one disease process? *Br. Med. J.* **280**, 66–8.

Cunningham, V.J. & Jones, T. (1993) Spectral analysis of dynamic PET studies. *J. Cerebr. Blood Flow Metab.* **13**, 15–23.

Cunningham, V.J., Ashburner, J. & Jones, T. (1993) Robust parametric images from dynamic PET studies. *J. Cerebr. Blood Flow Metab.* **13** (Suppl. 1), S728.

Dale, H.H. (1914) On the action of ergotoxine: with special reference to the existence of sympathetic vasodilators. *J. Physiol.* **65**, 219–300.

Dean, P.M. (1989) The development of theories about drug–receptor interaction. In *Molecular Foundations of Drug-receptor Interaction.* Cambridge University Press, Cambridge pp. 1–6.

Dewey, S.L., Wolf, A.P., Fowler, J.S. *et al.* (1988) The effects of central cholinergic blockade on [18F]-N-methyl-spiroperidol binding in the human brain using PET. *XVI CINP Congr.* **96**, 162.

Dewey, S.L., Logan, J., Wolf, A.P. *et al.* (1991) Amphetamine induced decreases in 18F-N-methyl-spiroperidol binding in the baboon brain using positron emission tomography (PET). *Synapse* **7**, 324–7.

Dewey, S.L., Smith, G.S., Logan, J. *et al.* (1992) GABAergic inhibition of endogenous dopamine release measured *in vivo* with 11C raclopride and positron emission tomography. *J. Neurosci.* **12**,. 3773–80.

Dewey, S.L., Smith, G.S., Logan, J., Brodie, J.D., Fowler, J.S. & Wolf, A.P. (1993) Striatal binding of the PET ligand 11C raclopride is altered by drugs that modify synaptic dopamine levels. *Synapse* **13**, 350–6.

Dobbeleir, A. & Dierckx, R. (1993) Quantification of Tch 99m HMPAO brain uptake in routine clinical practise using calibrated point sources as an external standard: phantom and human studies. *Eur. J. Nucl. Med.* **20**, 684–90.

Dolan, R., Bench, C. & Friston, K. (1990) Positron emission tomography in psychopharmacology. *Int. Rev. Psychiatry* **2**, 427–39.

Erlich, P. (1900) On immunity with special reference to cell life: Croonian Lecture. *Proc. Roy. Soc. London* **66**, 424–48.

Farde, L, Weisel, F.-A., Nordstrom, A.-L. & Sedvall G. (1989) D1 and D2 dopamine receptor occupancy during treatment with conventional and atypical neuroleptics. *Psychopharmacology* **99**, S28–S31.

Farde, L., Wiesel, F.A., Stone-Elander S. *et al.* (1990) D2 dopamine receptors in neuroleptic-naive schizophrenic patients. *Arch. Gen. Psychiatry* **47**, 213–19.

Farde, L., Nordstrom, A.L., Wiesel, F.-A. *et al.* (1992) Positron emission tomographic analysis of central D1 and D2 receptor occupancy in patients treated with classical neuroleptics and clozapine. *Arch. Gen. Psychiatry* **49**, 538–44.

Fowler, J.S., Volkow, N.D., Logan, J. *et al.* (1993) PET studies of reversible and irreversible MAO B inhibitors. *J. Nucl. Med.* **34**, 131P.

Frost, J.J., Rosier, A.M., Reich, S. *et al.* (1993) PET imaging of dopamine reuptake sites in Parkinson's disease by C-11-WIN 35 428 and PET. *J. Nucl. Med.* **34**, 31P.

Hierholzer, J., Cordes, M., Schelosky, L. *et al.* (1993) Functional receptor testing in patients with iodiopathic Parkinson's syndrome versus Parkinsons plus syndrome. *J. Nucl. Med.* **34**, 31P.

Holthoff, V.A., Koeppe, R.A., Frey, K.A. *et al.* (1993) Positron emission tomography measures of benzodiazepine receptors in Huntington's disease. *Ann. Neurol.* **34**, 76–81.

Innis, R.B., Malison, R.T., Al-Tikriti, M. *et al.* (1992) Amphetamine-stimulated dopamine release competes *in vivo* for (123)I IBZM binding to the D2 receptor in non-human primates. *Synapse* **10**, 177–84.

Innis, R.B., Seibyl, J.P., Scanley, B.F. *et al.* (1993) Single photon emission computed tomographic imaging demonstrates loss of striatal dopamine transporters in Parkinson's disease. *Proc. Nat. Acad. Sci. USA* **90**, 11965–9.

Iyo, M. & Yamasaki, T. (1993) The detection of age related decrease of dopamine D1, D2 and serotonin 5HT2 receptors in living human brain. *Prog. Neuropsychopharmacol. Biol. Psychiatry* **17** (3), 415–21.

Johnstone, E.C., Crow, T.J., Frith, C.D., Carney, M.W.P. & Price, J.S. (1978) Mechanism of the antipsychotic effect in the treatment of acute schizophrenia. *Lancet* i, 848–51.

Jones, A.K.P., Cunningham, V.J., Ha-Kawa, S. *et al.* (1993) Increases in central opioid receptor binding with relief of inflammatory pain in man demonstrated by PET and [11C]diprenorphine. *J. Cerebr. Blood Flow Metab.* **13** (Suppl. 1), S792.

Kessler, R.M., Scott Mason, N., Votaw, J.R. *et al.* (1992) Visualisation of extrastriatal D2 receptors in the human brain. *Eur. J. Pharmacol.* **223**, 105–7.

Kung, H.F., Pan, S., Kung, M.-P. *et al.* (1989) *In vitro* and *in vivo* evaluation of 123I IBZM: a potential CNS D-2 dopamine receptor imaging agent. *J. Nucl. Med.* **30**, 88–92.

Kung, H.F., Kung, M.P., Foulon, C. *et al.* (1993) D3 ligands for SPECT imaging: fantasy or reality? *J. Nucl. Med.* **34**, 132P.

Lammertsma, A., Bench, C.J., Gunn, K. & Frackowiack, R.S.J. (1993) Comparison of methods for routine analysis of clinical 11C raclopride studies. *J. Cerebr. Blood Flow Metab.* **13** (Suppl. 1), S727.

Langley, J.N. (1878) On the physiology of salivary secretion

II. On the mutual antagonism of atropin and pilocarpin having special reference to their relations in the submaxillary gland of the cat. *J. Physiol.* **1**, 339–69.

Laruelle, M., Al-Tikriti, M., Van Dyck, C.H. *et al.* (1993) D-Amphetamine displacement of ^{123}I IBF equilibrium binding in primates: a new paradigm to investigate D-amphetamine induced dopamine release. *Schizophrenia Res.* **9**, 201.

Lassen, N. (1992) Neuroreceptor quantitation *in vivo* by the steady state principle using constant infusion or bolus injection of radioactive tracers. *J. Cerebr. Blood Flow Metab.* **12**, 701–16.

Leenders, K.L., Salmon, E.P., Tyrrell, P. *et al.* (1990) The nigrostriatal dopaminergic system assessed *in vivo* by positron emission tomography in healthy volunteer subjects and patients with Parkinson's disease. *Arch. Neurol.* **47**, 1290–8.

Liddle, P.F., Friston, K.J. & Frith, C.D. (1992) Patterns of cerebral blood flow in schizophrenia. *Br. J. Psychiatry* **160**, 179–86.

Lundberg, T., Lindström, L.H., Hartvig, P. *et al.* (1989) Striatal and frontal cortex binding of ^{11}C labelled clozapine visualised by positron emission tomography in drug free schizophrenics and healthy volunteers. *Psychopharmacology (Berlin)* **99**, 8–12.

Mackay, A.V.P., Iversen, L.L., Rossor, M. *et al.* (1982) Increased brain dopamine and dopamine receptors in schizophrenia. *Arch. Gen. Psychiatry* **39**, 991–7.

Martinot, J.-L., Peron Magnan, P., Huret, J.D. *et al.* (1990) Striatal D2 dopaminergic receptors assessed with positron emission tomography and [76Br] bromospiperone in untreated schizophrenic patients. *Am. J. Psychiatry* **147**, 44–50.

Martinot, J.-L., Pailliere-Martinot, M.L., Loc'h, C. *et al.* (1991) The estimated density of D2 striatal receptors in schizophrenia—a study with positron emission tomography and 76Br Bromolisuride. *Br. J. Psychiatry* **158**, 346–50.

Martinot, J.-L., Pallere-Martinot, M.L., Loc'h, C. *et al.* (1994) Central D2 receptors and negative symptoms of schizophrenia. *Br. J. Psychiatry* **164**, 27–34.

Maziere, B. & Maziere, M. (1993) Studying *in vivo* brain chemistry with SPECT, receptors and neurotransmission. In Costa, D.C., Morgan, G.F. & Lassen, N.A. (eds) *New Trends in Nuclear Neurology and Psychiatry*. John Libbey, London, pp. 85–100.

Minoshima, S., Frey, K.A., Henry, T.R., Koeppe, R.A., Sackellares, J.C. & Kuhl, D.E. (1993) Regional alteration of benzodiazepine receptor distribution in refractory temporal lobe epilepsy revealed by group averaging techniques. *J. Nucl. Med.* **34**, 22P.

Nikkinen, P., Lewendahl, K., Sarolainen, S. & Lounes, J. (1993) Validation of quantitative brain dopamine D2 receptor imaging with a single head SPET camera. *Eur. J. Nucl. Med.* **20**, 680–4.

Nordstrom, A.-L., Farde, L. & Halldin, C. (1993a) High 5HT2 receptor occupancy in clozapine treated patients demonstrated by PET. *Psychopharmacology* **110**, 365–7.

Nordstrom, A.-L., Farde, L., Weisel, F.A. *et al.* (1993b) Central D2 dopamine receptor occupancy in relation to antipsychotic drug effects: a double blind PET study of schizophrenic patients. *Biol. Psychiatry* **33**, 227–35.

Nyberg, S., Farde, L., Eriksson, L., Halldin, C. & Eriksson, B. (1993) 5HT2 and D2 dopamine receptor occupancy in the living human brain. *Psychopharmacology* **110**, 265–72.

Patlak, C.S., Blasberg, R.G. & Ferstermacher, J.D. (1983) Graphical evaluation of blood to brain transfer constants from multiple time uptake data. *J. Cerebr. Blood Flow Metab.* **3**, 1–7.

Patlak, C., Dhawan, V., Takikawa, S. *et al.* (1993) Estimation of striatal uptake rate constant of FDOPA using PET: methodological issues. *J. Cerebr. Blood Flow Metab.* **13** (Suppl. 1), S282.

Peroutka, S.J. & Snyder, S.H. (1980) Relationship of neuroleptic drug effects at brain dopamine, serotonin, alpha adrenergic and histamine receptors to clinical potency. *Am. J. Psychiatry* **137**, 1518–22.

Pilowsky, L.S., Costa, D.C., Ell, P.J., Murray, R.M., Verhoeff, N.P.L.G. & Kerwin, R.W. (1992) Clozapine, single photon emission tomography and the D2 dopamine receptor blockade hypothesis of schizophrenia. *Lancet* **340**, 199–202.

Pilowsky, L.S., Costa, D.C., Ell, P.J., Murray, R.M., Verhoeff, N.P.L.G. & Kerwin, R.W. (1993) Antipsychotic medication, D2 dopamine receptor blockade and clinical response—a 123I IBZM SPET (single photon emission tomography) study. *Psychol. Med.* **23**, 791–9.

Pilowsky, L.S., Costa, D.C., Ell, P.J., Verhoeff, N.P.L.G., Murray, R.M. & Kerwin, R.W. (1994) D$_2$ dopamine receptor binding in the basal ganglia of antipsychotic free schizophrenic patients—a 123I IBZM single photon emission tomography (SPET) study. *Br. J. Psychiatry* **164**, 16–26.

Pizzolata, G., Chierichetti, F., Rossato, A. *et al.* (1993) Dopamine receptor SPET imaging in Parkinson's disease: a [123I] IBZM and [99mTc]-HM-PAO study. *Eur. Neurol.* **33**, 143–8.

Prevett, M.C., Lammerstma, A.A., Duncan, J.S. *et al.* (1993) Central benzodiazepine receptor quantitation (BZR) in normal subjects and in primary generalised epilepsy. *J. Cerebr. Blood Flow Metab.* **13** (Suppl. 1), S277.

Rinne, J.O., Hietala, J., Ruotsalainen, U. *et al.* (1993) Decrease in human striatal dopamine D2 receptor density with age: a PET study with ^{11}C raclopride. *J. Cerebr. Blood Flow Metab.* **13**, 310–14.

Rinne, U.K., Laihinen, A., Rinne, J.O. *et al.* (1990) Positron emission tomography demonstrates dopamine D2 receptor supersensitivity in the striatum of patients with early Parkinson's disease. *Movement Disorders* **5**, 55–9.

Ruottinen, H., Rinne, J.O., Laihinen, A. *et al.* (1993) The effect of COMT inhibition with entacapone on 18F-6-fluorodopa PET in Parkinson's disease. *J. Cerebr. Blood Flow Metab.* **13**, S359.

Savic, I. & Thorell, J.O. (1993) PET shows different pattern of benzodiazepine receptor changes in intractable compared with moderate partial epilepsy. *J. Cerebr. Blood Flow Metab.* **13** (Suppl. 1), S278.

Savic, I., Persson, A., Roland, P., Pauli, S., Sedvall, G. & Widen, L. (1988) *In vivo* demonstration of reduced benzodiazepine receptor binding in human epileptic foci. *Lancet* 15 Oct., 863–6.

Sawle, G. & Myers, R. (1993) Combined PET and MRI studies following neural cell transplantation for Parkinson's disease. *J. Cerebr. Blood Flow Metab.* **13**, S366.

Sawle, G.V., Brooks, D.J., Ibanez, V. & Frackowiack, R.S.J. (1990) Striatal D2 receptor density is inversely proportional to dopa uptake in untreated Parkinson's disease. *J. Neurol. Neurosurg. Psychiatry* **53**, 177.

Sawle, G.V., Playford, E.D., Brooks, D.J., Quinn, N. & Frackowiack, R.S.J. (1993) Asymmetrical pre-synaptic and post-synaptic changes in the striatal dopamine projection in dopa naive parkinsonism. *Brain* **116**, 853–67.

Schwarz, J., Tatsch, K., Arnold, G. *et al.* (1992) 123I iodobenzamide-SPECT predicts dopaminergic responsiveness in patients with *de novo* parkinsonism. *Neurology* **42**, 556–61.

Seibyl, J.P., Woods, S.W., Zohgbi, S.S. *et al.* (1992) Dynamic SPECT imaging of dopamine D2 receptors in human subjects with iodine 123-I IBZM. *J. Nucl. Med.* **33**, 1964–71.

Seibyl, J., Sybirska, E., Bremner, D. *et al.* (1993) [I-123] Iomazenil SPECT brain imaging demonstrates significant benzodiazepine receptor reserve in human and nonhuman primate brain. *J. Nucl. Med.* **34**, 102P.

Smith, M., Wolf, A.P., Brodie, J.D. *et al.* (1988) Serial [18F]*N*-methylspiroperidol PET studies to measure changes in antipsychotic drug D-2 receptor occupancy in schizophrenic patients. *Biol. Psychiatry* **23**, 653–63.

Snow, B.J., Tooyama, I., McGeer, E.G. & Calne, D.B. (1993) Premortem [18F] fluorodopa uptake correlates with postmortem dopaminergic cell counts and striatal dopamine in humans. *J. Cerebr. Blood Flow Metab.* **13**, S251.

Sokoloff, P., Giros, B., Martres, M.P. *et al.* (1990) Molecular cloning and characterization of a novel dopamine receptor (D3) as a target for neuroleptics. *Nature* **347**, 146–51.

Stocklin, G. (1992) Tracers for metabolic imaging of brain and heart: radiochemistry and radiopharmacology. *Eur. J. Nucl. Med.* **19**, 527–51.

Suhara, T., Inoue, O., Kobayashi, K., Suzuki, K. & Tateno, Y. (1993) Age-related changes in human muscarinic acetylcholine receptors measured by position emission tomography. *Neurosci. Lett.* **149** (2), 225–8.

Tatsch, K., Schwarz, J., Oertel, W.H. & Kirsch, C.-M. (1992) I-123 IBZM SPECT for imaging dopamine D2 receptors in iodiopathic Parkinson syndrome, Parkinsonian-like syndromes and Wilson's disease. In Schmidt, H.A.E. & Hofer, R. (eds) *Nuclear Medicine: Nuclear Medicine in Research and Practice.* Schattauer, Stuttgart, New York, pp. 406–10.

Taylor, P. & Insel, P.A. (1990) Molecular basis of pharmacological selectivity. In Pratt, W.B. & Taylor, P. (eds) *Principles of Drug Action: the Basis of Pharmacology.* Churchill Livingstone, London, pp. 1–103.

Tune, L.E., Wong, D.F. & Pearlson, G. (1992) Elevated dopamine 2 receptor density in 23 schizophrenic patients: a positron emission tomography study with 11C *N*-methylspiperone. *Schizophrenia Res.* **22** (6), 147.

van Isselt, J.W., Huffelen, A.C. & van Rijk, P.P. (1993) The value of I-123 iomazenil SPECT in the presurgical workup of patients with medically intractable focal epilepsy. *J. Nucl. Med.* **34**, 22P.

Van Royen, E.A., Verhoeff, N.P.L.G., Speelman, J.D., Wolters, E.Ch., Kuiper, M.A. & Janssen, A.G.M. (1993) Diminished striatal dopamine D2 receptor activity in multiple system atrophy and progressive supranuclear palsy demonstrated by 123I IBZM SPECT. *Arch. Neurol.* **50**, 513–16.

Van Tol, H.H.M., Bunzow, J.R., Guan, H.C. *et al.* (1991) Cloning of the gene for a human dopamine D4 receptor with high affinity for the antipsychotic clozapine. *Nature* **350**, 610–14.

Verhoeff, N.P.L.G. (1993) Imaging neurotransmission and neuroreceptors — physiological and pharmacological basis. In Costa, D.C., Morgan, G.F. & Lassen, N.A. (eds) *New Trends in Nuclear Neurology and Psychiatry.* John Libbey, London, pp. 25–36.

Volkow, N.D., Fowler, J.S., Wolf, A.P. *et al.* (1990) Effects of chronic cocaine abuse on postsynaptic dopamine receptors. *Am. J. Psychiatry* **147**, 719–24.

Volkow, N.D., Fowler, J.S. & Wolf, A.P. (1991) Use of positron emission tomography to study cocaine in the human brain. In Rapaka, R.S., Makriyannis, A. & Kuhar, M.J. (eds) *Emerging Technologies and New Directions in Drug Abuse Research.* Research Monograph 112, National Institute on Drug Abuse, Rockville, MA, pp. 168–79.

Volkow, N.D., Fowler, J.S., Wang, G.-J. *et al.* (1993) Decreased dopamine D2 receptor availability is associated with reduced frontal metabolism in cocaine abusers. *Synapse* **14**, 169–77.

Wang, G.-J., Volkow, N.D., Fowler, J.S. *et al.* (1993) Comparison of two PET radioligands for imaging extra striatal dopamine receptors in the human brain. *Synapse* **15**, 246–9.

Wolkin, A., Barouche, F., Wolf, A.P. *et al.* (1989) Dopamine blockade and clinical response: evidence for two biological subgroups of schizophrenia. *Am. J. Psychiatry* **146**, 905–8.

Wong, D.F., Wagner, H.N., Dannals, R.F. *et al.* (1984) Effects of age on dopamine and serotonin receptors measured by positron tomography in the living human brain. *Science* **226**, 1393–6.

Wong, D.F., Wagner, H.N., Tune, L.E., Dannals, R.F., Pearlson, G.D. & Links, J.M. (1986) Positron emission tomography reveals elevated D2 dopamine receptors in drug-naive schizophrenics. *Science* **234**, 1558–63.

Wong, D.F., Pearlson, G.D., Young, L.T. *et al.* (1989) Dopamine receptors are elevated in neuropsychiatric disorders other than schizophrenia. *J. Cerebr. Blood Flow Metab.* **9** (Suppl. 1), S593.

Wong, D.F., Wand, G., Yung, B.C.K. *et al.* (1993) The effects of intravenous ethanol on intrasynaptic dopamine measures in human basal ganglia. *J. Nucl. Med.* **34**, 132P.

Woods, S.W., Pearsall, H.R., Seibyl, J.P. & Hoffer, P.B. (1991) The Quinn essay: single photon emission computed tomography in neuropsychiatric disorders. In Hoffer, P.B. (ed.) *The Year Book of Nuclear Medicine*. Mosby Year Book, St Louis, pp. XIII–XIVII.

Wyper, D.J., Brown, D., Patterson, J. *et al.* (1993) Density of acetylcholine receptors in Alzheimer's disease measured in relation to regional cerebral blood flow. *J. Cerebr. Blood Flow Metab.* **13** (Suppl. 1), S1.

Yokoyama, H., Yanai, K., Iinuma, K. *et al.* (1993) Imaging of histamine H_1-receptors in human brain by PET analysed by graphical analysis on a pixel by pixel basis. *J. Cerebr. Blood Flow Metab.* **13** (Suppl. 1), S796.

Young, A.B., Frey, K.A. & Agranoff, B.W. (1986) Receptor assays, *in vitro* and *in vivo*. In Phelps, M.E., Mazziotta, J.C. & Schelbert H.R. (eds) *Positron Emission Tomography and Autoradiography: Principles and Applications for the Brain and Heart*. Raven Press, New York, pp. 73–113.

8: EEG Topographical Mapping

J. Gruzelier, A. Burgess
and T. Baldeweg

Introduction

When Hans Berger first recorded the alpha rhythm in 1929 he believed that electroencephalography (EEG) would come to be a 'window on the mind'. In the succeeding 60 years, although EEG has become a useful clinical tool, it is only in recent years that it has even begun to go some way towards fulfilling Berger's initial dream. For most of its history, the dominant form of presentation of EEG has been the familiar trace of potential against time (Fig. 8.1), one that is still very widely used today. Until relatively recently, most EEG recordings were made with a small number of electrodes and this meant that topographical mapping was not possible, even if the technology

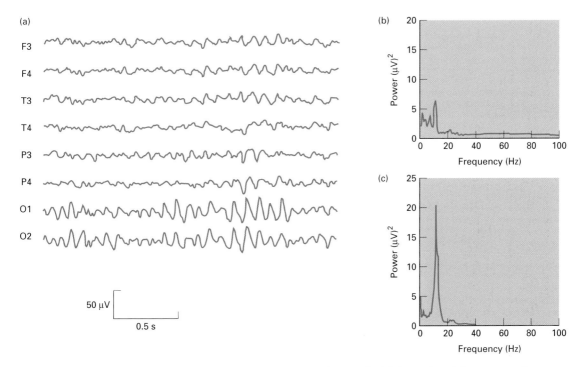

Fig. 8.1 EEG recording and power spectra. (a) EEG tracings from frontal (F3, F4), temporal (T3, T4), parietal (P3, P4) and occipital (O1, O2) derivations in a healthy subject during the eyes-closed resting state. Even electrode numbers refer to electrodes on the right hemisphere, odd numbers on the left hemisphere. The corresponding power spectra were computed over the whole recording period (1024 ms) in the frontal F3 (b) and right occipital (c) derivations. Power values are in $(\mu V)^2$. Note the posterior predominance of the alpha rhythm (10 Hz).

had been available. Nevertheless, from the early days of EEG attempts were made to produce topographical maps. The earliest known example of this was by the Japanese pioneer Motokawa, who in 1944 (cited in Petsche, 1989) produced a map of alpha potential recorded from 90 electrodes, averaged over 27 subjects. Even by today's standards, this was a Herculean effort. Unfortunately, Motokawa's work was not recognized by his contemporaries and made no lasting impact on EEG research.

In the post-Second World War period, several groups of researchers began to produce graphic displays of the EEG. Perhaps the most influential of these was the toposcope by Walter and Shipton (1951). The toposcope was made up of a series of cathode-ray tubes arranged such that each corresponded to one recording electrode on the scalp. The phase and amplitude of the EEG were represented by the angle and brightness of a line displayed on the cathode-ray tube. In this way, the EEG recordings from 22 electrodes were represented dynamically in a visual display for the first time. Unfortunately, because of technical and financial limitations, the work of the early pioneers like Walter and Shipton never entered widespread use and had relatively little permanent influence on EEG research.

Towards the end of the 1970s, advances in computer technology opened up new possibilities. Many researchers contributed towards the development of modern mapping, but two of the most influential have been Roy John and Frank Duffy. The paper by Duffy *et al.* (1979) was perhaps the first to introduce the use of topographical EEG, or what was called '*brain electrical activity mapping*' (BEAM), to a wider neuroscience audience. In addition, they developed statistical-probability mapping (Duffy *et al.*, 1981). At about the same time, John and his collaborators developed 'neurometrics', an EEG parallel to psychometrics. In the same way that psychologists have collected normative data on neuropsychological tasks, John collected normative data using EEG. In each case, an individual can be compared with normative data and

abnormalities detected by identifying features which were statistically rare in the standardisation sample. Using this technique, John *et al.* (1977) reported clear differences between healthy subjects and a wide range of psychiatric diagnoses, including alcoholic, phobic and schizophrenic patients. Although this technique is promising, there are drawbacks. In order to use normative data, the technique of EEG recording needs to be identical to that used during the collection of the standardisation data. In practice, because of variations in procedure, equipment and techniques at different centres, this is not easily achieved. An alternative is for each centre to collect its own database, but this is both time-consuming and expensive. For these reasons, the system of neurometrics has not been widely used.

Commercial EEG mapping systems are now widely available and, compared with magnetic resonance imaging (MRI), positron emission tomography (PET) or even single-photon emission tomography (SPET), very cheap. Most neurophysiology laboratories now have mapping systems, even if some electroencephalographers still prefer to use the raw EEG trace for clinical purposes. At the same time, interest among psychologists in topographical mapping of brain electrical activity has increased substantially as the technology has become more widely available. For the psychologist, the high temporal resolution of these methods provides the only way of examining the sequence of information flow in the brain and the interaction between different areas. Although conventional EEG recordings are still important, there has been a trend towards using techniques which capitalise on the temporal resolution of these systems. In most cases, this involves 'time-locking' recordings to the presentation of a stimulus or to a subject's response. The most widespread variation of this type of technique is the *event-related potential* (ERP). This involves recording changes in electrical potential from the scalp following the representation of a stimulus and averaging the measured signal over many trials. Averaging reduces the signal-to-noise ratio and emphasises consistent task-related changes in electrical potential, resulting in characteristic waveforms.

Functional neuroanatomy and the EEG

The electrical activity which can be recorded from the surface of the cortex (*electrocorticography* (ECoG)) referenced to an indifferent electrode, e.g. over the mastoids, reflects the spatial summation of two types of neuronal activity in the cortex. A cellular source produces slow synaptic potentials, which may be excitatory (*excitatory post-synaptic potential*, EPSP) or inhibitory (IPSP). Due to the long duration of these dendritic potentials (EPSP 10–30 ms and IPSP 70–150 ms), they are effective in producing coherent activity over an extended cortical area. Action potentials, which last only several milliseconds, do not make a significant contribution to the extracerebral electrical field.

Both EPSP and IPSP, although opposite in electrical polarity at the level of the cell membrane, can produce surface deflections of the same polarity. This depends on the location of the active synapse along the neuron. For example, an action-potential volley arriving in the superficial layers of the cortex and exciting the apical dendrites of a pyramidal cell produces a negative deflection of the surface ECoG. A deflection of the same polarity can, however, be the result of a physiologically different process, such as the inhibition (via an inhibitory interneuron) of a synapse in proximity to the cell soma.

Unilateral activation of a pyramidal cell leads to an electrical current flow both along the intracellular space of the dendrite and across the extracellular medium. This can be described as an elementary electrical dipole. The long dendrites of pyramidal cells represent the strongest dipole, and the parallel distribution of pyramidal dendrites within the cortex makes them the main contributor to the surface ECoG. Interneurons, in contrast, due to the nearly concentric form of their dendritic fields and the resulting cancellation of electrical fields, produce no external net electrical signal.

The magnitude of electrocortical activity ranges from $100\,\mu V$ to several hundred microvolts, and its frequency ranges from 1 to 50 Hz. During waking, a dominant posterior rhythmic activity between 8 and 13 Hz can be recorded (alpha rhythm).

Electrocortical activity as measured from the surface of the cortex can also be detected from the intact scalp—the electroencephalogram (EEG). However, it has considerably reduced amplitude (up to $100\,\mu V$). This is due to the increased distance of the recording electrode from the cortex and the diminishing influence of the intermediate tissues, especially the skull, with its high electrical resistance. This also leads to cancellation of high-frequency cortical activity, thereby reducing the upper frequency of the EEG.

Genesis of cortical rhythms

Microelectrode recordings have shown that electrocortical activity from a single cell spreads only 1–2 mm over the surface of the cortex. The source of coherent rhythmic activity which can be recorded from distant cortical electrodes is more likely to be caused by a common synchronising influence, rather than by the spread of the electrical field. Specific intracortical projections are thought to represent one synchronising mechanism, partly because isolated slices of cortex can produce rhythmic electrical activity after some time of reorganisation. A second mechanism which synchronises cortical activity, mainly in the 8–13 Hz (alpha rhythm) frequency range, involves multiple pacemakers in non-specific thalamic nuclei. The thalamic reticular nucleus, in particular, plays an essential role in pacemaking synchronised oscillations in the thalamus (Steriade *et al.*, 1990) through a system of excitatory and inhibitory connections. This rhythmicity spreads toward nearly all cortically projecting thalamic nuclei. Cortical neurons respond very specifically to thalamic input at given frequencies. These thalamocortical loops are being modulated by cholinergic projections of the mesopontine reticular formation. Stimulation of the latter disrupts synchronised oscillation in the thalamocortical systems, leading to desynchronisation of cortical activity and the blocking of the alpha rhythm. A similar desynchronising effect involves activation of the noradrenergic system arising in the locus ceruleus and projecting to the neocortex and hippocampus, as well as to the thalamus.

Genesis of sensory evoked potentials (EPs)

Stimulation of sensory pathways results in stimulus-related 'evoked' cortical activity, which can be extracted from the ongoing EEG. After the action potential volleys from the peripheral sensory organ pass the relay nuclei in the thalamus, they arrive at the cortical sensory projection areas. When large enough pools of cortical neurons have been activated, evoked electrical activity of several microvolts at the scalp can be detected. However, the ongoing spontaneous EEG activity is considerably larger in magnitude (up to $100\,\mu V$) and masks the evoked activity. This can only be detected by repeated stimulation and summation of stimulus-locked activity. Background EEG activity unrelated to the stimulus will cancel out after repeated stimulus presentations, e.g. several thousand trials for activity generated in the brainstem.

Brainstem evoked potentials (EPs) provide an example of the way EP recordings can monitor non-invasively the activation of different parts of a sensory pathway (Goff *et al.*, 1978). Click stimulation of the ears results in impulse activity along the acoustic nerve, which can be detected at a distant electrode (e.g. vertex) with reference to the ipsilateral mastoid (wave I). Subsequent activation of brainstem nuclei is reflected in further waves: II reflects activation in the nucleus cochlearis, wave III in the upper olive, waves IV and V in the inferior colliculus and wave VI activity at the level of the thalamus. Later waves up to 200 ms post-stimulus are being generated in the primary and secondary auditory projection areas in the temporal lobe. In experimental

conditions during which subjects have to perform complex reaction-time tasks, e.g. involving the discrimination between tones of different pitch, as in the popular P300 oddball paradigm, long-latency EP waves between 300 ms and 600 ms can be recorded. The anatomical origin of these 'cognitive' waves is not precisely known, and probably involves both temporoparietal and frontal regions.

Slow cortical potentials (SPs)

Another type of EEG activity, which is not normally recorded in the conventional EEG, is slow cortical potentials (SPs). With a special direct current (DC) amplifier, a transcortical steady-state potential of several microvolts magnitude can be recorded. This potential arises from the tonic depolarising influence of unspecific thalamocortical projections at the apical dendrites, which yields a cortical surface that is more negative than the subcortical white matter. During sleep, its absolute magnitude is markedly reduced, while seizure activity, oxygen deficit and hyperventilation cause an increase of the negative potential. The absolute value of the steady-state potential is difficult to measure in humans, a particular problem being the influence of skin and electrode potentials.

In many experimental situations, however, task-related changes in the steady-state potential can be recorded which only amount to several microvolts. Two typical examples of such an SP can be recorded in a warned reaction-time task. Depending on the pitch of the target tone (S2), the subject has to respond by pressing a key as quickly as possible with either the left or right hand. Negative slow-wave activity is recorded between presentation of a warning tone (S1) and the subsequent target tone (S2). This activity has a frontocentral maximum and is termed the *contingent negative variation* (CNV). The laterality of hand movements usually results in lateralised negative slow cortical activity, which is maximal over the contralateral motor areas and precedes the actual movement by several hundred milliseconds. This activity is labelled the readiness potential or *Bereitschaftspotential* (BP) (Kornhuber & Deecke, 1965) and is being used to study mechanisms of motor control and sensorimotor integration.

Localisation using EEG

In the early days of EEG, it was believed that changes in the electrical potential on the scalp reflected changes in activity in those brain regions immediately below the recording site. Unfortunately, this idea has proved to be far too simplistic. The most important limitation on localisation in this way is that potentials recorded at one point of the scalp may arise from electrical sources at some considerable distance. In addition, there is often quite a poor correspondence between scalp location and brain region. Although electrodes may be placed accurately on the scalp using standardised positioning systems, such as the international 10–20 system, the lie of the brain within the skull varies significantly between individuals. To overcome this problem, the correspondence between electrode placement and underlying brain structures may be evaluated using MRI scanning, but this is not always available. For these reasons, where accurate localisation of sources is important, more sophisticated techniques are required.

Dipole localisation

The pattern of electrical potential recorded on the scalp can be modelled as if it were the result of one or more electrical dipoles located within the head (Fender, 1987). If the head is assumed to be a uniform conducting sphere, it is a simple matter to show the pattern of potential that would be recorded from the surface from any combination of electrical dipoles. In practice, the head is not uniform, as the scalp, skull, cerebrospinal fluid (CSF) and brain all have different conductivities, and adjustments are needed to take this into account. This is the so-called forward-dipole problem and may be solved analytically. In EEG recordings, the problem is the reverse of this. Rather than determining the surface potential from given dipoles, the location of the dipoles must be determined from the scalp potential. This is the so-called reverse-dipole problem and there is no unique solution to it; any given pattern of scalp potentials might arise from any one of an infinite number of dipoles. Despite this, some solutions are more likely than others and in the case of a single dipole a unique solution does exist. The location and orientation of a dipole is found using standardised iterative methods, which work by systematically varying the dipole parameters until the predicted scalp potential matches the measured values. Where it is reasonable to assume that there is only one focus of electrical activity, such as in locating the focus of epileptic fits or in some EP paradigms, this system works quite well. Even so, because of simplifications in the model, such as assuming the head to be a sphere, and because of inhomogeneities in the conducting properties of the head, there are significant limitations to the accuracy of real anatomical localisation using this approach, even for a single dipole.

In many cases, however, the assumption of a single dipole is not realistic. Although the same methods may be used to locate multiple dipoles, the system only works well when there are clear expectations about the locations of the dipole: that is, for multiple sources dipole localisation may be useful to test out hypotheses about location, but it is less useful in exploratory analysis.

Current density

An alternative method to improve localisation using EEG is to calculate the *current density* from the recorded potential field (Nunez *et al.*, 1994). Current density is a measure of the amount of current passing through a defined area. It can be calculated relatively simply from the electrical potential. Current density gives greater spatial resolution because it is less smeared by passage through the skull than potential. In addition, current density emphasises near sources and minimises distant sources. The result is that current-density maps give sharper, more focused images of electrical activity on the cortical surface. Indeed, it can be shown that current density is directly proportional to the electrical potential on the cortex.

Figure 8.2(a) shows a topographical map where the contours reflect differences in alpha potential between subjects performing a simple hand-movement task and an inactive baseline condition. Compare this with Fig. 8.2(b), which shows the same data transformed to current density. The current-density map shows clearer, more focused areas of attenuation during the motor task. Current-density maps are also more reproducible and are less sensitive to residual artefacts in the EEG recordings than potential maps. In the past, increasing the number of electrodes was the only way of improving spatial resolution in EEG and this was relatively ineffective. Because of the degree of smearing of electrical potential through the scalp, the resolution of a system with 64 or 128 electrodes was little better than a system with only 32 electrodes. With the availability of current-density

transformations, increasing the number of electrodes offers the chance of making significant improvements in the spatial resolution of the EEG.

Image construction

Traditional EEG was recorded in analogue form and the output consisted of plots of electrical potential over time, as shown in Fig. 8.1. Analysis of the traces was a difficult, time-consuming and highly specialist role, and it involved a substantial amount of subjective interpretation. Data in this format were not easily subjected to quantitative analysis and it was not until digital computers had become widely available that topographical mapping in its current form was possible. Modern EEG recordings are digitised and the potential between each electrode and a reference point is sampled, usually at a rate of 100–200 times per second.

The reference electrode

Recordings from each electrode are taken against a reference point, such that the voltage recorded

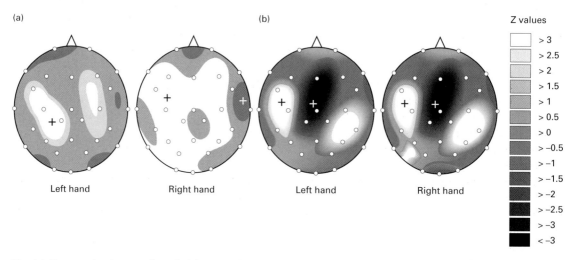

Fig. 8.2 Topographical maps of simple left- and right-hand motor tasks depicting differences between task and resting baseline for (a) alpha potential and (b) alpha current density.

at each electrode is a measure of the difference in electrical potential between the electrode and reference. This poses a dilemma, because the measured potential may say more about electrical activity at the reference than at the point of interest. Many attempts have been made to find a neutral reference point for recording, but no such ideal exists. Reference electrodes placed at a distance from the head are particularly sensitive to extraneous electrical noise, including the electrocardiogram (ECG). For this reason, references are nearly always cephalic, with the most commonly used ones being the nose tip, ear lobes or the apex of the scalp (electrode CZ). The most widely used references are also the most controversial: linked ears or linked mastoids. The main criticism of these references is that the linkage across the scalp creates a short circuit between the two sides which distorts the electrical field (Nunez, 1981). Although this problem may be more theoretical than real, it is best to avoid using linked ears or linked mastoids as a reference point, particularly when laterality issues are being addressed. One of the common attempts to reduce the reference problem is to calculate a mathematical reference point—most commonly, the average reference. This involves calculating the mean potential difference between each electrode and a reference site (e.g. nose tip) and then recalculating each electrode value as a deviation from this mean value. This method has the advantage that it reduces the vulnerability of the recording to electrical activity at the reference point. It has the disadvantage, however, that it makes the recordings insensitive to global changes in electrical activity, which may sometimes be of interest. Another solution is to calculate the Laplacian transformation of the potential (i.e. the current-source density, which measures the entering and exiting current at each location). Although this is computationally more extensive, not only are the resulting values 'reference-free' but they also show better spatial resolution than potential values. However, they are insensitive to the regional potential generated by endogenous EP components, such as the P300.

Artefact elimination

Once the recordings have been made, the first step in data analysis is to eliminate those sections of the EEG which include artefact. The most problematic artefacts are caused by electrical activity from the eyes or muscles, although other sources of contamination, such as ECG, may sometimes be a problem. These artefacts may produce electrical changes that can be very much stronger than the signal of interest. Although there are algorithms which can automatically eliminate contaminated sections or which can remove artefacts, selection by a suitably trained observer is generally the most reliable filter. Sections of EEG which include significant amounts of artefact should be discarded.

Analysis of EEG: identifying the components

With EEG, the most common form of analysis is to perform a spectral analysis, using the *fast Fourier transform* (FFT). The FFT is an algorithm that can analyse any continuous waveform into a sum of sine and cosine waves of different amplitudes and frequencies. From the FFT it is possible to calculate the power (i.e. the measure of the energy output of the EEG in a defined time period) in the EGG signal at different frequencies. FFT is typically calculated from sections of EEG, called *epochs*, lasting only a few seconds. Longer epochs are difficult to obtain because of contamination by artefact, and sections shorter than 1 s make it impossible to get reliable estimates of power at low frequencies. Power values in the awake EEG usually show a peak in the delta (0–4 Hz) and alpha (8–12 Hz) ranges, as shown in the spectrogram in Fig. 8.1(b,c). Other frequency ranges that are commonly used are theta (4–7 Hz) and beta (12–30 Hz). Delta, theta, alpha and beta are the classic frequency ranges first identified from visual inspection of EEG traces, although increasingly these bands are being subdivided into narrower bands. In each case, the power in each frequency band is averaged over a number of epochs. Although power is the most commonly used measure, frequency measures, such as the peak frequency, are also sometimes used.

Statistical analysis and parametric mapping

Once the mean power or mean peak frequency for each electrode has been calculated, it is possible to start the statistical analysis. One major problem for EEG analysis is that the signal is not stationary over long periods; even under constant conditions, the mean and variance of the EEG power may fluctuate over time. Sophisticated time-series analyses are available to deal with this difficulty, but in most cases the problem is overcome by using relatively short time periods. As stationarity cannot be assumed with EEG, it is good practice to show that the EEG in a baseline condition has been relatively stable over the course of an experiment.

EEG variables, such as power, are not normally distributed and a transformation of the data, such as square-root or logarithmic transformations, is often needed before parametric statistical analyses may be used. Once transformed, a wide range of analytical techniques can be applied. In a typical analysis, EEG recordings are compared for each electrode, either between subject groups or within the same subjects under different conditions. In theory, as the values at each electrode are not independent, a multivariate analysis of variance (MANOVA) would be appropriate. In practice, however, the number of variables (i.e. electrodes) often exceeds the number of subjects, and in these situations MANOVA is not applicable, as there are too few degrees of freedom. To overcome this problem, many researchers reduce the number of variables, either by averaging groups of variables or by selecting a priori only a limited subset of the possible comparisons. This is equivalent to the region-of-interest (ROI) methods used in SPET and PET and allows the size of the type I error (false positives) to be controlled. The main limitation of this method is that it does not allow

for the comparison of complete topographical maps.

The alternative is to calculate multiple statistical comparisons between maps, using univariate statistics. Figure 8.2(a) shows such a topographical map, where the contours reflect differences in alpha current density between subjects performing the simple hand-movement task compared with an inactive baseline condition. In this case, the differences are represented as z-scores; with univariate statistics, differences greater than 1.96 would be considered statistically significant at the $P < 0.05$ level (two-tailed). Unfortunately, although this method allows for the comparison of complete maps, it results in an inflated type I error. There are many ways of correcting this, such as with the Bonferroni method. Figure 8.3(b) shows the same data as Fig. 8.3(a) but highlighting only those areas which are significantly different after using the Bonferroni correction procedure. Using this method with 28 electrodes, the z-score difference required for statistical difference at $P < 0.05$ is 3.12. However, although this correction procedure is straightforward, it is far too conservative, thus resulting in inflated type II errors (false negatives). Randomisation methods may also be used to give more realistic correction values. Figure 8.3(c) shows the same data as Fig. 8.3(a) but highlighting only those areas which were significantly different following the randomisation procedure. Using this method a z-value of 2.67 provides the 0.05 level of significance. Unfortunately, randomisation procedures are extremely time-consuming and for this reason are not widely used.

There is, in short, no satisfactory solution to the method of statistical comparison between maps. For this reason, some researchers emphasise the importance of reproducibility of findings: that is, a first study is used to locate probable regions of difference and a second study is conducted to determine whether the same pattern is found in a replication of the first study. This is most appropriate when the initial study is exploratory in nature and there is no clear hypothesis to test.

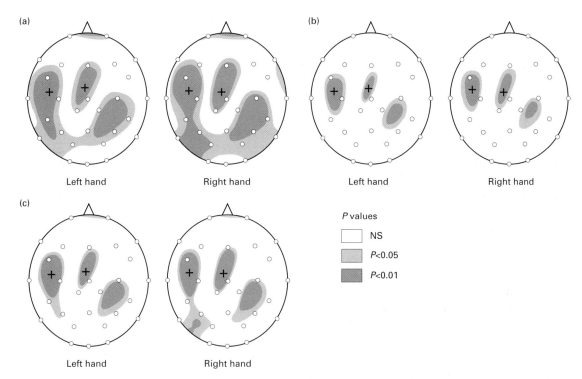

Fig. 8.3 Statistical probability maps of alpha current density comparing resting baseline with left- and right-hand motor tasks for (a) univariate *P* values, (b) after Bonferroni correction and (c) after randomisation correction.

Interpolating the maps

The main issue in the construction of topographical maps of EEG is how to draw accurate maps from a relatively small number of recording points. Older systems used fewer than 20 electrodes and the most commonly used commercial systems now have between 20 and 32 channels. EEG recordings using 64 or 128 electrodes are uncommon and usually only available in research settings (Tucker, 1993).

Once the electrical potential at each electrode site has been recorded, a topographical map can be drawn by interpolating potential values at sites between electrodes. The most commonly used interpolation method is the *nearest neighbours* (*k*-NN) or barycentric method. In this algorithm, the potential at any point on the map is calculated from the mean of the *k* nearest electrodes (where *k* is usually 3 or 4), weighted by a function of the distance between the point and each electrode. The distance function is usually the distance squared or cubed, although other functions are sometimes used. While these methods require minimal computation, the resulting maps tend to lack smoothness and the maxima and minima points are constrained to be at electrode sites. Such restraints are not realistic, and for this reason other interpolation methods have been proposed. One of these is polynomial interpolation; unfortunately *polynomial* interpolation methods do not perform well in simulation studies, which casts doubt on their accuracy. A better method uses so-called *spherical splines*. This technique has been adapted from meteorology, where it is used to plot global maps of air pressure and temperature on the basis of noisy data collected from widely separated recording sites. The parallels between the meteorologists' needs and those of the psychophysiologist are close in this case. Spherical splines show acceptable smoothness and perform well in simulations. In addition, the technique allows for smoothing of the data and the calculation of statistical confidence intervals. The major problem with splining techniques is that they are very computationally intensive and time-consuming. For this reason, barycentric methods, despite their limitations, remain the most commonly used interpolation procedures for producing topographical maps.

Cognition and EEG

The very earliest EEG recordings showed a correlation between behaviour and the EEG. The most obvious case was opening and closing the eyes. With eyes closed, most individuals show a high-amplitude alpha rhythm, which is maximal in occipital regions and which is attenuated as soon as the eyes are opened. Alpha is also attenuated during movement, and motor tasks have been investigated from the earliest days of EEG. Jasper and Andrews (1938) reported that the precentral alpha and beta rhythms were blocked during movement. Jasper and Penfield (1949) found that blocking of rhythmic EEG was highly localised and that movement of different parts of the body had an effect at different locations on the scalp. More recently Burgess and Gruzelier (1993) investigated the changes in EEG associated with voluntary hand movements, using a 28-electrode system. They found bilateral decreases in alpha, beta-1 and beta-2 during the motor task compared with the eyes-open baseline condition at the electrode sites corresponding to the motor and premotor cortex. Although the bilateral changes during unimanual tasks seem counterintuitive, similar findings have also been reported with PET, SPET and functional MRI (fMRI).

Voluntary movement has also been studied using EPs. Two main potentials associated with voluntary movement have been found: the BP preceding movement (Kornhuber & Deecke, 1965) and the motor potential (MP) concurrent with the movement itself (Deecke, 1987). The BP is maximal at the vertex and shows asymmetry,

with the most negative electrical potential occurring contralateral to the side of the movement (Shibasaki *et al.*, 1980). In contrast, the MP amplitude is symmetrical, although the onset of the MP is earlier with the non-dominant hand (Tarkka & Hallett, 1990). Pfurtscheller and colleagues have reported compatible findings using the paradigm of event-related EEG desynchronisation for both alpha (Pfurtscheller & Aranibar, 1977) and beta (Pfurtscheller, 1981) activity. Pfurtscheller and Berghold (1989) have found that the maximum desynchronisation prior to movement is localised to the contralateral motor areas (C3 and C4, respectively), with bilateral desynchronisation after movement onset.

Reliable EEG changes associated with higher cognitive processes have been more difficult to establish. In the last 20 years, much interest has focused on detecting lateralised changes in the EEG in response to different cognitive activities. In principle, it seems a simple matter to investigate this. One simply measures the EEG during a task which is believed to be a function of the left hemisphere and compares that with recordings of a right-hemisphere task. Although there have been many reports of lateralised changes in EEG over the years, in many cases these may have been attributable to differences between the tasks that were not directly related to the cognitive processes of interest. Gevins and Schaeffer (1983), reviewing the literature on lateral specialisation, concluded that most of the reports of lateral differences in the EEG during cognitive tasks could be attributable to artefacts in the procedures used, such as differences in demands (eye and hand movement), in task difficulty and in the stimuli presented. Once these factors are controlled for, lateralised changes in the EEG prove elusive. Whether this is because of limitations in the system of recording or because the idea that cognitive tasks are performed solely in a localised region of the brain is often mistaken is unclear. Even very simple tasks result in quite widespread changes in the EEG, and the notion that limited brain regions are independently activated during a task is probably too simplistic.

Cognition and ERPs

While EEG recordings remain useful and may be the only appropriate psychophysiological mapping system for some cognitive processes, when information about temporal sequence is required ERPs are generally more useful. ERPs have been used to explore many cognitive domains, including language, memory and sensory processes. To take one domain, memory, ERP studies have helped explore and delineate the cognitive processes identified from conventional experimental techniques. A number of recent studies have compared the ERPs during continuous-recognition tasks for words, in which a series of words is presented to a subject, some of which have been previously seen. It has been found that repeated words which are subsequently recognised show a different ERP pattern from those which are not recognised (Sanquist *et al.*, 1980). This suggests that part of the failure to recognise a word may be due to differences in the initial encoding of that word. There is also a difference between the ERPs of words which are recognised as having been seen previously and those which have been seen for the first time.

While ERP studies have proved of use in studies of cognitive functioning, they only use a little of the potential of this type of functional imaging. Over the last 10 years Alan Gevins and colleagues have developed sophisticated ERP methods which not only examine the temporal change in potential at one site, but also examine the temporal relationship between different sites. These methods show where the primary sites of activation are, and also show the direction and sequence of information flow between them. Gevins and co-workers have published several studies of this type on both motor and cognitive tasks (e.g. Gevins & Cutillo, 1993). At present, the main limitation is that the richness and quantity of information produced by these methods are very great, which makes it difficult to represent the results in a concise and clear form.

Clinical applications

Quantitative EEG (qEEG) has proved to be a powerful clinical research tool, despite having only a limited clinical utility beyond the standard routine EEG (Nuwer, 1988; AAN, 1989). The American Psychiatric Association (1991) concluded that its most valuable clinical role appears to be the assessment of pathological conditions characterised by slow-EEG-wave abnormalities, such as stroke, dementia, delirium and intoxication. The advantage of qEEG in detecting slow-wave activity may justify its use in controlled treatment studies in patients with neurodegenerative disorders. While EEG changes in these conditions are not specific to particular types of dementia, recently EEG-coherence measures have been used to assess different types of white-matter involvement. Multi-infarct dementia has been associated with decreased EEG coherence between interconnected cortical regions, while Alzheimer's disease has been characterised by a decrease in maximum coherence between regions connected by distant tracts passing through subcortical white and grey matter (Leuchter *et al.*, 1992).

The technique has a high sensitivity for the detection of ischaemia-related cerebral impairment, and a number of parameters are closely correlated with regional blood flow. The qEEG approach has been found to be superior to xenon-133 measures of regional cerebral blood flow in detecting transient ischaemic attacks (Jonkman *et al.*, 1985). However, determination of the lateralisation and localisation of the lesion was not very accurate. EEG changes are unable to differentiate infarction from haemorrhage, tumour or other focal cerebral lesions. Currently, qEEG is being successfully explored for intra-operative central nervous system (CNS) monitoring during cardiothoracic surgery. Recent applications of dipole-model analysis have proved useful in localising focal seizure activity, although qEEG mapping is not useful in diagnosing epilepsy (AAN, 1989).

Applications in psychiatry

P300 abnormalities in schizophrenia

Possibly the best-known application of EEG topographical mapping in psychiatry concerns the P300 in schizophrenia, measured to auditory stimuli (Pritchard, 1986; Friedman, 1991). Duffy and collaborators (Morstyn *et al.*, 1983) reported an early application of statistical-probability mapping with 10 long-hospitalised schizophrenic patients. Support was found for a reduced P300 amplitude, which they were able to locate to the midtemporal and posterior temporal regions of the left hemisphere, and which they used as a benchmark for subsequent studies. A replication (Faux *et al.*, 1987) with 11 patients of the same type confirmed a left-sided temporal reduction, which here extended to the parietal region. In both studies, P300 amplitude was calculated with a subtraction formula, which involved not only the conventional condition of attending for infrequent among frequent tones, but also an 'inattention' condition, where the same stimuli were presented while the subject read a book. When they calculated P300 amplitude in the conventional way without the inattention condition, the maximum deficit was in the right temporal region (Faux *et al.*, 1987), a result not taken up in subsequent studies.

A subsequent investigation with 20 patients (Faux *et al.*, 1990) compared the conventional linked-ear reference with a nose reference and restricted analysis to the customary 'infrequent–attend' condition. Significant effects with the linked-ear reference were found in the midtemporal site, this time extending anteriorly to the frontotemporal region. With the nose reference, the effect took in the centroparietal region. ROI analyses of bilateral midtemporal areas and the band connecting them confirmed the relatively greater left-sided reduction in amplitude. Bearing in mind the attention condition analysed, the asymmetry was in fact the opposite to the one found in the previous study. In a further investigation, using a larger, 28-electrode system,

Faux *et al.* (1993) examined 14 unmedicated schizophrenic patients; in all previous investigations, patients were medicated. With the larger array, the maximal difference was more narrowly located to the left temporocentroparietal region.

The main emphasis the present authors have placed upon such results has been evidence of a left temporal deficit, a long-standing hypothesis in schizophrenia research (Gruzelier, 1991). Nevertheless, there were inconsistencies between the studies as to which hemisphere was implicated. The extent of the effect beyond the temporal lobe also varied between studies, an issue somewhat obscured by the ROI approach adopted. Nevertheless, this series of experiments is commendable in its concerns with replication and with both methodological and statistical reliability; it thereby serves to illustrate some of the stringent requirements in mapping.

The heterogeneity of the localisation of the P300 attenuation in schizophrenia, not to mention the heterogeneity of the P300 process itself, is likely to become a source of contention. From another laboratory Pfefferbaum *et al.*, (1989) failed to find asymmetries of topographical distribution, and in fact Shenton *et al.* (1989) went on to report opposite temporal-lobe asymmetries in P300 amplitude in two patients of the Faux *et al.* (1987) sample. The patients with the right-sided deficit had more positive symptoms—thought disorder, poorer premorbid history and earlier age of onset, poorer response to neuroleptics and more diffuse neuropsychological deficits. Strik *et al.* (1993), with a group fulfilling the same diagnostic criteria for schizophrenia (DSM III-R) as Faux and colleagues, have also explored heterogeneity. They subcategorised patients according to Leonhard's (1979) classification as core schizophrenia (*n* = 11) or as having cycloid psychosis (*n* = 7), i.e. with remitting illnesses and a typically paranoid or catatonic character. Reference-free global-field power methods were used to calculate P300 parameters (Lehmann, 1987). Considering the group as a whole, there were no differences in P300 amplitude or latency when compared with controls, but, regarding the subgroups, the schizophrenic subgroup had lower amplitudes than both other groups and only in the schizophrenic group was there a lateral displacement of the peak to the right when compared with the controls. Further comparisons with other psychiatric disorders are awaited to determine the specificity of the findings for schizophrenia.

Sensory evoked potentials

Over a decade, Shagass and collaborators have marshalled the most comprehensive body of data on sensory EPs in psychiatric patients. Shagass and Roemer (1991) compared 72 schizophrenic subjects (DSM II and III) who were unmedicated for a median of 10 days with 57 who were medicated, and with 127 age- and sex-matched normal controls. Multimodal EPs were recorded from 15 electrodes to left and right median-nerve stimulation, checkerboard pattern flashes and binaural clicks. The conventional principal-component factor analysis was applied to the EP waveforms, and spatial maps were made of the factor scores for earlier and later components separately. The major finding was for the topographical differences between unmedicated patients and normal controls, which were located: (i) in the posterior temporoparietal region of the left hemisphere, where activity was found to be augmented in patients; and (ii) in the frontocentral temporal region, where activity was reduced. The axis of left posterior hyperactivity–right anterior hypoactivity was most marked for somatosensory EPs, although the visual and auditory EPs also contributed; the later EP components, which were those involving association cortex, were the more commonly represented. Medicated patients did not share this topography.

The same investigators have also examined, with similar procedures, 73 patients with major depression, the majority of whom were unmedicated for at least 7 days, and compared them with normal controls and unmedicated schizophrenic patients (Shagass & Roemer,

1992a). While there were a number of principal-component factor scores that distinguished the affective disorders from the controls, there was little topographical convergence in these effects and none in terms of laterality. In depressives, in the auditory modality, there was evidence of augmented earlier components (55 and 150 ms) and reduced posterior components. Conversely, when depressives were compared with schizophrenic patients, later cognitive components measured in a P300 procedure were augmented in posterior regions in depressives and were reduced in anterior regions.

In order to determine whether subtypes of depression influenced the results, a comparison was made between 20 unipolar and 20 bipolar patients matched for age and sex. Few differences were found, and, in the absence of a priori hypotheses and in view of the large number of comparisons made, these could have occurred by chance. In a companion paper (Shagass & Roemer, 1992b), relations were examined between the EP components of the affective disorders and scales of the Brief Psychiatric Rating Scale. Subdividing the patients on the basis of the depressive mood rating disclosed bidirectional differences for some components of somatosensory and auditory EPs. Bilateral frontal negativity was highest for patients with low depression ratings, intermediate for controls and lowest for patients with high ratings. The effects concerned midlatency EP components, which represent attentional processes and which appear impaired in severely depressed cases and hyperresponsive in those with low ratings of depression. Different pathologies may be represented by the results, all of which justify further investigation with a more comprehensive electrode montage, especially in the anterior regions, where the chosen montage was limited.

EEG spectral activity

EEG mapping of spectral bandwidths has confirmed earlier reports, based on more limited recordings, of increased slow- and fast-wave activity in schizophrenia. Morihisa *et al.* (1983) reported that slow delta-wave activity was particularly excessive in the frontal lobe, more so in unmedicated patients, whereas fast beta activity in the range 28–31.5 Hz was elevated in posterior regions. While raised frontal delta has also been reported by Morstyn *et al.* (1983) and Guenther *et al.* (1986a), the significance of frontal delta has been called into question by Karson *et al.* (1987) as a possible artefact of eye movements. When traces contaminated with eye movements were eliminated, unmedicated schizophrenic patients did not differ from controls in resting levels of delta. Similarly, Dierks *et al.* (1989), who carried out a careful eye-movement-rejection procedure, failed to find evidence of enhanced frontal delta, as was the case with two investigations from our laboratory, using stringent artefact-rejection procedures (Gruzelier *et al.*, 1990, 1994). A conundrum nevertheless remains. Because an abnormally high incidence of eye movements may be a feature of schizophrenic pathology, one which may in part be underpinned by frontal abnormalities, a functional abnormality may be removed along with the EEG artefacts. Accordingly, evidence of raised slow-wave activity in frontal regions would benefit from correlation with measures of 'hypofrontality' from other imaging procedures. Then, evidence of lateral asymmetry in frontal delta is unlikely to be artefactual, assuming no lateral bias in direction of gaze in the recording chamber. Gattaz *et al.* (1992) reported that increased delta power in the left frontal region was the best discriminating variable in a discriminant analysis of 15 controls and 17 DSM-III-R patients, 11 of whom were first-onset cases without treatment with neuroleptic medication. This finding, incidentally, calls into question the explanation for the heterogeneity of hypofrontality findings in schizophrenia, which associates hypofrontality with chronicity.

Functional activation studies in schizophrenia have also been carried out with concurrent monitoring of EEG spectra, which has advantages over many other functional imaging procedures in terms of the number of tasks that can be included in a single session. Guenther and colleagues compared 10 schizophrenic patients in a relaxation condition with performance on sensorimotor tasks involving the right hand (Guenther & Breitling, 1985) and motor tasks of increasing complexity (Guenther *et al.*, 1986a). Considering the task-related results, whereas the controls showed increases in slow-wave activity over the resting state, schizophrenic patients failed to show the same increases in power in the left hemisphere compared with the right. Power throughout the beta range (12–30 Hz) decreased in both groups but, as with the other bandwidths, changes in patients were asymmetric, with a lack of change in the left primary sensory and motor areas. In a subsequent study of predominantly chronic, negative-symptom schizophrenic subjects, Guenther *et al.* (1989) found different results from before, which included no systematic changes during the sensorimotor task. A parallel was found in a complementary cerebral-blood-flow (xenon-133) investigation, in which there was hyporeactivity in those patients with negative symptoms; positive-symptom patients showed diffuse bilateral hyperactivation (Guenther *et al.*, 1986b).

Syndromes in schizophrenia

The importance of subdivision by syndrome in psychiatric disorders is becoming increasingly apparent. We have conducted two mapping studies with a 28-electrode montage. In the first, 10 dextral schizophrenic patients were examined who had positive symptoms which, in addition to Schneiderian symptoms, included those belonging to an 'active' syndrome, characterised by raised activity levels, including cognition, positive affect and affective delusions (Gruzelier *et al.*, 1990). This is a syndrome which in a series of studies has been associated with an imbalance in activity in the direction of higher activation of the left hemisphere compared with the right, the latter having been found to be hypofunctional on tests of learning and memory (for a review, see

Gruzelier, 1991). In the mapping study, tasks involved recognition memory for words (left hemisphere) compared with faces (right hemisphere) and a left- and right-hand finger–thumb apposition task. Consistent with predictions the active syndrome patients were poorer at the faces- than the word-memory task. Of the task conditions, it was those that involve predominantly right hemispheric functions—faces memory and the left-hand motor task—that differentiated the EEG of patients from those of controls. In the faces-recognition condition, there was an abnormal elevation in fast beta in the right temporo-parietal region, the region which when damaged in neurological patients results in deficiencies in faces memory. In the motor task, there were two foci: the left supplementary motor region involved in the sequencing component of the task and the right parietal region compatible with sensorimotor task requirements. In both tasks, beta activity failed to show the focal reductions found in controls, such as that accompanying thalamo-cortical desynchronisation.

In the second investigation, comparisons were made between another group of active syndrome patients and a group with predominantly negative symptoms, who were examined with the recognition-memory procedures. The active-syndrome patients showed the advantage for word over faces memory as before, while the negative syndrome patients showed a faces memory advantage. Regarding the EEG, the active syndrome was again best characterised by fast beta activity. As shown in Fig. 8.4, again the effect was maximal in the faces recognition memory condition, the one in which neuropsychological performance was impaired. On this occasion, the effect was spread throughout the left hemisphere. Such an abnormal activation of the left hemisphere is in keeping with the hypothetical lateral imbalance that characterises the active syndrome. The left is also the hemisphere less appropriate for the faces task, and the abnormal activation may contribute to the impairment on the task. In all other conditions, the active syndrome was characterised by an elevation in

beta restricted to the left posterior temporal region, as shown in Fig. 8.4. This region is one frequently associated with electrocortical abnormalities in schizophrenia (see the studies of Faux described above), but was here restricted to patients with a positive syndrome.

The patients with negative symptoms were characterised differently. The memory tasks produced an abnormal posterior elevation biased to the right hemisphere, particularly in fast beta, as shown in Fig. 8.5, but also in slow beta in an addition-word recognition, as shown in Fig. 8.6. There were abnormal reductions in activity in fast and slow beta—one in the frontal region extending rightwards in slow beta and the other in the left parietal region. The reductions in beta were found in the resting condition and both acquisition (passive) conditions, indicating an

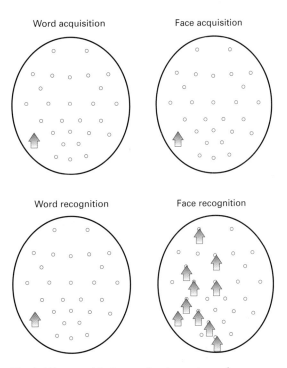

Fig. 8.4 Topographical maps showing regions where active-positive-syndrome schizophrenics had elevated fast beta amplitudes in word and face-recognition memory conditions when compared with controls.

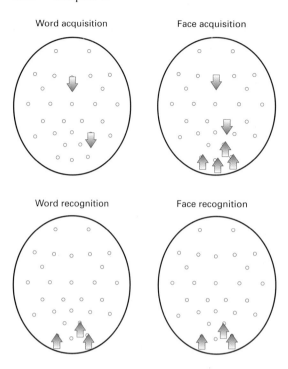

Word acquisition   Face acquisition

Word recognition   Face recognition

Fig. 8.5 Topographical maps showing regions where negative-symptom schizophrenic patients had elevations or reductions in fast beta when compared with controls.

association with symptoms rather than task-induced activation. Although many of the patients were medicated, comparisons between medicated and unmedicated groups did not alter the results.

It is important to note that the features characterising the two syndromes of schizophrenic patients were lost if the two groups were pooled, in which case the only difference from controls was a reduction in alpha in patients.

Future directions

In basic clinical science, further advances in technology and computer science will increase the utility of the EEG and lead to more microscopic insights into the neurophysiological abnormalities underlying mental illness. These will include microstate analysis (Wackermann *et al.*, 1993) and the application of deterministic chaos theory (Rapp *et al.*, 1989) and artificial neural nets

(Anderer *et al.*, 1994; Pritchard *et al.*, 1994). High-resolution EEG is being developed which may incorporate as many as 128 electrodes and which permits three-dimensional mapping (Tucker, 1993). A more complete characterisation of cerebral electrical activity can be achieved by simultaneously recording both EEG and magnetoencephalogram (MEG). The latter can be recorded at a short distance from the scalp, avoiding practical problems such as electrode resistance, polarisation and skin potentials and the blurring of the skull. However, the MEG is blind to radial source dipoles in gyri; hence the complementary need for the EEG. An integrated approach to brain imaging is developing which combines different technologies, such as PET, MRI, fMRI, EEG and MEG.

In terms of clinical practice pharmaco-EEG offers exciting prospects. Pharmaco-EEG has been

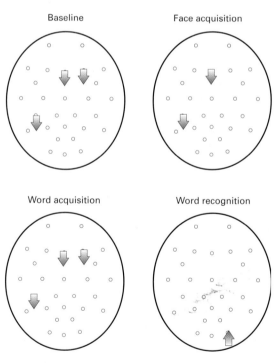

Baseline   Face acquisition

Word acquisition   Word recognition

Fig. 8.6 Maps of slow beta amplitudes showing regions where schizophrenia patients with negative symptoms differed from controls.

an established tool for the monitoring of the pharmacokinetics of a particular compound or to classify its central effects according to differential amplitude changes in various frequency bands. A promising development is the accumulating evidence that drug responders can be differentiated from drug non-responders. Czobor and Volavka (1992) reported that, while in acutely exacerbated schizophrenic patients there was no difference between responders and non-responders to haloperidol in plasma levels after 6 weeks of treatment, there was a significant relationship between haloperidol plasma levels and increases in theta activity for treatment responders but not for non-responders. Clinical responders also showed increases in alpha and decreases in delta on drugs, which were maximal at frontal placements and which were not shown by non-responders. Predictions as to clinical response could also be made; baseline alpha was significantly related to a reduction in Brief Psychiatric Rating Scale (BPRS) total scores at 3 and 6 weeks (Czabor and Volavka, 1991). Of particular importance are the findings that, on the basis of a single test dose, predictions can be made as to drug responder status (Gaebel *et al.*, 1988; Galderisi *et al.*, 1994).

Finally, the neurometric (qEEG) approach, which has shown promising results with regard to the ability to classify different disorders (John *et al.*, 1992), is potentially very useful. This is by virtue of the fact that within diagnostic categories patients may belong to different neurometric subtypes, which, apart from drug response, may be clinically important. Examples of such differences might be between those comatose head-injured patients who will regain cognitive competence and those who will not, or between those mildly impaired elderly patients who will show significant cognitive deterioration within 5 years and those who will not. Furthermore, clusters of patients who are characterised by a complex EEG profile typically contain patients with different diagnoses. Preliminary evidence indicates that different clusters respond differently to treatment, which suggests different biochemical

underpinnings. If this holds true, BEAM would revolutionise clinical practice.

Acknowledgement

Torsten Baldeweg is supported by a Medical Research Council (MRC) project grant to John Gruzelier.

References

American Academy of Neurology (AAN) (1989) EEG brain mapping. *Neurology* 39, 1100–1.

American Psychiatric Association (1991) Quantitative electroencephalography: a report on the present state of computerized EEG techniques. *Am. J. Psychiatry* 148, 961–4.

Anderer, P., Saletu, B., Kloppel, B., Semlitsch, H.V. & Werner, H. (1994) Discrimination between demented patients and normals based on topographic EEG slow wave activity: comparison between z statistics, discriminant analysis and artificial neural network classifiers. *Electroencephalogr. Clin. Neurophysiol.* 91, 108–17.

Burgess, A.P. & Gruzelier, J. (1993) Localisation of cerebral function using topographical mapping of EEG: a preliminary validation study. *Electroencephalogr. Clin. Neurophysiol.* 87, 254–7.

Czabor, P. & Volavka, J. (1991) Pretreatment EEG predicts short-term response to haloperidol treatment. *Soc. Biol. Psychiatry* 30, 927–42.

Czabor, P. & Volavka, J. (1992) Level of haloperidol in plasma is related to electroencephalographic findings in patients who improve. *Psychiatry Res.* 42, 129–44. Elsevier.

Deecke, L. (1987) *Bereitschaftspotential* as an indicator of movement preparation in supplementary motor area and motor cortex. *Ciba Found. Symp.* 132, 231–50.

Dierks, T., Mauer, K., Hil, R. & Schmidtke, A. (1989) Evaluation and interpretation of topographical EEG data in schizophrenic patients. In Mauer, K. (ed.) *Topographical Brain Mapping of EEG and Evoked Potentials.* Springer, London, pp. 507–17.

Duffy, F.H., Burchfiel, J.L. & Lombroso, C.T. (1979) Brain electrical activity mapping (BEAM): a method for extending the clinical utility of EEG and evoked potential data. *Ann. Neurol.* 5, 309–21.

Duffy, F.H., Bartels, P.H. & Burchfiel, J.L. (1981) Significance probability mapping: an aid in the topographic analysis of brain electrical activity. *Electroencephalogr. Clin. Neurophysiol.* 51, 455–62.

Faux, S.F., Torello, M.W., McCarley, R.W., Shenton, M.E. & Duffy, F.H. (1987) P300 topographical alterations in schizophrenia: a replica study. In Johnson Jr, R., Rohrbaugh, J.W. & Parasuraman, R. (eds) *Current*

Trends in Event Related Potential Research Electroence-phalography (Suppl. 40). Elsevier Science Publishers BV.

Faux, S.F., Shenton, M.E., McCarley, R.W., Nestor, P.G., Marcy, B. & Ludwig, A. (1990) Preservation of P300 event-related potential topographic asymmetries in schizophrenia with use of either linked ear or nose reference sites. *Electroencephalogr. Clin. Neurophysiol.* **75**, 348–91.

Faux, S.F., McCarley, R.W., Nestor, P.G. *et al.* (1993) P300 topographical asymmetries are present in unmedicated schizophrenics. *Electroencephalogr. Clin. Neurophysiol.* **88**, 32–41.

Fender, D.H. (1987) Source localisation of brain electrical activity. In Gevins, A.S. & Rémond, A. (eds) *Handbook of Electroencephalography and Clinical Neurophysiology*, Vol. 1. Elsevier, New York.

Friedman, D. (1991) Endogenous scalp-reduced brain potentials in schizophrenia: a methodological review. In Steinhauer, S.R., Gruzelier, J.H. & Zubin, J. (eds) *Handbook of Schizophrenia*, Vol. 5: *Neuropsychology, Psychophysiology and Information Processing*. Elsevier Science Publishers BV, pp. 91–127.

Galderisi, S., Maj, M., Mucci, A., Bucci, P. & Kemali, D. (1994) The QEEG alpha1 changes after a single dose of high potency neuroleptics as a predictor of short term response to treatment in schizophrenic patients. *Biol. Psychiatry* **35**, 367-74.

Gattaz, W.F., Mayer, S., Ziegler, P., Platz, M. & Gasser, T. (1992) Hypofrontality on topographic EEG in schizophrenia: correlations with neuropsychological and psychopathological parameters. *Eur. Arch. Psychiatry Clin. Neurosci.* **241** (6), 328–32.

Gevins, A.S. & Cutillo, B. (1993) Spatiotemporal dynamics of component processes in human working memory. *Electroencephalogr. Clin. Neurophysiol.* **67**, 128–43.

Gevins, A.S. & Schaeffer, R.E. (1983) Critical review of EEG correlates of higher cortical functions. *CRC Crit. Rev. Bioengineering* **4**, 113–64.

Goff, W.R. Allison, T. & Vaughan, H.G. (1978) The functional anatomy of event related potentials. In Callaway, E., Tueting, P. & Koslow, St H. (eds) *Event-related Potentials in Man*. Academic Press, New York.

Gruzelier, J. (1991) Hemispheric imbalance: syndromes of schizophrenia, premorbid personality, and neurodevelopmental influences. In Steinhauer, S.R., Gruzelier, J. & Zubin, J. (eds) *Handbook of Schizophrenia*, Vol. 5: *Neuropsychology, Psychophysiology and Information Processing*. Elsevier Science Publishers BV, pp. 599–650.

Gruzelier, J.H., Liddiard, D., Davis, L. & Wilson, L. (1990) Topographical EEG differences between schizophrenic patients and controls during neuropsychological functional activation. *Int. J. Psychophysiol.* **8**, 275.

Gruzelier, J.H., Laws, K., Liddiard, D. *et al.* (1994) Topographical EEG during words and faces memory tasks in syndromes of schizophrenia. Presented at the International Seventh Swiss Brain Mapping Meeting (SMM 7), Zurich, Switzerland.

Guenther, W. & Breitling, D. (1985) Predominant sensorimotor area left hemisphere dysfunction in schizophrenia measured by brain electrical activity mapping. *Biol. Psychiatry* **20**, 515.

Guenther, W., Breitling, D., Banquet, J.P., Marcie, P. & Rondot, P. (1986a) EEG mapping of left hemisphere dysfunction during motor performance in schizophrenia. *Biol. Psychiatry* **21**, 249.

Guenther, W., Moser, E., Muller-Spahn, F., Ofele, K., Bull, U. & Hippins, H. (1986b) Pathological cerebral blood flow during molar functions in schizophrenic and endogenous depressed patients. *Biol. Psychiatry* **21**, 889–99.

Guenther, W., Steinburg, R., Petsch, Streck, P. & Kugler, J. (1989) EEG mapping in psychiatry: studies on Type I/II schizophrenia using motor activation. In Maurer, K. (ed.) *Topographic Brain Mapping of EEG and Evoked Potentials.* pp. 438–50.

Jasper, H.H. & Andrews, H.L. (1938) Electro-encephalography III. Normal differentiation of occipital and precentral regions in man. *Arch. Neurol. Psychiatry* **39**, 96–115.

Jasper, H.H. & Penfield, W. (1949) Electrocorticograms in man: effect of voluntary movement upon the electrical activity of the pre-central gyrus. *Arch. Psychiatr. Z. Neurol.* **183**, 163–74.

John, E.R., Karmel, B.Z., Corning, W.C. *et al.* (1977) Neurometrics: numerical taxonomy identifies different profiles of brain functions within groups of behaviourally similar people. *Science* **196**, 1393–410.

John, E.R., Prichep, L.S. & Almas, M. (1992) Subtyping of psychiatric patients by cluster analysis of QEEG. *Brain Topogr.* **4** (4), 321–6.

Jonkman, E.J., Poorvliet, D.C., Veering, M.M., Weerd, A.M. & John, E.R. (1985) The use of neurometrics in the study of patients with cerebral ischaemia. *Electroencephalogr. Clin. Neurophysiol.* **61**, 333–41.

Karson, C.N., Coppola, R., Morihisa, J.M. & Weinburger, D.R. (1987) Computed electroencephalographic activity mapping in schizophrenia. *Arch. Gen. Psychiatry* **44**, 514.

Kornhuber, H.H. & Deecke, L. (1965) Hirnpotentialänderungen bei Willkürbewegungen und passivem Bewegungen des Menschen: Bereitschaftspotential und reafferente Potentiale. *Pflügers Arch.* **284**, 1–17.

Lehmann, D. (1987) Principles of spatial analysis. In Gevins, A.S. & Remond, A. (eds) *Methods of Analysis of Brain Electrical and Magnetic Signals: EEG Handbook*, revised edn, Vol. 1. Elsevier, Amsterdam, pp. 335–81.

Leonhard, K. (1979) *The Classification of Endogenous Psychoses*. Irvington Publications, New York.

Leuchter, A.F., Newton, T.F., Cook, I.A. *et al.* (1992) Changes in brain functional connectivity in Alzheimer-type and multi-infarct dementia. *Brain* **115**, 1543–61.

Morihisa, J.M., Duffy, F.H. & Wyatt, R.J. (1983) Brain electrical activity mapping (BEAM) in schizophrenic patients. *Arch. Gen. Psychiatry* **40**, 719.

Morstyn, R., Duffy, F.H. & McCarley, R.W. (1983) Altered P300 topography in schizophrenia. *Arch. Gen. Psychiatry* **40**, 729–34.

Nunez, P.L. (1981) *Electrical Fields of the Brain: the Neurophysics of EEG.* Oxford University Press, New York.

Nunez, P.L., Silberstein, R.B., Cadusch, P.J., Wijesinghe, R.S., Westdorp, A.F. & Srinivasan, R. (1994) A theoretical and experimental study of high resolution EEG based on surface Laplacians and cortical imaging. *Electroencephalogr. Clin. Neurophysiol.* **90**, 40–57.

Nuwer, M.R. (1988) Quantitative EEG: I. Frequency analysis and topographical mapping in clinical settings. *J. Clin. Neurophysiol.* **5**, 45–84.

Petsche, H. (1989) From graphein to topos: past and future of mapping. In Maurer, K. (ed.) *Topographic Brain Mapping of EEG and Evoked Potentials.* Springer-Verlag, Berlin, Heidelberg.

Pfefferbaum, A., Ford, J.M., White, P.M. & Roth, W.T. (1989) P3 in schizophrenia is affected by stimulus modality, response requirements, medication status, and negative symptoms. *Arch. Gen. Psychiatry* **46**, 1035–44.

Pfurtscheller, G. (1981) Central beta rhythm during sensory motor activities in man. *Electroencephalogr. Clin. Neurophysiol.* **51**, 253–64.

Pfurtscheller, G. & Aranibar, A. (1977) Event related cortical desynchronisation detected by power measurements of scalp EEG. *Electroencephalogr. Clin Neurophysiol.* **42**, 817–26.

Pfurtscheller, G. & Berghold, A. (1989) Patterns of cortical activation during planning of voluntary movement. *Electroencephalogr. Clin. Neurophysiol.* **72**, 250–8.

Pritchard, W.S. (1986) Cognitive event-related potential correlates of schizophrenia. *Psychol. Bull.* **1**, 43–66.

Pritchard, W.S., Duke, D.W., Coburn, K. *et al.* (1994) EEG-based, neural-net predictive classification of Alzheimer's disease versus control subjects is augmented by non-linear EEG measures. *Electroencephalogr. Clin. Neurophysiol.* **91**, 118–30.

Rapp, P.E., Bashore, T.R., Martinerie, J.M., Albano, A.M., Zimmerman, I.D. & Mees, A.I. (1989) Dynamics of brain electrical activity. *Brain Topogr.* **2**, 99–118.

Sanquist, T.F., Rohrbaugh, J.W., Syndulko, K. & Lindsley, D.B. (1980) Electrocortical signs of levels of processing: perceptual analysis and recognition memory. *Psychophysiology* **17**, 568–76.

Shagass, C. & Roemer, R.A. (1991) Evoked potential topography in unmedicated and medicated schizophrenics. *Int. J. Psychophysiol.* **10**, 213–24.

Shagass, C. & Roemer, R.A. (1992a) Evoked potential topography in major depression. 1. Comparisons with nonpatients and schizophrenics. *Int. J. Psychophysiol.* **13**, 241–54.

Shagass, C. & Roemer, R.A. (1992b) Evoked potential topography in major depression. II. Comparisons between subgroups. *Int. J. Psychophysiol.* **13**, 255–61.

Shenton, M.E., Faux, S.F., McCarley, R.W. *et al.* (1989) Correlations between abnormal auditory P300 topography and positive symptom in schizophrenia: a preliminary report. *Biol. Psychiatry* **25**, 710–16.

Shibasaki, H., Barrett, G., Halliday, E. & Halliday, A.M. (1980) Components of the movement-related cortical potential and their scalp topography. *Electroencephalogr. Clin. Neurophysiol.* **49**, 213–26.

Steriade, M., Gloor, P., Llinas, R.R., Lopes Da Silva, F.H. & Mesulam, M.M. (1990) Basic mechanisms of cerebral rhythmic activities. *Electroencephalogr. Clin. Neurophysiol.* **76**, 481–508.

Strik, W.K., Dierks, T., Franzek, E., Maurer, K. & Beckmann, H. (1993) Differences in P300 amplitudes and topography between cycloid psychosis and schizophrenia in Leonhard's classification. *Acta Psychiatr. Scand.* **87**, 179–83.

Tarkka, I.M. & Hallett, M. (1990) Cortical topography of premotor and motor potentials preceding self-paced voluntary movement of dominant and non-dominant hands. *Electroencephalogr. Clin. Neurophysiol.* **75**, 36–43.

Tucker, D.M. (1993) Spatial sampling of head electrical fields: the geodesic sensor net. *Electroencephalogr. Clin. Neurophysiol.* **87**, 154–63.

Wackermann, J., Lehmann, D., Michel, C.M. & Strik, W.K. (1993) Adaptive segmentation of spontaneous EEG map series into spatially defined microstates. *Int. J. Psychophysiol.* **14**, 269–83.

Walter, W.G. & Shipton, H.W. (1951) A new toposcopic display system. *Electroencephalogr. Clin. Neurophysiol.* **3**, 281–92.

9: Magnetoencephalography

H. Andrews

Introduction

The first demonstration of the possibility of recording biomagnetic fields originating from current movements occurring spontaneously in the brain (Cohen, 1972)—like the demonstration 10 years earlier of magnetic electrocardiography (ECG) (Baule & McFee, 1963)—created something of a stir, not least because of the *coup de théâtre* involved where the recording apparatus was not attached to the body of the subject producing these fields. Unlike electrical fields, it was apparent that magnetic fields could be measured directly and, with some qualifications, were largely unaffected by the tissue surrounding the electrically active sources of the fields. At the time of the original demonstration, it should be recalled that the only technique for examining the physiological workings of the spontaneously active brain was the electroencephalogram (EEG); with this apparatus the brain electrical signal was captured by simultaneously recording a variable number of channels—configured into one of several standard montages—consisting of the continuously varying potential differences between pairs of electrodes sited over the (rough) hemisphere of the cranium, using the positioning rules of the recently internationally adopted 10–20 placement system.

Since that time, technical and theoretical advances in the two techniques, magnetoencephalography (MEG) and EEG, have been, broadly, in terms of enlarging the advantages of the one in the direction of the other: for MEG, the obvious advantage of the EEG was the large (and increasingly larger) array of recording electrodes; for EEG, the obvious advantage of MEG was its capacity to demonstrate the dipole generators of electrical fields within the cerebral cortex. With the recent announcement of a project in Japan to construct a 200-magnetometer MEG and the recent demonstration of deblurring algorithms for a 128-electrode EEG (Gevins *et al.*, 1994), the comparability of the two techniques in their modern forms can be assessed without regard to the partisan claims of the proponents of each (e.g. Balish *et al.*, 1991, vs. Cohen *et al.*, 1990).

With respect to forming images of cortical activity, the two techniques are theoretically similar in terms of: (i) the spatial and temporal resolutions of the images; (ii) their reliance on high-quality structural images of the cortical mantle immediately below the recording sites.

Both techniques share a preoccupation with artefacts; typically, EEG recordings rely on uniform and low electrode impedances at the electrode/scalp junction, and MEG recordings rely on the construction of screening rooms. What is being recorded in both instances is minute; EEG data are presented against a milli- and microvolt scale and MEG against a picotesla scale.

For much of the period of development of MEG, the technique has been vaunted as a means of overcoming the intractable difficulties seemingly inherent in the interpretation of EEG: namely, the distortion of electrical fields from the cortex by enveloping and intervening tissue, and the inability of scalp-recorded EEG to 'model' the underlying generators of the scalp fields.

Electroencephalographic localisation

At this point, some of the terms to be used in the rest of this account should be introduced and defined, so that the similarities and differences in the uses made of MEG and EEG to provide an explanation of the activity can be understood. Both techniques address and attempt to overcome the problem of inferring the position and strength of 'generators' of brain activity where some distance intervenes between the generator location and the recording instrument. The fact of there being a distance means that the properties of what intervenes between the generator and recorder have to be taken into account.

Montage

This refers to the pattern of interconnection of electrodes placed over the scalp. The cranium is, to a first approximation, a hemisphere, and the standard 10–20 electrode placement arrangement is a polar coordinate system referred to four fixed bone features of the skull—the nasion, the inion and the left and right promontories behind the left and right ear—which fall on the largest circular plane of an idealised sphere, of which the cranium is an idealised hemisphere. The placement system puts 20 electrodes at equal distances from each other over the hemisphere. A variety of patterns of connection between the electrodes so placed are employed, each of which accentuates certain features of the polygraphic EEG record, so that EEG phenomena can be elicited as part of a clinical investigation. These patterns of connection—the montage—are described at length in standard EEG textbooks; only one need be considered here, the *average* reference montage. In this, the EEG channel—all polygraphic EEG output is a record of the continuous variation in electrical potential between two electrodes—is made up of one exploring electrode and one reference electrode, whose potential is the average potential of all the other electrodes in the montage. This configuration of channels means that no electrode elsewhere on the scalp is

'privileged' with respect to any other. With other configurations, particularly *common* referencing, where each exploring electrode in each channel is coupled with the same single electrode in all channels, the intention is to accord the privilege to what is assumed to be the most 'silent' electrode, the one least affected by the generator the exploring electrode is responding to. This is, for localisation of generators in the vast majority of instances, an unrealisable intention.

As the sum of potential differences between the channels configured for average reference will be zero, the polygraphic output from an average reference montage provides a description of the relative distribution of potential across the hemisphere.

Current-source density

From the relative distribution of potential across the scalp, it becomes possible to leave the polygraphic channel output form of the traditional EEG in order to plot as a map the recorded-channel voltage outputs. Average referencing produces channel outputs which have high correlations between channels where exploring electrodes are close to each other. The explanation for this principally resides in the 'smearing' effect on scalp potential distribution of the intervening tissues, particularly as a result of the differences in resistivity of the skull and the dura mater and, to a lesser extent, the differences in conductance of neural tissue and cerebrospinal fluid. The extent to which this 'smearing' can be removed is a current and controversial topic in EEG mapping (see Chapter 8), but, whatever the effects of 'smearing' amounts to, because the field is being continuously deformed as a result of resistivities of intervening tissue, the distribution of the field may be computed in terms of gradients between electrodes. In other words field voltage values might be interpolated for points between electrodes on the basis of the recorded electrode values.

Various 'nearest-neighbour' interpolation algorithms have been developed to create, among other outputs, isopotential maps, where field lines connecting real and computed points of equal potential can be produced. The assumption here is that, beyond a certain level of density of electrode coverage of the scalp, no new information can be gained. However, the biophysics of cortical currents allows us to deduce that the density of coverage of the scalp at that point of no new information is approximately where there is an interelectrode distance of 2.5 cm: electrode montages in excess of 200 are therefore likely to be required before interpolation of values becomes free of the risk of spatial aliasing (see below, section on system error). This is an order of magnitude greater than most electrode montages typically employed, so it is clear that interpolation algorithms employed with 10–20 electrode montages are susceptible to undetectable spatial aliasing.

EEG mapping

The importance of this becomes apparent when what is done with isopotential field maps is understood. In order to infer the location of the movement of electrical charge which may account for the electrical-field distribution, the electrode values are integrated. The first spatial integration produces a map of the gradients of the field (in microvolts per unit length) and the second spatial integration produces a map of the changes in gradients of the field (in microvolts per unit area) in each case producing an identical location of field reversal, and in most cases producing similar locations of field maxima and minima. As current is a measure of the rate of charge passing a point (1 ampere = 1 coulomb per second), the rate of change of potential field is an indirect measure of current. From second-spatial-integration maps, also called Laplacian maps, the location and orientation of 'current-dipole equivalents' can be inferred. Charge flows from the 'source' (area of high charge, voltage field maximum) to the 'sink' (area of low charge, voltage field minimum) over the period of time for which the field contours remain sufficiently stable to support the inference

of current flowing in one direction at one location.

In summary, electrical-field data can provide indirect measurement of the location of current flow by inference from perturbation of the potential field recorded from the scalp. It is indirect in the definitional sense that rate of change of voltage gradient in a conducting medium is proportional to the rate of movement of charge. However, because it is an indirect measure, limitations in the field data will produce misleading descriptions of current-dipole equivalents, which may not be obvious.

Magnetoencephalographic localisation

The above concerns are only applicable to the problem of deducing current flow from voltage fields. With magnetic-field measurement at some distance from the current source, the deduction is direct, but with some important qualifications, to which we now turn.

A (standard) ampere is defined in terms of the force in newtons per metre (2×10^{-7} N/m) existing between two parallel conductors a standard distance apart (1 m in a vacuum) with constant current. The force is attractive when current flows in the same direction in both conductors, and repulsive if in different directions. This establishes the relationship between current flowing in one direction, the distance from the conductor and the strength of the magnetic field, and the relationship between direction of current and direction of magnetic field. Accordingly, any measure of magnetic-field strength and direction will be directly related to the size and direction of current flow.

Because it is the size and direction of current flow which directly interests us in terms of the production of images of brain function, the problems of quantifying these from measures of magnetic-field strength need to be addressed. These are problems, like those associated with the scalp electrical field, caused by the intervening tissues, but of a rather different nature. The first difference is that biological tissue is *diamagnetic*;

that is, the meningeal layers, the skull and skin and the cerebrospinal fluid do not deform a magnetic field in the way that they deform an electrical field. The second difference is that, because the magnetic-field strength is being measured directly, the need to have an elaborate montage covering the hemisphere in order to integrate voltage values to produce field-strength relativities can be dispensed with. This does not diminish the problem of spatial aliasing, but it does provide a more direct relationship between the number of sample points and the confidence with which current-flow position can be estimated. The third difference is that the distance between the magnetometer and the current generator is measured directly, as they are both in the same geometric coordinate space—that is, their coordinate locations are given with respect to the same origin. We now need to consider what is meant by current flow in a hemisphere made up of concentric layers which have heterogeneous conductivities, each layer of which is a conducting medium.

Magnetic fields of current dipoles in the cortex

We know that the cytoarchitecture of the cerebral cortex is impressively columnar, and that the organisation of the relatively large-bodied pyramidal cells, which make up the majority of active cells in the cortex, is such that intracellular currents associated with transient postsynaptic membrane conduction changes will be largely in the two directions normal to the cortical surface at that point. A volume of cortical cells with subthreshold membrane potential charges will therefore, on activation from other sources, be functionally a current dipole. Currently density in a cortical-cell volume (A/m^2) is the aggregate of current dipoles in a volume. The moment of a current dipole (Am) is a product of the current density, the length and the cross-sectional area of the dipole (i.e. current dipole (Am) = current density (A/m^2) × length (m) × cross-sectional area (m^2)). The current dipole whose strength and position is being estimated from measures of the magnetic field associated with it is referred to as the *primary source*. Its dipolar nature means that the flux density of the magnetic field it produces diminishes as the square of the distance between its centre and the detection point. (Flux density is expressed in teslas, which are newtons/ampere. metre or, as here, force per current dipole.)

MEG insensitivity to radially orientated dipoles

In addition to primary sources, where the dipolar nature of the cells and the dipolar nature of current flow are clearly connected, there are secondary sources, which are also dipolar, but for different reasons. The brain and its layers together constitute an inhomogeneous volume conductor of electrical charge. At boundaries between two regions with large differences in electrical conductivity, such as the dura mater and the skull, the effect can be modelled by considering such boundaries as made up of current dipoles normal to the boundary. These current dipoles are the *secondary* sources of current. The boundaries of relevance here can be thought of as concentric with the skull over the hemispheric recording plane, and they are principally made up of the skull–dura junction. Radially orientated *primary* source current dipoles, as a result of volume conduction, will create radially orientated *secondary* boundary-layer conduction dipoles of moments which exactly cancel those of the primary (radial) dipoles (Geselowitz, 1970). As we are measuring vector fields with the magnetometer, the situation generalises so that the *radial* component of a *primary* current dipole will produce *no* detectable magnetic field in a conducting hemisphere beyond the secondary source dipolar layer. Applying the same reasoning, the *tangential* component of a *primary* current dipole will not produce secondary source boundary current dipoles between it and the magnetometer; therefore the radial magnetic field will be unaffected. The measurement of the radial magnetic field therefore directly records the movement of charge in a primary source current dipole, orientated tangentially to the skull. From consideration of the columnar cytoarchitecture of the convolutions of the cortical mantle, these current dipoles will be the cortical cells in the sulci.

The magnetic field tangential to the skull will be made up of the magnetic effects of tangentially orientated secondary sources of primary radial dipoles, and boundary perturbation of volume current set up by tangential components of the primary source dipoles. It is therefore inherently ambiguous, particularly in situations as at present, when only small areas of skull are surveyed by magnetometers. With large-array magnetometer montages in the future, the ambiguity in terms of dipole-moment strength and orientation of the tangential magnetic field may be reduced.

In summary, the radial magnetic field directly measures current dipole moment, location and direction of current flow of the tangentially orientated vector of the primary source. Radially orientated current dipoles produce no external magnetic field in a closed spherical conductor, such as the head. The measurement is direct, in that the coordinate location of the dipole centre is below the recording plane, one-half of the distance between the two centres of the isomagnetic-field map and perpendicular to the magnetic polarity-reversal boundary.

MEG sensitivity

Having reviewed the techniques of derivation of primary current dipoles by measuring the magnetic field external to the head in which they are produced, we are in a position to estimate the sensitivity of the technique under certain assumptions. These assumptions are that: (i) the external field is 'graded': that is, for relatively low-frequency magnetic fields (less than 100 Hz) the fields arise from postsynaptic transient membrane-potential charges; and (ii) the field is exclusively produced by parallel pyramidal-cell bodies in the cerebral cortex. In circumstances where these assumptions are most likely to hold—

the early involvement of the cortex in the processing of sensory information, movement preparation and initiation—the resolution of MEG is astonishing. The typical dipole moments deduced in evoked-field studies are 2–20 µAm, which, assuming some cancellation within the cortical column, is a current dipole made up of between 10^4 and 10^5 cells, occupying between 0.5 and 5 mm^2. These fields have gradients in the picotesla and femtotesla range, which is near the maximum sensitivity of superconducting quantum interference devices (SQUIDs; see next section). The resolution of location of the primary current dipole is to between the fingers in the Penfield sensory homunculus (Brenner *et al.*, 1978; Okada *et al.*, 1982), and the direct measure of location of the current dipole has shown that the auditory evoked potential N100 (see below, section on evoked brain activity), which has a common-reference-derived symmetrical scalp distribution around the vertex, is in fact generated by dipoles located within the primary auditory cortex in the temporal lobes asymmetrical with respect to ear of stimulation (Hari *et al.*, 1980; Elberling *et al.*, 1982). The imaging of generators of various sorts of brain activity will be returned to later (section on the interpretation of EEG and MEG waveform differences), as matters are not quite as straightforward as this. We now briefly consider how magnetic fields around the head are detected, given the impressive results which can be achieved.

How magnetic fields of the head are measured

The tiny biomagnetic fields from the cortical mantle are detected by a unique (in biological sciences) kind of signal detection apparatus known as a SQUID. Unlike other, more commonly encountered detection devices, its sensitivity to phenomena of interest resides in the physics of the apparatus, rather than the construction of the detector. This becomes apparent once what is contained within the acronym is unpacked.

Superconducting

The electrical, and therefore magnetic, properties of materials cooled to below their superconducting threshold temperature change dramatically, so that phenomena present at normal temperatures disappear and others emerge. Of relevance here are the electrical property of resistance and the magnetic property of inductance. With the latter, the phenomena described by Lenz's law—current induced in a conductor as a result of movement through a magnetic field will in turn induce a magnetic field which opposes its flow—no longer apply. Therefore, once current has started to flow in a superconducting loop as the result of an external imposed magnetic field, it will not stop flowing when the field is switched off.

Quantum

The explanation for this persistence of current flow in a superconducting medium when the magnetic field is switched off lies in a change in the behaviour of the electrons in the medium. At normal temperatures, electrons are in a variety of energy states: these energy states are not continuously distributed, but are discrete. The various energy states occupied are quantum states, and the thermal energy of the material is the aggregate of these states. As thermal energy is withdrawn, by cooling, the number of different quantum states occupied by the electrons falls, so that, as superconducting temperatures are approached, the energy quanta of the electrons come progressively to resemble each other. At supercooled temperatures the electrons cease to repel each other, and instead pair up to form Cooper pairs. In a supercooled conducting medium, virtually all electrons are in Cooper pairs, and therefore have the same energy and can be described by one wave function. This wave property of superconducting electrons is of importance when one considers what happens to the wave function as it collapses at the boundary of the superconducting state.

Interference

The behaviour of the wave function of Cooper pairs as it decays to zero was predicted in the 1960s by Josephson: apparatus which exploits this behaviour is known as a Josephson junction. In SQUIDs, two separate loops of superconducting material are brought into extremely close proximity, separated only by an insulating layer micrometres thick. The insulating layer, by definition, does not allow electron-pair particles to pass from one superconducting medium to the other; however, Cooper pairs are both particles and waves, and the collapse of the wave function across the insulating membrane cannot occur abruptly, and so occurs over a physical distance within the thickness of the insulating layer. The collapse of the wave function causes current to flow in the layer, which is referred to as 'tunnelling' current. This is current not caused by the flow of charged particles, but by the loss of Cooper-pair wave energy. The magnitude of the tunnelling current is proportional to the phase difference of the wave functions on either side of the junction. Also, the presence of a voltage across the junction is proportional to the rate of change of the phase difference.

The tunnelling current in the junction is an alternating current (as a consequence of the alternating negative and positive values of the phase differences on either side) and the frequency of the alternating current is affected by the magnitude of the voltage across the junction. Accordingly, any change to the magnetic flux in the superconducting loop will affect the phase in the junction.

Device

A phase-sensitive detector receiving input from the junction, coupled with a device integrating the rectified output from the detector, will produce a voltage proportional to the change in the magnetic flux in the superconducting loop. This can then generate magnetic flux in a coil which exactly opposes the change, restoring the phase relationships across the junction to the status quo ante.

For the purposes here, clearly we wish the change in the magnetic flux of the superconducting loop to come only from the biomagnetic fields generated in the cortical mantle. A detecting coil near to the head coupled to an input coil within the SQUID will produce alteration in the magnitude of the loop flux. The detecting coil will also be sensitive to other small magnetic fields in the vicinity, to larger fields nearby and to the Earth's magnetic field. To overcome the effects of these other sources of magnetic flux, detection coils can be wound as *gradiometers*. First-order gradiometers reject spatially uniform ambient fields, and second-order gradiometers (two first-order gradiometers in series and wound separately) reject spatially uniform field gradients in addition.

In summary, a SQUID can be thought of as a three-component magnetic-field change-detection device: a detection coil arrangement; a superconducting loop with a junction, the electrical properties of which are affected by external magnetic-field change; and electronics which maintain the sensitivity of the junction to the field changes and produce calibrated output describing the field changes.

Electroencephalographic and magnetoencephalographic images of brain activity

In order to consider recent studies of brain activity using MEG, some other principles and problems should be introduced at this point. To recap, as imaging techniques, both EEG and MEG capture variation in electromagnetic fields over or near (respectively) the surface of a sphere (the head) and attempt to infer the geometry of the generating sources of these field variations. The source geometry in both cases is computed as the location, orientation and strength of an idealised dipole. The columnar nature of the cortical neuronal architecture renders this dipole modelling plausible in those circumstances where, from

physiological principles, the neuronal assemblages involved anatomically approximate to local dipoles. The modelling of dipoles becomes increasingly problematic when there are reasons to think that the neuronal assemblages are dispersed. Under these circumstances, dipole 'solutions' to recorded fields will be spurious. This is a perfectly general problem, affecting both MEG and EEG, and is not solved by developing techniques for greater accuracy of dipole localisation. Dipole modelling from surface field data is therefore an acceptable imaging technique only for certain sorts of bioelectric phenomena. We can call this the *imaging-limit* problem.

System error

Both EEG and MEG data make assumptions about the conducting properties of the head, which feature in the methods of deducing dipole position and strength from the data. Let us reconsider the problem of volume currents, and their 'smearing' with respect to scalp-recorded electric fields (see above, section on current-source density). We know that the vector *magnetic* field at a sample point, from the Biot–Savart law is given by the product $(\mu_0 / 4\pi R^3)QR$, where μ_0 is the permeability of free space ($4\pi \times 10^{-7}$ N/A^2), Q is the current-dipole moment and R is the distance between the centre of the current dipole and the sample point. We also know that the vector *electrical* field is given by the product $(4\pi\sigma R^3)^{-1}QR$, where σ is the term for the conductivity of the medium. The indirect nature of the measurement of current-dipole moment, and therefore the equivocation between dipole moment and dipole location which dipole-equivalent modelling from electrical field data concerns itself with, is solely due to uncertainties concerning the quantification of the deformation of the electrical field. In a closed spherical conducting medium, the relationship between the electric-field strength and current density is given as $E = \tau J$, where E is the electrical field strength gradient (in V/m), J is current density (in A/m^2) and τ is the resistivity of the medium in ohm metres (or its reciprocal, δ, conductivity (i.e. $1/\Omega$m, or siemens/m)). What is usually referred to as the 'inverse problem' states that there is no unique dipole solution to any surface field. The head models therefore deal with the 'smearing' by rendering plausible certain locations for dipoles over others, and they employ statistical techniques which promote single-dipole solutions over more complex ones. Head models must therefore be judged by their *adequacy* in approximating the resistivities of surrounding tissue, and on the *appropriateness* of their dipole solution algorithms.

The tissue comprising the head varies considerably (for the present purpose) so it is unlikely that any given head model will faithfully reproduce the actual field distortions produced by any individual's head. However, if a sufficiently detailed image of these tissues can be made, together with an accurate record of the position of the electrodes or detecting coils producing the data, then a more realistic calculation of dipole position can be contemplated. Magnetic resonance imaging (MRI) provides this (as in EEG studies by Gevins *et al.*, 1994, and MEG studies by Rogers *et al.*, 1991) and thus allows a pragmatic resolution of the inverse problem. The difficulty over the unique dipolar solution remains, but, if the surface field is recorded in sufficient detail and the anatomy of the relevant tissue is sufficiently well characterised to show that any dipole solution resides in a plausible location, then this is an important advance in the fidelity of the image. We can call this combined field and tissue definition task the *system-error* problem.

For completeness, we can consider the term '*spatial aliasing*' here, as the contribution to system error which inadequate definition of the surface field makes. As is clear from the discussion (see above, section on EEG mapping) of field gradients, the greater the density of recording points, the less the reliance on interpolation of field values in the surface map. For dipole-modelling purposes, if we consider the identification of field extrema as the principal issue of location accuracy, then field maps from sample points at greater distances from each other than is required to record all of the possible field variations produced by the cortex will be suboptimal. The ersatz values produced by interpolation algorithms will produce locations of field extrema from 'missing' data, which will 'mislead' the dipole-location computations. Because what is at present feasible is a pragmatic resolution of the inverse problem, it is important to be as clear as possible about the various sources contributing to the system-error problem. Field sampling density for various purposes will need to be established both from theoretical considerations concerning point spread and from empirical studies of data redundancy, but what is already clear is that sampling densities conforming to the traditional 10–20 system of EEG electrode placement require to be increased at least sixfold.

Evoked brain activity

Having dealt with two important problems concerning image fidelity, we can now turn to what we would hope MEG will provide us with an image *of*. Considerable progress has been made over the past two decades in the electrophysiological understanding of the cortex and subcortical structures in the functioning brain, using various signal-enhancing techniques. The most productive one to consider here is the technique of averaging, where the field-strength values are repetitively sampled over epochs time-locked to the presentation of stimuli. For each channel, the averaging produces a trace where the amplitude of each point reflects the difference from zero of brain activity evoked by the stimulus. This is based on the assumption that all brain activity not associated with the stimulus will progressively cancel out if the average of a sufficient number of epochs is taken. Numbers of epochs required to separate background from time-locked brain activity can be established empirically, and will depend on a number of considerations: the amplitude of the time-locked 'signal' compared with the amount of random 'noise'; the changes over time of the time-locked 'signal'—refractory periods, habituation and dishabituation to stimulus sequences—and the physical and psychological properties of the stimuli themselves. Within this area of enquiry several features of time-locked evoked brain activity have become clear:

1 There is a transition from short and middle latency (less than 100 ms post-stimulus) values of the average, to long latency (greater than 150 ms post-stimulus) values, where short-latency waveforms are largely dependent on the physical properties of the stimulus—intensity, luminance—and long-latency waveforms are largely dependent on psychological properties—salience, relevance, expectability.

2 The roles of attention and understanding play an increasingly important and complex part in determining the amplitude of all values with latencies after 80 ms or so post-stimulus.

If we consider the general type of experiment referred to as 'oddball'—pay attention to the rare stimulus and ignore the common stimulus—and make separate averages for the two sorts of stimulus, certain patterns of amplitude variation can be reliably demonstrated. These patterns of amplitude variation are usually referred to using peak-description terminology, as there is a common peak-and-trough pattern to most evoked responses between 100 and 400 ms post-stimulus. Accordingly we have N100, N200 and P300, referring to the negative (N) and positive (P) amplitudes of a peak at roughly 100, 200 and 300 ms, respectively. In addition, we have N200a and b, and P300a and b, the a and b referring to different types of contrasts or tasks between the two stimulus sorts in the oddball.

Long-latency responses which are not evoked by oddball tasks comprise N400, principally evoked by semantic tasks; and slow and late potentials in the average—positive slow wave (PSW), contingent negative variation (CNV), postimperative negative variation (PINV), the readiness potential (RP)—are evoked by a variety of aspects of task performance, such as expectation, preparation to respond, selecting a response and so forth, which do not have reliably recognisable peaks.

This nomenclature has evolved from experience of scalp-recorded EEG, but what has been suspected for several years is now finally established by the use of depth electrodes. Halgren's group (Baudema *et al.*, 1995; Halgren *et al.*, 1995a,b) found that the scalp-recorded waveforms also occur in other brain structures—within the frontal and parietal cortices, within the hippocampal formation and the amygdala, within the medial temporal pole—and that there is only a loose relationship between the latencies of the peak features of the average recorded from the scalp and the same features recorded from depth-implanted electrodes.

The separate oddball averages demonstrate that the depth electrodes record time-locked activity which preserves the differences between the different sorts of oddball-evoked activity recorded with scalp electrodes. The fact that the scalp-recorded evoked responses persist following removal of, or damage to, the deeper structures (e.g. Polich & Squire, 1993) which depth-electrode recordings show produce these evoked responses, implies that the 'cortical' evoked responses are not caused by passive propagation from deeper structures, but are in fact generated in the cortex. Also, the variability in the latencies of the oddball-evoked waveform strongly suggests that there is a substantial amount of autonomy between different brain structures in terms of oddball-evoked activity. We can be reasonably clear on the functional significance of oddball responses originating in the cortex, and we can infer that oddball-response activity in other parts of the brain means that the distinctions between sorts of stimuli in the oddball are being preserved, but we do not know, at present, how to interpret this. Nor do we have an explanation for the differences in latencies.

The most parsimonious explanation is that the various brain structures involved in stimulus processing do, broadly speaking, the same thing at somewhat different rates. This has important consequences in the enterprise of correlating EEG and MEG phenomena, and more generally in providing an interpretation of what the image is an image of. This becomes clearer when we consider two papers correlating electrical and magnetic evoked responses.

The interpretation of
EEG and MEG waveform differences

Sherg and von Cramon (1985), reworking Vaughan *et al.*'s (1980) paper, provide a four-dipole solution to the auditory evoked potential (AEP) between 60 and 250 ms. This consists of symmetrical dipoles activated successively, the first in or near the primary auditory cortex, vertically orientated and perpendicular to the superior temporal plane, and the second radially orientated in the secondary auditory cortex, perpendicular to the lateral surface of the superior temporal gyrus. There is a close agreement between EEG and MEG data contributing to the dipole solution in primary cortex but less for the secondary cortex dipole. This is seen in the differences in the latency shift across the electrode chain (coronally across the head), compared with the corresponding detecting-coil locations. There was a greater latency shift of N100M (magnetic) across the head than was found in the electrical N100. The radial dipole, from first principles, would not produce a magnetic field outside the head; hence the MEG field data would be composed largely of the tangential dipole in or near the primary cortex. This is their explanation for the difference in EEG and MEG waveforms.

Rogers *et al.* (1991) found that the P300M had a later peak latency and was a broader wave than the P300. Their dipole solution was a sequence of dipole activations moving medially to laterally in the auditory cortex, and their interpretation of the difference between the magnetic and the electrical P300 came from considerations of a dipole reducing in moment (hence producing a smaller P300) but moving laterally towards the MEG detecting coil, hence minimising the apparent rate at which the moment of the dipole was, in fact, reducing. (Magnetic-field strength is a function of the square of the distance (see above, section on magnetic fields of current dipoles in the cortex), whereas electrical field strength is a function of the distance.)

From these two papers, clearly there is broad agreement (as might be expected) between EEG and MEG data concerning dipole solutions. However, given what we know about the lack of magnetic-field distortion by the brain layers and skull compared with their effects on the electrical field, we may wonder to what extent the underlying brain structures, also producing evoked responses, contribute to the magnetic average. Okada *et al.* (1983) identified the hippocampal formation as a source for the P300 on the basis of a dipole solution modelling the effects on the magnetic field of surrounding brain structures, which are substantially different from their effect on electrical fields (see above, section on system error). It would therefore be reasonable to keep open the possibility that different aggregates of neural tissue are involved in generating magnetic and electrical average evoked responses, and that it will be undecidable whether the different latencies of the features of the response will be due to: (i) differential sensitivity to dipole orientation (as in Sherg & von Cramon, 1985); (ii) differential sensitivity to effective dipole movement (as in Rogers *et al.*, 1991); (iii) differences in aggregate neuronal sources; or (iv) various combinations of all of these.

The limits of 'dipolar' solutions

It should be noted that Halgren's group's conclusion from their enormous series of depth-electrode oddball recordings of evoked responses is that these are widely dispersed in underlying structures, and hence the phenomena are not well described as equivalent dipoles occupying a space point. Dipole solutions are, of course, solutions in a dipole model, and the limits of a model need to be established.

Consider the situation where a large sheet of cortical tissue is involved in the generation of an electromagnetic-field component and there is a large degree of cancellation involved in the various membrane-potential charges. The current dipole will be weak (because of cancellation) and will accordingly appear further from the recording plane because of the distance separating the field extrema, which has been caused, in this instance, by the widespread cortical activity. If we assume that current-dipole length does not change, there is a reciprocal relationship between current density and dipole cross-sectional area (Q (current-dipole moment) = J (current density) × length × cross-sectional area), so that the dipole moment remains invariant as current density falls and cross-sectional area increases. Therefore, the apparent dipole location will emerge as further from the recording plane than the neural tissue generating the field. This generalises to the problem of dipole location from surface data, where the activity in the generating neural tissue in deeper structures is dispersed. Thus we encounter another version of the 'inverse problem'.

MEG is clearly impressive in source-location studies, where, for physiological reasons, a dipolar solution in the cortical mantle is expected, such as the initiation of movement in the sensorimotor cortex (Okada *et al.*, 1984; Cheyne & Weinberg, 1989; Kristeva *et al.*, 1991; Toro *et al.*, 1993). It can also contribute to widely suspected but hitherto undemonstrated distinctions in brain regional differential activation involved in the generation of the CNV (Basile *et al.*, 1994). The nature and extent of cortical interconnection, together with the evolving understanding of the relationships between the cortical mantle and deeper brain structures, clearly place limits on the scope for meaningful dipole modelling from surface data. MEG and EEG can clearly cooperate with adequate brain-structure imaging in reducing the size of the *system-error* problem in functional brain imaging. However, the *imaging-limit* problem will require a better theory of cortical activity than we have at present. A better theory will allow clearer distinctions between a model and an image.

References

Balish, M., Sato, S., Connaughton, P. & Kurta, C. (1991) Localisation of implanted dipoles by magnetoencephalography. *Neurology* **41**, 1072–6.

Basile, L.F.H., Rogers, R.L., Bourbon, W.T. & Papanicolaou, A.C. (1994) Slow magnetic flux from human frontal cortex. *Electroencephalogr. Clin. Neurophysiol.* **90**, 157–65.

Baudema, P., Halgren, E., Heit, G. & Clarke, J.M. (1995) Intracerebral potentials to rare target and distractor auditory and visual stimuli. (iii) Frontal cortex. *Electroencephalogr. Clin. Neurophysiol.* **94**, 251–64.

Baule, G.M. & McFee, R. (1963) Detection of the magnetic field of the heart. *Am. Heart J.* **66**, 95–6.

Brenner, D., Lipton, J., Kaufman, L. & Williamson, S.J. (1978) Somatically evoked magnetic fields of the human brain. *Science* **199**, 81–3.

Cheyne, D. & Weinberg, H. (1989) Neuromagnetic fields accompanying unilateral finger movements: pre-movement and movement evoked fields. *Exp. Brain Res.* **78**, 604–12.

Cohen, D. (1972) Magnetoencephalography: detection of the brain's electrical activity with a superconducting magnetometer. *Science* **175**, 664–6.

Cohen, D., Currin, B.N., Yunokuchi, K. *et al.* (1990) MEG versus EEG localisation testing using implanted sources in the human brain. *Ann. Neurol.* **28**, 811–17.

Elberling, C., Bak, C., Kofoed, B., Lebech, J. & Saermark, K. (1982) Auditory magnetic fields from the human cerebral cortex: location and strength of an equivalent current dipole. *Acta Neurol. Scand.* **65**, 553–69.

Geselowitz, D.B. (1970) On the magnetic field generated outside in homogeneous volume conductor by internal current sources. *IEEE Trans. Magnetism* **MAG-6**, 346–7.

Halgren, E., Baudema, P., Clarke, J.M. *et al.* (1995a) Intracerebral potentials to rare target and distractor auditory and visual stimuli. (i) Superior temporal plane and parietal lobe. *Electroencephalogr. Clin. Neurophysiol.* **94**, 191–220.

Halgren, E., Baudema, P., Clarke, J.M. *et al.* (1995b) Intracerebral potentials to rare target and distractor auditory and visual stimuli. (ii) Medial, lateral and posterior temporal lobe. *Electroencephalogr. Clin. Neurophysiol.* **94**, 229–50.

Hari, R., Atitowiemi, K., Järvinen, M.-L., Katila, T. & Varpula, T. (1980) Auditory evoked transient and sustained magnetic fields of the human brain. *Exp. Brain Res.* **40**, 237–40.

Kristeva, R., Cheyne, D. & Deecke, L. (1991) Neuromagnetic fields accompanying unilateral and bilateral voluntary movements: topography and source analysis. *Electroencephalogr. Clin. Neurophysiol.* **81**, 285–98.

Okada, Y.C., Williamson, S.J. & Kaufman, L. (1982) Magnetic field of the human sensorimotor cortex. *Int. J. Neurosci.* **17**, 33–8.

Okada, Y.C., Kaufman, L. & Williamson, S.J. (1983) The hippocampal formation as a source of the slow endogenous potentials. *Electroencephalogr. Clin. Neurophysiol.* **55**, 417–26.

Okada, Y.C., Tanabaum, R., Williamson, S.J. & Kaufman, L. (1984) Somatotopic organisation of the human somatosensory cortex revealed by neuromagnetic measurements. *Exp. Brain Res.* **56**, 197–205.

Polich, J. & Squire, L.R. (1993) P300 from amnesic patients with bilateral hippocampal lesions. *Electroencephalogr. Clin. Neurophysiol.* **86**, 408–17.

Rogers, R.L., Baumann, S.B., Papanicolaou, A.C., Bourbon, T.W., Alagarsammy, S. & Eisenberg, W.M. (1991) Localisation of the P3 sources using magnetoencephalography and magnetic resonance imaging. *Electroencephalogr. Clin. Neurophysiol.* **79**, 308–21.

Sherg, M. & von Cramon, D. (1985) Two bilateral sources of the late AEP as identified by a spatio-temporal dipole model. *Electroencephalogr. Clin. Neurophysiol.* **62**, 32–44.

Toro, C., Matsumoto, J., Deusch, G., Roth, B.J. & Hallett, M. (1993) Source analysis of scalp-recorded movement-related electrical potentials. *Electroencephalogr. Clin. Neurophysiol.* **86**, 167–75.

Vaughan, H.G., Ritter, W. & Simpson, R. (1980) Topographic analysis of auditory event-related potentials. In Kornhuber, H.H. & Deecke, L. (eds) *Motivation, Motor and Sensory Processes of the Brain*. Progress in Brain Research 54, Elsevier, Amsterdam, pp. 279–85.

10: Structural Brain Imaging in Schizophrenia

P. W. R. Woodruff and S. W. Lewis

Introduction

In contrast to the organic psychoses such as delirium and dementia, the functional psychoses have traditionally been seen essentially as disorders of mind rather than brain. In so far as there were, at some level, assumed to be brain abnormalities, these were a considerable way downstream, comprising disturbances of software rather than hardware. This view was not the one held by Emil Kraepelin when he first delineated schizophrenia. Post-mortem investigations in schizophrenia were frequent in the first half of the twentieth century but the lack of a clear hypothetical focus to direct investigations and the absence of proper control groups led to the abandonment of this approach in the 1950s. The idea that obtaining a visual image of brain structure during life was at about the same time becoming a possibility, largely through the technique of pneumoencephalography (PEG) (see Chapter 1). PEG essentially used the low electron density of air to act as an X-ray contrast medium. The procedure was lengthy, painful and hazardous. Nonetheless, during the 1950s and early 1960s a handful of European studies used PEG to measure ventricular size in schizophrenia (Haug, 1962). These studies suggested that, in chronic schizophrenia, some degree of lateral-ventricular enlargement was present. These studies attracted relatively little attention. It was not until the second half of the 1970s that *in vivo* structural brain imaging, using non-invasive, painless, relatively safe techniques, became available. The use of X-ray computed tomography (CT) in schizophrenia research was central to confirming a biological focus for investigations into causal mechanisms in schizophrenia. As well as the importance of structural imaging in redrawing the proper focus for investigation, the findings have also been critical in generating hypotheses about the nature of brain abnormalities in schizophrenia.

CT studies in schizophrenia

Methodology

Early on, it became clear that any differences seen in CT measures between patient and control groups were in the main quantitative rather than qualitative. Moreover, these changes were usually minor in degree, with considerable overlap between groups. Studies were soon seen to vary widely in the reported prevalence of abnormal findings and the most reasonable explanation of this lay in variation in the selection of patients, the choice of controls and the methods of measurement. The most commonly measured structures were the lateral ventricles, partly because they were easily visualised on transverse CT slices.

A major source of variation between earlier (prior to about 1988) studies was in the techniques of measurement used. The most popular index of lateral ventricular size was the ventricle: brain ratio (VBR). The VBR expresses the area of the lateral ventricles as a percentage of the brain area measured on the same slice, multiplied for convenience by 100. Its rationale was that, since people with large heads will normally have large ventricles, this ratio would control for differences in head size. It assumes first that there is a linear relationship between ventricle size and head size in the general population, and second that head size in schizophrenic patients is no different from that in controls. In fact, neither assumption is watertight (Harvey *et al.*, 1990), although VBR does seem to be a valid indicator of the total volume of the lateral ventricles.

Actual measurement of areas was performed in one of two ways. Mechanical planimetry used an articulated device to trace manually around the edge of the structure on the photographic film. However, this relies on visual inspection and, particularly where ventricles are small, the grey areas at the interface between fluid and brain can give rise to real problems in deciding where the edges of the ventricle actually lie: the so-called partial-volume effect. This method was largely superseded by various automated or semiautomated techniques. These have theoretical and practical advantages in that they use the original

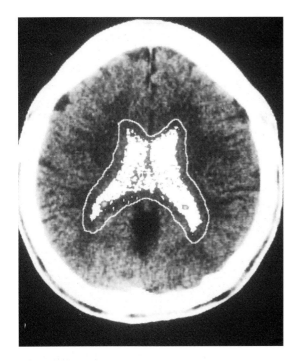

Fig. 10.1 Transverse CT image of normal brain with interactive image analysis program identifying the area occupied by CSF in the lateral ventricles.

digital CT data and, although the partial-volume problem is not wholly overcome, have very high inter-rater reliability (Fig. 10.1).

Most studies used operational diagnostic criteria to define the patient group, but still differed widely in patients' demographic and treatment characteristics. There is now much evidence that these factors do influence the prevalence of abnormalities found, and epidemiological samples, such as first-episode patients (Turner *et al.*, 1986) or consecutive admissions from a defined catchment area (Iacono *et al.*, 1988), are to be preferred. The rigorous selection of controls is at least as important. The ideal control group would seem to be healthy volunteers matched at least for age and sex, prospectively scanned on the same machine during the same period. Psychiatric screening and determination of alcohol consumption is needed. Any exclusion criteria used in the patient group should also be used in the controls. Those more commonly applied are histories of neurological disease, mental retardation, an upper age limit and concurrent physical illness. Evidence of heavy alcohol consumption is also a common exclusion criterion, although some studies only excluded alcohol abuse if of 'aetiological significance to the psychiatric disorder' (Williams *et al.*, 1985), despite evidence that it is a potent confounding variable, however defined (see below).

By 1994 there were over 60 controlled studies in the world literature which had examined some aspect of brain structure in schizophrenic patients using CT. The review of Lewis (1990) considered only those studies in which controls were prospectively ascertained healthy volunteers, scanned concurrently with the patient group. There were 21 studies meeting these criteria. Most of these were the most recent studies. In comparison with less well-controlled studies, a relatively high proportion of these studies failed to show significant CT abnormalities in schizophrenic patients. Of the 21 studies considered, nine could not demonstrate lateral ventricular enlargement in the patient group and a further three showed this at only marginal degrees of statistical significance. The largest study since that review to fulfil these methodological criteria is that of Jones *et al.* (1994). In this study, 67 community volunteers were matched to 161 consecutively admitted patients with research diagnostic criteria (RDC) schizophrenia or schizoaffective disorder. The thorny issue of how to define the limits of normality in ventricular size was approached by using the distribution of ventricular size in the controls as the unit of measurement. In a logistic regression model, head size, sex, social class and ethnicity all exerted significant effects on ventricular volume, a finding which stresses the importance of taking these demographic factors into account. After adjusting for each of these variables, the resulting differences between cases and controls, previously just at the trend level, increased markedly. Head-size differences between cases and controls were seen to be entirely due to the effects of ethnicity and childhood social class. Lateral- and third-ventricle size was largest in family-history-negative men. These measures were one-third to one-half larger in males with, compared with males without, a first-degree family history of schizophrenia. No relationships with obstetric complications, age at onset, length of illness or sex *per se* were seen. Odds ratios were used to estimate levels of risk, and both enlargement of lateral and third ventricles carried an odds ratio of about 2.0 for schizophrenia. There was no evidence for a bimodal distribution of these measures in schizophrenia, in agreement with other studies. The concept of a subgroup of patients with ventricular enlargement is therefore misleading: all schizophrenic subjects seem to have slightly larger ventricles than they should.

This study stresses how vital it is to take into account non-illness confounding factors. Control groups should comprise prospectively scanned healthy volunteers, although the decision about which variables should be matched between patients and controls is still at issue. Certainly, age and sex should be matched. In addition, evidence is accruing that other demographic factors can influence measures of brain structure: social class (Pearlson *et al.*, 1989), height, ethnicity

(Nimgaonkar *et al.*, 1988) and educational level (DeMeyer *et al.*, 1988), for example. The effect of such variables has been highlighted by the controversial claims of reduced head size in schizophrenic patients. The initial report of this proved to be explainable on the basis of difference in height (Andreasen *et al.*, 1986). Although a subsequent study which controlled for height still found smaller head size, significant social-class effects were present (Pearlson *et al.*, 1989).

Besides lateral-ventricular size, studies increasingly looked for difference in other cerebral-fluid spaces, in particular enlargement of the third ventricle and cerebral cortical sulci. Several later studies reported an enlarged third ventricle or enlarged cortical sulci in the absence of significant lateral-ventricular changes (Lewis, 1990). Other claims, such as enlarged cerebellar sulci, widened Sylvian and interhemispheric fissures and

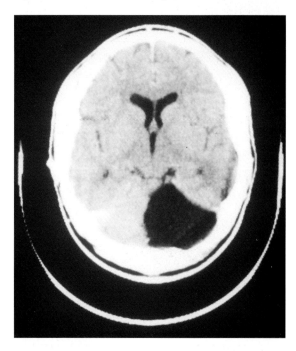

Fig. 10.2 CT showing a clinically unsuspected occipitotemporal porencephalic cyst, probably the aftermath of an ischaemic event *in utero*, in a 25-year-old man with paranoid schizophrenia. Unsuspected neurodevelopmental lesions occur in 5% of schizophrenic patients on brain imaging.

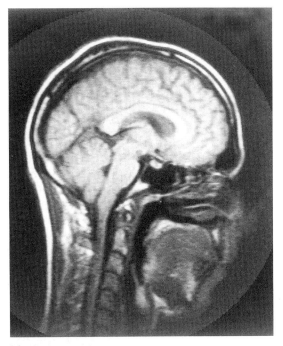

(a)

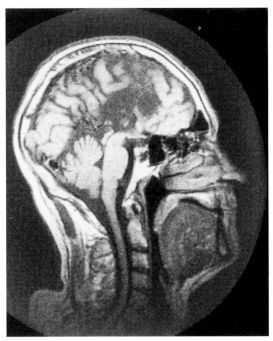

(b)

Fig. 10.3 (a) Midsagittal MRI in a normal subject. (b) Midsagittal MRI showing clinically unsuspected agenesis of the corpus callosum in a 50-year-old man of normal intelligence with chronic schizophrenia.

asymmetry of occipital pole size, have not been well replicated, although these measures are not reliably measured with CT.

Focal CT lesions in schizophrenia

As well as the minor degrees of enlargement of ventricles and sulci found in the majority of studies, there are a handful of reports in the literature of gross focal brain lesions in schizophrenia, as demonstrated by CT: aqueduct stenosis (Reveley & Reveley, 1983), arachnoid and septal cysts (Kuhnley *et al.*, 1981; Lewis & Mezey, 1985) and agenesis of the corpus callosum (Lewis *et al.*, 1988). Examples of these lesions are given in Figs. 10.2 and 10.3.

Three larger studies enable an estimate to be made of the prevalence of such focal lesions on

CT in schizophrenia. Owens *et al.* (1980), in their series of 136 schizophrenic patients, found 'unsuspected intracranial pathology' as a focal finding on CT in 12 cases (9%), excluding lesions due to leucotomy. Five of these 12 were aged over 65. Lewis (1987) examined a series of 228 Maudsley Hospital patients who met RDC for schizophrenia and who had been consecutively scanned for clinical reasons. Patients with a history of epilepsy or intracranial surgery or who were aged over 65 at the time of scan were excluded. The original scan reports were examined and the films of those not unequivocally normal were reappraised by a neuroradiologist blind to the original report. In 41 patients the scan showed a definite intracranial abnormality. This was in the nature of enlarged fluid spaces in 28 cases, but in 13 patients (6%) there was a discrete focal lesion. These 13 lesions varied widely in location and probable pathology, although left temporal and right parietal regions were most commonly implicated. The third study was an attempt to examine a geographically defined sample of schizophrenic patients, ascertained as part of a large, multidisciplinary survey (Brugha *et al.*, 1988). All Camberwell residents who, on a particular census day, were aged 18–65 and were in regular contact with any psychiatric day service were approached. Of 120 eligible people, 83 consented to CT and psychiatric interview. Of these, 50 met RDC for schizophrenia of schizoaffective disorder. In four of these 50 patients were found clinically unsuspected focal lesions: low density regions in the right caudate head; a left occipitotemporal porencephalic cyst; low-density regions in the right parietal lobe; agenesis of the corpus callosum (described further by Lewis *et al.*, 1988). None of 50 matched healthy volunteers showed focal pathology on CT. One magnetic resonance imaging (MRI) study has examined the prevalence of neurodevelopmental lesions in schizophrenia and found unsuspected lesions in four out of 47 cases (O'Callaghan *et al.*, 1990).

Given the differences in the nature of the patient samples, these three studies are in rough agreement about the prevalence of unexpected focal abnormalities on CT: between 6% and 9%. From the practical viewpoint of the referring clinician, it should be noted that the discovery of these abnormalities led to no change in the management of the patient in the great majority of cases. This was because most of the lesions appeared to be non-progressive and in the nature of developmental anomalies.

Despite intriguing case reports of familial association (Francis, 1979), the prevalence of basal ganglia calcifica-tion on CT was not found to be raised in schizo-phrenia in two large studies (Casanova *et al.*, 1990; Philpot & Lewis, 1990).

Clinical correlates of CT abnormalities

Given that a minority of schizophrenic patients do have modest enlargement of lateral and third ventricles and cortical sulci on CT compared with controls, can such cases be identified in terms of a particular clinical picture? For most clinical variables mooted at one time or another to be related to ventricular enlargement, there is little in the way of convincing replication. The appealing notion that negative symptoms and poor treatment response are characteristics of schizophrenia with ventricular enlargement does not have much objective support from CT studies. The only associations that have more positive than negative replications are those of tardive dyskinesia and, most particularly, impaired performance on neuropsychological tests, although the specific areas of cognitive impairment tend to vary from study to study. There is some evidence that abnormalities on CT scans are actually predicted by an atypical clinical picture. Harvey *et al.* (1990) found that their subgroup of unspecified functional psychoses had particularly enlarged ventricles, and unusual symptoms such as delusional misidentification are commonly reported with CT abnormalities. In the CT study of 228 schizophrenic patients referred to earlier (Lewis, 1987), the subgroup with unequivocally abnormal scans had a significantly greater frequency of changing clinical diagnosis, suggesting an atypical presentation.

One determinedly negative association worth noting is that of duration of illness. The degree of ventricular enlargement is convincingly not a function of how long the patient has been ill or of how long he/she has been treated. The lack of an association between length of illness and degree of lateral-ventricular enlargement suggests that this enlargement is not progressive, either in the sense of reflecting a neurodegenerative disorder or as being an artefact of continuing treatment or institutional care. This view receives support from the demonstration of significant ventricular enlargement in young, first-episode patients (Turner *et al.*, 1986). Direct evidence for the non-progressive nature of ventricular enlargement is now available from several follow-up CT studies, which have rescanned patients after periods of up to 7 years. Three such studies have reported no change in ventricular size (Nasrallah *et al.*, 1986; Illowsky *et al.*, 1988; Reveley *et al.*, 1988), although a fourth did find a significant enlargement from baseline VBR in rescanned schizophrenic patients versus healthy controls (Kemali *et al.*, 1989). Obviously, it is important in such studies to control for known confounding variables, such as heavy drinking.

The implication from the apparently non-progressive nature of the CT scan changes, which is reinforced by the increasing number of reports of congenital focal lesions, as noted above, is that they represent early neurodevelopmental abnormalities. These could result from the action of inherited factors or from environmental insults, or from a combination of the two. Clues about this have been sought by trying to show an association between CT abnormalities and indicators either of a genetic diathesis or of early neurodevelopmental damage—specifically, manifest family history of psychiatric disorder or a history of pregnancy and birth complications.

With regard to genetic factors, the original hypothesis, that ventricular enlargement was largely confined to those patients with no evident family history (Murray *et al.*, 1985), has received mixed support. In 1990, there had been 13 studies looking for this association, of which four had reported a significant inverse correlation between ventricular size and positive family history (Reveley *et al.*, 1984; Cazullo *et al.*, 1985; Turner *et al.*, 1986; Romani *et al.*, 1987). Most reports found no relationship (Kemali *et al.*, 1983; Pearlson *et al.*, 1985, 1989; Farmer *et al.*, 1987; Nimgaonkar *et al.*, 1988; Johnstone *et al.*, 1989; Kaiya *et al.*, 1989). However, many of these studies lacked adequate statistical power, and all are open to the problems of the family-history method—varying definitions, uncertain reliability and variable family sizes. In a meta-analysis of this area, Vita *et al.* (1994) were able to show a statistically significant effect across published studies. The study of Jones *et al.* (1994) also found an effect of family history. In a study designed to overcome the problem of limited power, Owens *et al.* (1989) compared ventricular size in 48 schizophrenic patients with a history of major affective disorder or schizophrenia in first-degree relatives, 48 schizophrenic patients with no such history in first- or second-degree relatives

and the same number of healthy controls. The three groups were matched for age and sex. Significant ventricular enlargement was found in those without a family history, as predicted. However, those patients with a family history positive for schizophrenia also showed significant enlarge-ment, against expectations, whereas a family history of affective disorder was associated with normal ventricular size.

Several studies have demonstrated a raised rate of obstetric complications in the histories of schizophrenic patients compared with other psychiatric patients, well siblings or unrelated controls (Lewis, 1989; Eagles *et al.*, 1990). This has led to the hypothesis that obstetric complications could be a risk factor for schizophrenia with abnormal CT findings. Like the assessment of family history, the assessment of past obstetric complications is dogged by problems of definition and, in most cases, relies on the memory of an informant, although a validation study has shown that such data can be reliable (O'Callaghan *et al.*, 1990). Thus, although a small number of studies have reported a positive association between a history of obstetric complications and ventricular size (Turner *et al.*, 1986; Pearlson *et al.*, 1989), frontal-horn area (De Lisi *et al.* 1986) and combinations of ventricular enlargement with sulcal (Owens *et al.*, 1988) or third-ventricle widening (Cannon *et al.*, 1989), a larger number of studies have shown no association.

In summary, the story of X-ray CT in schizophrenia research is at the same time enlightening and salutary. As a technique, its inception coincided with the renaissance of biological psychiatry in the 1970s, and a torrent of early studies were more or less agreed that ventricular enlargement characterised a large proportion of patients with schizophrenia. More recently, there have been several large, properly controlled studies, which have signalled caution about the initial enthusiasm. It is still fair to conclude that relative enlargement of third and lateral ventricles and cortical sulci is found in some schizophrenic patients, but the extent of these changes is probably not as marked as first thought. The failure of several rigorous studies to demonstrate these changes has yet to be explained. Variation in sampling methods of patients seems increasingly to be an important factor when appropriate control groups are used. What factors determine the various structural brain parameters in the general population remains an under-researched area and it is becoming obvious that a range of interacting demographic factors, such as age, sex, socioeconomic status, race, educational level and alcohol consumption, are important.

Magnetic resonance imaging

MRI is now the definitive *in vivo* structural brain-imaging technique. MRI has the advantages of not using ionising radiation, and its high resolution, good tissue contrast and multiplanar abilities make it the technique of choice in looking at detailed brain structure. Contraindications to MRI include: (i) metallic implants, e.g. aneurysm clips or orthopaedic screws; (ii) metallic foreign bodies, e.g. metal-lathe eye injuries or shotgun injuries; and (iii) pregnancy (potential risk unknown).

As noted in Chapter 3, MRI is a means of detecting a spatially localised signal which arises from the magnetic property of atomic nuclei. The most commonly used sequences for structural imaging are those called *spin–echo* and *inversion recovery*, as noted in Chapter 3. The disadvantage of inversion recovery is long imaging time and hence the potential for movement artefact. Reducing imaging time by lessening the number of data acquisitions is at the expense of the signal-to-noise ratio. Physiological movement can be taken into account by cardiac or respiratory gating. Faster imaging techniques, e.g. gradient echo-pulse sequences, have particular uses in blood-flow angiography and for detecting cerebrospinal fluid (CSF) pulsation. Ultrafast techniques, such as echo-planar imaging, are increasingly being applied for functional imaging. The T1 and T2 values for CSF, white and grey matter are shown in Table 10.1. In a heavily T1-

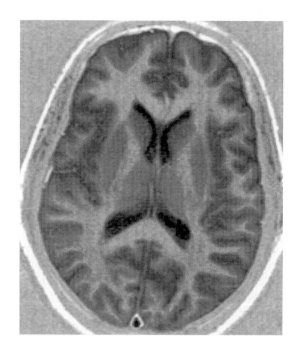

Fig. 10.4 An inversion-recovery, highly T1-weighted, MR image of the brain in the axial plane. This image shows maximal contrast between white matter and cortical and subcortical grey matter.

Table 10.1 T1 and T2 relaxation times for the three main tissues (in seconds).

Tissue	T1	T2
Cerebrospinal fluid	4.0	2.0
Grey matter	1.0	0.08
White matter	0.6	0.03

weighted image of the brain, white matter appears lighter than grey matter and CSF (Fig. 10.4). In a T2-weighted image, white matter is darker than grey matter and CSF. The high resolution of brain anatomy now possible using MRI, together with new computerised measuring techniques, have enabled researchers to refine their exploration of brain abnormalities in schizophrenia. Using MRI, it is now possible to examine the size of constituent brain regions and, with the aid of advanced computer-analysis techniques, it is possible to determine the relative contributions to those regions of grey matter, white matter and CSF.

Volumetric analysis

Many research studies using MRI in psychiatry measure volume or areas of anatomical regions. High resolution plus appropriate imaging sequences are required to maximise contrast. In general, resolution has improved considerably in recent years with the use of more powerful magnets and more refined hardware. Early studies using planimetry and simple linear or area measures have evolved to more accurate volume measurements with computer-outlining techniques. Usually slices of 1–10 mm thick are taken and the anatomical region is outlined and volume estimated from the area multiplied by slice thickness. The thinner the slice, the better the estimate of volume as long as resolution is adequate. However, as the slice becomes thinner, the signal:noise ratio is reduced. There is therefore the need to balance these factors, which depend on the technology available.

It was soon realized that the sensitivity of MRI allowed more interesting hypotheses to be tested in schizophrenia. With CT research, the ventricular system had been the centre of scientific attention, largely because it was one of the only things which could be measured objectively on CT. The ability of MRI to image in several planes and to differentiate between different compartments of brain tissue led on to measurement of discrete brain structures rather than fluid spaces. The different dispositions of hydrogen atoms in grey and white matter, largely dictated by differences in water content, allowed volumetric measurements of the two compartments independently. This has not been possible with CT, partly because the electron density of the two tissues was similar, and partly because artefacts generated by nearby bone stopped realistic measurement of the cerebral cortex.

Some artefacts of area and volume measure-ments applicable to CT are still constraints with MRI. In particular, the partial-volume artefact can still be a difficulty, especially when measuring small structures or convoluted surfaces. The increasing use of very thin, contiguous slices down to 1–2 mm and image-analysis techniques which allow for resegmentation and reconstruction in other planes are important in overcoming partial-volume measurements in measuring small structures.

MRI studies: influences on normal anatomy

The importance of MRI in psychiatric research is to enable extension of post-mortem brain studies by providing the means to measure neuroanatomical regions *in vivo*. As noted above, MRI can detect boundaries between grey and white matter within anatomical regions. Combining structural MRI with information using clinical, neuropsychological, neurophysiological and functional neuroimaging techniques provides a powerful means of detecting important relationships between brain structure and function in psychiatry. Before conclusions can be drawn in psychiatric disease states, we must understand how some demographic and other factors can influence normal variations.

Normal brain asymmetry

In the normal brain, the left occipital pole is larger and extends more posteriorly than the right, whereas the right frontal region is often larger and protrudes more anteriorly than does the left. The right temporal region is usually larger than the left. Compared with the right, on the left side the planum temporale is larger and the Sylvian fissure ascends more steeply and extends more posteriorly (Jack *et al.*, 1988). In general, men show more hemispheric asymmetry than women (Bear *et al.*, 1986). The corpus callosum is possibly larger and more bulbous posteriorly in women and non-right-handers (De Lacoste-Utamsing & Holloway, 1982; Witelson, 1989). Right-handed persons have more cerebral asymmetry than left-handers. Cerebral size in women is less than in men. This difference is probably related to factors determining height (Andreasen *et al.*, 1986).

Age

Brain shrinkage occurs as age advances. This shrinkage becomes more prominent after the age of 55. Studies using MRI have demonstrated age-related decreases in volume of cerebral-cortical grey matter, basal ganglia and anterior dien-cephalic grey matter (Jernigan *et al.*, 1990; Jernigan *et al.*, 1991d). Murphy *et al.* (1992) compared two groups of normal subjects aged <35 and >60 and found specific reduction in lenticular and caudate nuclei, after taking reduced cerebral size into account. Volume of lateral ventricles, third ventricle and CSF were all greater in the older group. Normal brain asymmetry was preserved. Even in people less than 45 years old, age probably accounts for 25–45% of the variance in the proportion of grey matter in the brain (Zipursky *et al.*, 1992).

Social class

A negative association has been reported between socioeconomic status and brain size (Pearlson *et al.*, 1989). It has been suggested that this association may be due to poor nutrition adversely affecting brain growth. The association may also be partly due to the fact that people with conditions that result in brain shrinkage 'drift' down the social scale as a result of their condition. Using paternal social class to match subject groups may take account of social drift.

Intelligence and education

Intelligence accounts for about 12–30% of the variance in brain size of normal individuals, which is greater the higher the intelligence quotient (IQ). Andreasen *et al.* (1993) found IQ correlated with volumes of cerebrum, cerebellum, temporal lobe, hippocampus and grey matter. There was no such correlation with white matter,

CSF, caudate or lateral-ventricular volume. The finding of decreased frontal lobe size in schizophrenic subjects was later attributed to the choice of a control group with more years of education (Andreasen *et al.*, 1986). Comparison of the same patient group with a control group matched for education did not reveal differences in frontal lobe size (Andreasen *et al.*, 1990).

MRI is very sensitive to lesions which may persist after full clinical recovery from trauma. There may, for example, be distinct foci or more generalised atrophy observed. Special care needs to be exercised in evaluating individuals likely to have such lesions before including them in research study groups.

Alcohol and the brain

Alcohol is a common drug of misuse with potential to affect brain structure. We will therefore consider it in a little detail. Chronic alcoholism is the source of considerable psychiatric and social morbidity. The prevalence of alcohol dependence in the UK is about 3.5% (Edwards *et al.*, 1972). Up to 60% of patients from alcoholism units have a detectable abnormality on CT brain scan (Ron, 1983). It is therefore possible that as many as 2% of adults suffer alcohol-related brain damage.

Post-mortem studies have demonstrated reduced brain volume and enlarged ventricles (Harper & Kril, 1990). The extent to which cerebral changes due to alcoholism are a result of white-matter loss or cortical neuronal loss is still debated. Harper & Kril (1987) reported neuronal death in brains or alcoholic subjects, whereas Jensen and Pakkenberg (1993) did not. Reduced brain volume in the latter study was accounted for by diminution in white matter.

Neuroimaging studies *in vivo* have also found generalised brain abnormalities in alcoholism. CT scan studies reported ventricular enlargement and widening of cerebral sulci and Sylvian and interhemispheric fissures, which partially reversed after abstinence (Carlen *et al.*, 1978; Ron, 1983). MRI studies have provided a more detailed picture of neuroanatomical disruption in alcoholics. For instance, highly significant increases of cerebral (particularly cortical) and ventricular CSF have been associated with generally decreased cortical and subcortical grey matter (Jernigan *et al.*, 1991a). These findings were confirmed by Pfefferbaum *et al.* (1992), who also noted generalised white-matter loss.

A rarer form of alcohol-induced white-matter pathology affecting the corpus callosum is Marchiafava–Bignami disease. Recently MRI studies have indicated that chronic forms of corpus callosum atrophy may occur in alcoholism (Chang *et al.*, 1992), and that these changes are, to some extent, reversible (Izquierdo *et al.*, 1992).

Using MRI it has been demonstrated that alcoholic subjects who developed Wernicke–Korsakoff's syndrome (WKS) had more damage to anterior diencephalon, orbitofrontal cortex and medial-temporal lobes than those unaffected by this syndrome (Jernigan *et al.*, 1991b; Blansjaar *et al.*, 1992). Mamillary nuclei measured using MRI were smaller in patients with alcohol-induced Korsakoff's amnesia when compared with non-Korsakoff's amnesic patients (Squire *et al.*, 1990). Patients with WKS may also exhibit more generalised brain abnormalities, such as ventricular enlargement and cerebral shrinkage similar to that found in non-WKS alcoholic patients (Jacobson & Lishman, 1990). Like WKS patients, non-WKS chronic alcoholics may additionally develop regional abnormalities, such as those in the caudate and lenticular nucleus, diencephalon, medial-temporal region, dorsolateral prefrontal cortex and parieto-occipital cortex (Jernigan *et al.*, 1991a).

Preliminary evidence provided by CT studies that the frontal lobes are preferentially affected in alcoholism (Jacobson & Lishman, 1990) has been confirmed by some MRI studies (Jernigan *et al.*, 1991a), but not others (Pfefferbaum *et al.*, 1992). Reversible and irreversible brain shrinkage have both been demonstrated in alcoholism using MRI. Short-term abstinence (4–6 weeks) may reverse changes seen on earlier scans (presumably through rehydration) (Zipursky *et al.*, 1989), although this is not a universal finding (Kroft *et al.*, 1991).

Like the CT studies before (e.g. Ron, 1983), brain changes showed only a modest relationship to drinking history in some studies, but alcoholism did appear to accelerate the cerebral effects of ageing (Pfefferbaum *et al.*, 1992). Other studies, however, have shown that length of drinking history was associated with increased cerebral CSF (Mann *et al.*, 1989). The cerebral changes in alcoholic subjects (e.g. increased CSF volume and raised T1) have been associated with poorer performance on a number of cognitive tasks, although in studies so far these appear to be relatively non-specific (Ron, 1983; Chick *et al.*, 1989; Jernigan *et al.*, 1991a). There is some evidence that females are more vulnerable to cerebral changes due to alcoholism (Mann *et al.*, 1992).

Opiates, cocaine, solvents, benzodiazepines and other drugs or chemicals may also be related to brain abnormalities (Schmauss & Krieg, 1987; Strang & Gurling, 1989; Leira *et al.*, 1992) although the evidence is far less consistent than for alcohol. It is therefore prudent to take account of drug abuse in studies designated to investigate brain abnormalities from other causes.

Iatrogenic causes

There is little evidence that neuroleptic medication *per se* alters brain structure detectably using MRI, except perhaps the basal ganglia. Studies in psychotic patients do not generally find correlations between brain size and length of exposure to, or dose of, antipsychotics (Suddath *et al.*, 1990). However, at least two careful studies, one in first-episode patients followed up and rescanned at 18 months (Chakos *et al.*, 1994), have now shown that antipsychotic drug treatment seems to cause a modest (5–10%), cumulative, dose-related increase in caudate-nucleus volume. This effect has also been shown in animal studies. It may be due to neuronal hypertrophy in the striatum as a result of dopamine blockade.

On the evidence available, it is unlikely that electroconvulsive therapy (ECT) results in brain abnormalities (Coffey *et al.*, 1991). T1 values may rise acutely after ECT and return to normal within hours. The rise in T1 level probably represents temporary disruption of the blood–brain barrier (Mander *et al.*, 1987).

MRI in schizophrenia

Ventricular size

One of the most consistent findings using structural brain imaging of schizophrenic patients has been that of increased lateral-ventricular size (Table 10.2). Increased third- and fourth-ventricular size has also been demonstrated in schizophrenia. Ventricular size in normal subjects varies regionally such that left occipital and right posterotemporal horns are largest (Degreef *et al.*, 1992), so studies that only take measurements from a few slices can give misleading results. For these reasons, it is better to measure whole-ventricular size and covary statistically for the effects of whole-brain volume (Arndt *et al.*, 1991). Using such a technique, Kelsoe (Kelsoe *et al.*, 1988) found a 62% greater lateral-ventricular volume and 73% larger third-ventricular volume in schizophrenics, compared with normal controls. Degreef *et al.* (1992) measured the entire ventricular system in 40 patients with their first episode of schizophrenia. Lateral-ventricular volume was 26% greater than in normal controls, particularly in the left temporal and frontal horns. Left temporal-horn volumes correlated with positive and negative symptoms, including hallucinations, bizarre behaviour, affective flattening, attention deficit and anhedonia. Other studies have found correlations between lateral- and third-ventricular enlargement and positive symptoms (Young *et al.*, 1991). Increased ventricular size has been related to poor outcome (Shenton *et al.*, 1992).

Ventricular enlargement, when noted, tends to be more pronounced on the left side. Of at least four studies that commented on lateralised differences of ventricular size in schizophrenia, all reported more ventricular enlargement on the left, particularly in the temporofrontal region (Kelsoe

et al., 1988; Johnstone *et al.*, 1989; Degreef *et al.*, 1992; Harvey *et al.*, 1993). This fits in with neuropathological studies that noted enlargement of the temporal horn of the left ventricle in brains of schizophrenics (Bogerts *et al.*, 1990). It was suggested that such enlargement might be associated with a regional brain abnormality, such as tissue loss of surrounding medial-temporal structures, (*vide infra*).

To address the issue as to whether ventricular and sulcal CSF volume are directly related, Gur *et al.* (1994) measured both sulcal CSF and VBR in a large group of schizophrenic patients. Patients with predominantly negative symptoms had significantly greater VBR but only marginal differences in cerebral volume or whole-brain sulcal CSF volume compared with controls. This, they argued, was a pattern consistent with degenerative brain atrophy. Schizophrenic patients with positive symptoms have also been found to have enlarged lateral and third ventricles (Degreef *et al.*, 1992). This contrasts with further observations of Gur *et al.* (1994) that raised VBR in patients with predominantly Schneiderian positive symptoms was due to significantly reduced cranial and brain volumes and not increased ventricular or CSF volume. For this, cerebral developmental abnormality was a suggested explanation. Paranoid patients had a reduced sulcal CSF : brain ratio, explained by late developmental problems in these patients. The latter contention was based on Jernigan *et al.* (1991c), who state that throughout normal brain development in adolescence the sulcal CSF volume increases. Figure 10.5 illustrates the coexistence of enlarged ventricles without increased sulcal CSF, consistent with an early developmental brain pattern according to Gur *et al.* (1994).

As noted with CT, ventricular enlargement is found even in patients in their first psychotic illness. This suggests that these brain abnormalities are long-standing. The lack of correlation between ventricular size and duration of illness further suggests non-progression of structural brain abnormalities once symptoms develop

Table 10.2 MRI studies of cerebral and ventricular size in schizophrenia versus normal controls.

Study	Patients/ controls	Male/female patients	Brain[1] area (a) or vol. (v)	Sulcal CSF	Ventricular area (a) or vol. (v)	VBR
Matthew *et al.*, 1985	18/18	11/7	< (a)	–	–	–
Andreasen *et al.*, 1986	38/49	28/10	m < (a)	–	–	–
Stratta *et al.*, 1989	20/20	15/5	< (a)	–	–	>*, 4=
Kelsoe *et al.*, 1988	27/14	22/5	< (v)	–	L > * R < (v)	–
Rossi *et al.*, 1988	15/15	15/0	< (a)	–	–	>
Hauser *et al.*, 1989	24/25	11/9	> (a)	–	–	–
Johnstone *et al.*, 1989	21/21	15/6	> (a)	–	R < L > (a)	–
Rossi *et al.*, 1989	12/12	8/4	< (a)	–	–	>* 4 >
Barta et al. 1990	15/15	15/0	< (v)	–	3 > (v)	
Casanova *et al.*, 1990[2]	12/12	5/7	< (a)	–	–	–
Dauphinais *et al.*, 1990	28/21	15/13	< * (v)	–	>*, 3 > (v)	>*
Nasrallah *et al.*, 1990	56/35	41/15	< (a)	–	3f >* (a)	m <f >*
Raine *et al.*, 1990	15/18	9/6	f < (a)	–	–	–
Rossi *et al.*, 1990	17/13	10/7	> (a)	–	> (a)	>
Suddath *et al.*, 1990[2]	15/15	8/7	–	–	>*, 3 >* (v)	–
DeLisi *et al.*, 1991[3]	15/20	9/6	< (v)	–	>*4 (v)	–
Gur *et al.*, 1991	42/43	27/15	m < f < (v)	m >* f<	m= f > (v)	>*
Jernigan *et al.*, 1991d	42/24	28/14	< (v)	>	>*4 (v)	–
Young *et al.*, 1991	31/33	24/7	–	–	–	> 3>
Bornstein *et al.*, 1992	72/31	49/23	–	–	–	L >* 3>
Degreef *et al.*, 1992	40/25	25/15	–	–	L > R 3 > (v)	–

(Continued)

[1] Whether intracranial or cerebral measurements performed was not specified.
[2] Twins.
[3] Neurological controls.
[4] Controlled for head size.
L, left; R, right; m, males; f, females; GM, grey matter; WM, white matter; *, statistically significant; <, less than in controls; >, greater than in controls; =, equal to that in controls.

Table 10.2 *Continued*

Study	Patients/ controls	Male/female patients	Intracranial area (a) or vol (v)	Cerebral area (a) or vol. (v)	Sulcal CSF	Ventricular area (a) or vol (v)	VBR
Breier *et al.*, 1992	44/29	29/15	< (v)	–	–	–	–
di Michele *et al.*, 1992	25/17	13/12	> (a)	–	–	–	–
Shenton *et al.*, 1992	15/15	15/0	> (v)	GM> WM > (v)	<	> 3 =, 4 = (v)	>
Zipursky *et al.*, 1992	22/20	22/0	= (v)	GM <* WM > (v)	>*	>* (v) 3 > (a)	–
Harvey *et al.*, 1993	48/34	37/11	< (v)	GM <* WM = (v)	m >*	Rm<, RF> Lm> Lf>*	–
Woodruff *et al.*, 1993	30/44	23/7	–	m <* (a)	–	–	–
Gur *et al.*, 1994	81/81	50/31	–	<* (v)	m>	>* (v)	f >*

[1] Whether intracranial or cerebral measurements performed was not specified.
[2] Twins.
[3] Neurological controls.
[4] Controlled for head size.
L, left; R, right; m, males; f, females; GM, grey matter; WM, white matter; *, statistically significant; <, less than in controls; >, greater than in controls; =, equal to that in controls.

(Young *et al.*, 1991). As fetal brain tissue expands, the ventricle: brain volume ratio decreases.

The implication of ventricular abnormalities for the aetiology of schizophrenia. As the normal brain develops, the VBR decreases. It has therefore been argued that increased VBR in schizophrenia may represent immaturity of the brain, although ventricular volume itself may not be increased. Raised VBR may also be due to sequelae of periventricular haemorrhage, with consequent effects on cortical development. Brain abnormalities in schizophrenia could be consequent upon early brain insult, together with a genetically predetermined process (Jones & Murray, 1991). If so, the brain abnormalities should be detectable at or before the onset of symptoms, and show little progression thereafter. To answer this question properly, long-term prospective follow-up studies need to be performed to monitor the effect of illness on ventricular size. These studies are very difficult, not least because rapidly advancing MRI techno- logy makes the comparison of scans taken years apart unreliable. The studies that have collected prospective MRI data have not so far demonstrated a clear pattern. Therefore we have to rely on evidence provided by cross-sectional data. Evidence of ventricular enlargement in schizophrenic patients at first presentation suggests that these abnormalities are of long-standing (DeLisi *et al.*, 1992). Also the lack of correlation between ventricular size and length of illness favours non-progression in these brain abnormalities (Young *et al.*, 1991), although this is not a universal finding. It would, therefore, be premature on the MRI evidence so far available to discount progressive brain abnormalities in schizophrenia.

The ventricular system does not *itself* contain the neurons whose defective function mediates clinical features of schizophrenia. However, during early brain development, neurons are formed by proliferation from the ventricular lining and a subventricular zone, from which they later migrate to cortical regions. From here, axons grow, myelinate and form synaptic connections.

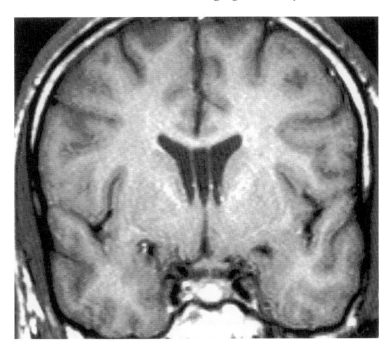

Fig. 10.5 Ventricular enlargement with relatively preserved cerebral structure in a schizophrenic patient: a coronal view. (Note also septun pellucidum.)

The final neuronal configuration is then modified by a process of axonal elimination. Therefore, enlarged ventricles in schizophrenia may be the result of abnormal early neurodevelopment, which also results in aberrant neuronal connections in cortical regions. It is important therefore to look closely at evidence for abnormalities in cortical regions that may be linked to ventricular abnormalities and may explain connections between these and the clinical features of schizophrenia.

Frontal lobe

There are both clinical and theoretical reasons why the frontal lobe should be considered important in our understanding of schizophrenia. Schizophrenics may exhibit symptoms similar to patients with frontal-lobe lesions, e.g. deficits of attention, abstract thinking and judgement, motivation and volition, fluency of speech and impulse control. A wealth of neuropsychological data have demonstrated that schizophrenic subjects perform particularly poorly on tests that draw upon neural networks concentrated in the frontal lobes (Goldberg *et al.*, 1990). Much of the functional neuroimaging data using tests such as the Wisconsin Card Sort Test provides further support for the idea that the frontal lobe is underactive in schizophrenia (Weinberger *et al.*, 1992).

Because the frontal lobe is structurally an ill-defined region and consists of complex neural networks, it may be simplistic to assume that changes in its gross structure are related to the clinical expression of schizophrenia. But, as techniques improve, so the more subtle links between structural and functional abnormalities in schizophrenia can be examined. Early attempts with MRI were suggestive of reduced frontal-lobe size in schizophrenic subjects compared with normal controls (Andreasen *et al.*, 1986). A later failure to replicate these findings with a control group better matched for educational level cast doubt on the validity of previous findings (Andreasen *et al.*, 1990). However, some more recent studies, using high-resolution MRI, have demonstrated specific grey- and white-matter reduction in the frontal lobes of schizophrenic patients (Breier *et al.*, 1992; Zipursky *et al.*, 1992). Reasons for these early inconsistencies may include difficulty of reliably measuring an area so dependent on head tilt (Fig. 10.6a,b), different selection criteria for controls and high variability of frontal-lobe size within the schizophrenic sample. It may be that only a subgroup of schizophrenic subjects with deficient frontal-lobe function exhibit abnormalities of frontal-lobe structure. For instance, deficient common-sense judgement, well recognised in those with frontal-lobe lesions, was related to reduced frontal-lobe size in schizophrenia (Woodruff *et al.*, 1994b).

Can frontal-lobe abnormalities in schizophrenia be further localised? Functional neuro-imaging findings in schizophrenia have focused attention on the dorsolateral prefrontal cortex (Weinberger *et al.*, 1992). In addition to post-mortem evidence that neurons are abnormally organised in the prefrontal region of schizophrenic brains (Benes *et al.*, 1991), membrane abnormalities in the dorsolateral prefrontal cortex

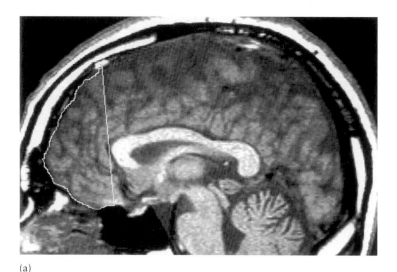

(a)

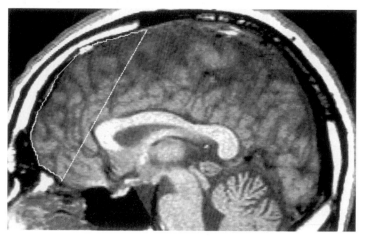

(b)

Fig. 10.6 Midsagittal images of the brain with the frontal lobe region outlined in white. Most studies take sections coronal to the plane shown, and, by adding the areas together, it is possible to calculate the frontal-lobe volume. The two images demonstrate the importance of taking account of head tilt. The volume calculated on the frontal lobe defined in (a) is significantly less than in (b).

(reduced nicotinamide adenine dinucleotide phosphate (NADP) diaphorase concentration) have recently been described (Akbarian *et al.*, 1993a,b). The latter is consistent with the MRI spectroscopic finding of abnormal phospholipid metabolism in this region (Pettergrew *et al.*, 1991).

Structural MRI studies have also provided some evidence for lateralised frontal-lobe abnormalities. Increased T2 levels in the left frontal region were described by Williamson *et al.* (1991). More recently, structural abnormalities in the left dorsolateral prefrontal cortex have been reported which correspond to deficits in shifting cognitive set, abstract reasoning and vigilance (functions thought to be performed in this part of the brain) (Seidman *et al.*, 1994). But the frontal lobe, like the rest of the brain, does not work in isolation. For instance, underactivity of the dorsolateral prefrontal cortex in schizophrenia during a working-memory task was linked to hippocampal volume (Weinberger *et al.*, 1992). Such volume changes may be reflected in function. Preliminary evidence has linked reduced dorsolateral prefrontal cortex activity with increased hippocampal activity in schizophrenics (Berman *et al.*, 1994).

Temporal lobes, hippocampus and related brain regions

The temporal lobes have been the focus of much MRI work in schizophrenia for a number of reasons. It has long been recognised that patients with temporal-lobe epilepsy, perhaps particularly on the left, may experience psychotic states indistinguishable from schizophrenia, and electrical stimulation of the temporal lobe can elicit psychotic symptoms. Therefore, one hypothesis in schizophrenia has been that the primary symptoms of auditory hallucinations, thought disorder and delusions are due to temporal-lobe abnormalities and might be reflected in reduced size, perhaps particularly on the left side. At least 13 MRI studies have compared temporal-lobe volume between patients and controls; 12 find

less volume on the left (statistically significant in seven studies) and nine on the right (statistically significant in three studies) (Table 10.3). Three studies measured grey and white matter separately; all found temporal-lobe grey-matter reduction in schizophrenic subjects, one found white-matter reduction bilaterally and another white-matter reduction on the left and increase on the right.

In order to interpret accurately these findings it is necessary to focus even more closely on constituent regions within the temporal lobe, such as the hippocampus, concerned with memory. A discordant identical twin study reported both lateral-ventricular enlargement and reduced temporal-lobe grey matter (including hippocampal volume) in schizophrenic probands (Suddath *et al.*, 1990). More specifically, reduced left hippocampal volume and its association with impaired verbal memory scores distinguished affected from non-affected cotwins (Goldberg *et al.*, 1990). A number of other studies have also reported reduced hippocampal volumes in schizophrenic subjects on both left and right sides (Table 10.3).

Another area within the temporal lobe of interest in schizophrenia is the superior temporal gyrus (STG), concerned with auditory association and perception. Stimulation of this area can result in auditory hallucinations. Therefore it was of especial interest when Barta *et al.* (1990) found that schizophrenic subjects had less STG volume than controls and that this decrease was associated with auditory hallucinations. In addition, Shenton *et al.* (1992) described localised reduction of left posterior STG volume in schizophrenia which correlated with the degree of thought disorder. These important studies indicate that in schizophrenia the tendency to experience specific symptoms (auditory hallucinations) is associated with the volume of a brain region functionally related to the symptom (auditory association). However, the true situation is likely to be much more complex and these findings need to be replicated. For instance, a recent study did not find an association between thought disorder or

Table 10.3 MRI studies of brain regions in schizophrenics versus normal controls.

Study	Left temporal lobe	Right temporal lobe	Corpus callosum	Frontal lobe	Hippocampus/ amygdala
Matthew *et al.*, 1985			>		
Nasrallah *et al.*, 1986			>		
Andreasen *et al.*, 1986				<*	
Smith *et al.*, 1987					
Kelsoe *et al.*, 1988	<	<	<	R >, L =	>
Rossi *et al.*, 1989			<		
Bogerts *et al.*, 1990	>	>			L < m*
Hauser *et al.*, 1989[1]			<		
Johnstone *et al.*, 1989[1]	<, L < R*	<			
Rossi *et al.*, 1989			<*		
Stratta *et al.*, 1989			<*		
Barta *et al.*, 1990	STG <*	STG <*			<, < L*
Casanova *et al.*, 1990			>		
Dauphinais *et al.*, 1990	<	<			R, L < m L < f
Nasrallah *et al.*, 1990				<	
Raine *et al.*, 1990			< m		
Rossi *et al.*, 1990	<*	<*	=	<	
Suddath *et al.*, 1990	WM < GM <*	WM > GM <		WM < GM <	R <* L < *
DeLisi *et al.*, 1991[2]	<	<			<
Young *et al.*, 1991	<	>	<	>	=
Breier *et al.*, 1992				WM < *	<*
di Michele *et al.*, 1992	<*				
Shenton *et al.*, 1992	< STG*	NS			<*
Zipursky *et al.*, 1992	GM <*	GM <*		GM <*	
Harvey *et al.*, 1993	GM < WM <	GM < WM <			
Woodruff *et al.*, 1993			< *m		

[1] Studies that included an affective disorder patient group.
[2] Neurological controls.
L, left; R, right; m, males; f, females; GM, grey matter; WM, white matter; STG, superior temporal gyrus; *, statistically significant; NS, not significant; <, less than in controls; >, greater than in controls; =, equal to that in controls.

auditory hallucinations and STG size in first-episode schizophrenia (DeLisi *et al.*, 1992). One problem may be difficulty in defining the functionally relevant gyrus throughout its length in different subjects. Figure 10.7(a,b) illustrate how the STG anatomy changes along its length. This observation highlights the potential difficulty in choosing anatomically equivalent slices in different individuals.

Language is an asymmetrical cerebral function.

Much MRI research has therefore focused on structural asymmetry of the temporal lobes in schizophrenia. Recent work has concentrated on the planum temporale, a region of superior temporal cortex near Heschl's gyrus and beneath the Sylvian fissure. Here, sexual dimorphism of the brain is particularly pronounced. A recent MRI study has confirmed *in vivo* post-mortem observations that in normal males the planum temporale is more asymmetrical (left larger than

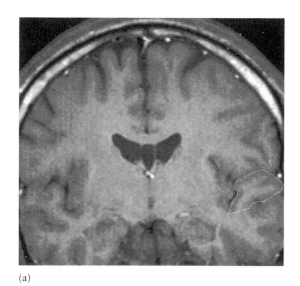

(a)

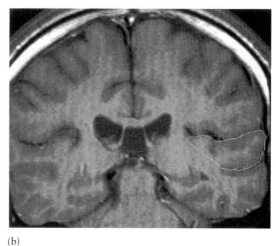

(b)

Fig. 10.7 The superior temporal gyrus (STG) changes shape considerably along its axis. (a) The 'finger-like' anterior STG (outlined in white). (b) The posterior STG and adjoining Heschl's gyrus medially (outlined). Studies of auditory association cortex would normally exclude Heschl's gyrus from the region of interest.

right) than in females (Kulynych *et al.*, 1994). Using groups matched by sex, several studies have reported differences in asymmetry of the planum temporale between schizophrenic subjects and controls. For instance, Rossi *et al.* (1992) reported that schizophrenic patients exhibited reduced asymmetry of the planum temporale, an observation associated with thought disorder. DeLisi *et al.* (1992) found a similar pattern without an association with thought disorder. Other studies have not found differences in asymmetry (Falkai *et al.*, 1994; Kleinschmidt *et al.*, 1994).

The left temporal lobe normally develops later than the right. So processess leading to abnormalities of late fetal brain development might have more impact on left than right temporal-lobe development (Woodruff & Murray, 1994a). As the left planum temporale is usually larger than the right, the net effect of a disruption to normal development would be reduced asymmetry up to the point when both sides were of equal size. Thereafter asymmetry would increase in the reverse direction. The work that demonstrated

mainly left temporal-lobe diminution (particularly the STG) in schizophrenic subjects compared with controls is therefore compatible with reduced planum temporale asymmetry.

The corpus callosum

Many studies using MRI have examined the corpus callosum in schizophrenia. A consistent pattern of abnormality is now emerging (Woodruff *et al.*, 1995).

The corpus callosum has long been considered important in studies of insanity (Clarke, 1987). One model of schizophrenia was that of splitting of psychic functions. The corpus callosum is the largest brain tissue which connects corresponding regions of the two hemispheres. Therefore, abnormalities of hemispheric connection would be likely to involve the corpus callosum. A number of neuropsychological studies provide supporting evidence for interhemispheric dysconnection in schizophrenia (Coger & Serafetinides, 1990).

The first demonstrated association between psychosis and dysgenesis of the corpus callosum, by Lewis *et al.* (1988), has been confirmed by others in a large series of schizophrenic patients (Swayze *et al.*, 1990). Another anomaly related developmentally to the corpus callosum is cavum septum pellucidum, where a congenital cystic space is found in the midline fibrous panel that separates the frontal horns, the septum pellucidum (see Fig. 10.5). An association between this and schizophrenia was also first noted in six patients, all male and with histories of developmental delays, on CT (Lewis and Mezey, 1985). In a later MRI study, this lesion was detected in 21% of schizophrenic patients compared with 2% of controls (Degreef *et al.*, 1992). These associations suggest that neurodevelopmental damage to the corpus callosum and related midline structures may predispose to the later onset of psychosis.

Several early post-mortem studies, suggesting that the corpus callosum size was marginally increased in a small sample of schizophrenic brains, stimulated MRI studies to determine the *in vivo* structure of the corpus callosum in schizophrenia (Rosenthal & Bigelow, 1972; Bigelow *et al.*, 1983). Early studies using linear measures of width and length of the corpus callosum found few significant differences between schizophrenics and controls, although there was a suggestion that length was increased (Woodruff *et al.*, 1993). The corpus callosum has

an extremely variable shape as defined with MRI (Casanova *et al.*, 1990). This variable shape may lead to misleading results using width measures (Fig. 10.8). For instance, Woodruff *et al.* (1993) found that group differences in corpus callosum widths varied depending on whether widths were drawn perpendicularly or vertically to the corpus callosum surface. This prompted the authors to suggest that area measures were more suitable for detecting differences between groups.

Other possible reasons for the lack of differences observed in early studies may have included small sample size and inadequate correction for the effects of sex and handedness on corpus callosum size. Normally, females have a more bulbous and thicker posterior corpus callosum than males (De Lacoste-Utamsing & Holloway, 1982). Greater corpus callosum widths in schizophrenic subjects than controls reported by Nasrallah *et al.* (1986) and Raine *et al.* (1990) were in females. This was counter to the finding of Hauser *et al.* (1989). Although there was no difference in corpus callosum area between right-handed male schizophrenic subjects and equivalent controls, Nasrallah *et al.* (1986) found that, compared with left-handed male controls, left-handed male schizophrenic subjects had statistically significantly reduced corpus callosum area. Later studies found reduced corpus callosum area more generally in male schizophrenic

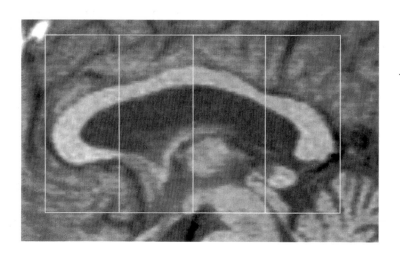

Fig. 10.8 The shape of the corpus callosum varies considerably between individuals. This makes measurement of widths, as opposed to areas, unreliable. Reduced area measures have been found in schizophrenia, particularly in the central isthmus (bisected by the fourth perpendicular from the left), which transmits fibres between the two superior temporal gyri.

subjects (Woodruff *et al.*, 1993). The pattern of handedness and corpus callosum size in schizophrenia may be different from that in controls. Normally, left-handed individuals have a larger corpus callosum isthmus than right-handed subjects (Witelson & Goldsmith, 1991). The opposite pattern was observed in MRI measurements of the corpus callosum area in schizophrenic subjects (Nasrallah *et al.*, 1986).

In order to clarify whether or not corpus callosum structure is abnormal in schizophrenia, a recent meta-analysis of 13 published MRI studies of the corpus callosum was carried out. Together, the studies comprised 313 patients and 281 controls. The results revealed that corpus callosum area was indeed significantly smaller in schizophrenics than in controls ($P < 0.02$) (Woodruff *et al.*, 1995). It was not possible from these studies to ascertain the specificity of reduced corpus callosum size in schizophrenia. Most take account of brain size by calculating a ratio of corpus callosum area to brain area, data constrained by similar problems as apply to VBR (*vide supra*) (Harvey *et al.*, 1990; Arndt *et al.*, 1991). However, one study, which made statistical adjustments to account for effects of brain size, also found significantly reduced corpus callosum area in schizophrenia (Woodruff *et al.*, 1993). In this study, reduced corpus callosum area was particularly marked in the central region of the corpus callosum, which transmits fibres between the two STGs. This provided some circumstantial support for the hypothesis that immature development of the STG is accompanied by fewer homotopic fibres connecting it with the STG on the opposite side. This study also reported a possible association between reduced corpus callosum size in schizophrenic patients and delusions. David *et al.* (1995) also described an association between auditory hallucinations in schizophrenia and reduced anterior corpus callosum area. In contrast, Gunther *et al.* (1991) found that larger corpus callosum size in schizophrenic subjects was associated with positive symptoms and smaller corpora callosa with negative symptoms. The relationship between corpus callosum size and shape and cerebral asymmetry of the superior temporal cortex (e.g. planum temporale), and the expression of these abnormalities as symptoms and neuropsychological deficits in schizophrenia requires much further research.

Whole brain

Reduced cerebral size has been reported in many MRI studies of schizophrenia (Table 10.2). Alterations in whole-brain size are not necessarily equal to those of constituent regions. For example, Barta *et al.* (1990) found a 2% decrease in whole brain as opposed to a decrease of 7–10% in temporal lobes. Whole-brain volumes were slightly greater in patients than in controls, despite reductions in STG gyrus volume in the study of Shenton *et al.* (1992). The normal relationship between height and brain size may be lost in schizophrenia: cerebral size is less despite preservation of height. One study has reported a loss of normal hemispheric asymmetry (larger right frontal, left occipital) in a group of 70 first-episode patients (Bilder *et al.*, 1994). This finding echoes some early CT studies but needs replication.

The questions remain as to whether the small but definite decreases in temporal-lobe grey matter are truly limited to the temporal lobe in schizophrenia and which brain compartment underlies the apparent reduction in overall volume. Theoretical considerations have focused attention on the medial temporal lobe, but recent MRI volumetric studies have suggested that more widespread volumetric decreases in grey matter are present. Harvey *et al.* (1993) controlled for a variety of anthropometric and demographic variables, including height, parental social class, age and gender, to show a small (9%) but highly significant reduction in diffuse cerebral-cortical grey-matter volume, but not white-matter volume, in schizophrenic patients compared with controls. Zipursky and colleagues (1992) in a careful study reported the same finding, that of a generalised reduction in grey-matter volume in schizophrenia compared with controls. Zipursky and colleagues had a second control group of age-matched alcohol-dependent subjects. In this group, grey matter volume was also reduced but in the presence of a proportional reduction in white matter volume also. This finding suggests that a global neurodegenerative process is not at work. Importantly, the findings seem to be specific to schizophrenia rather than psychosis in general. Harvey *et al.* (1993) found the grey-matter volume reduction in schizophrenic patients, but not in bipolar patients. Schlaepfer and colleagues (1994), in 46 schizophrenic subjects and 60 controls, found a 4.6% reduction in total grey-matter volume in patients. The volume reduction was most marked in hetero-modal association cortex in prefrontal, superior temporal and inferior parietal regions. This finding was not present in bipolar comparison subjects.

These most recent findings with structural MRI in schizophrenia support a hypothesis that it is a disorder of development of cerebral cortex, perhaps particularly association cortex.

Other psychoses: affective disorders

Imaging findings, particularly functional imaging, in affective disorders are described in Chapter 12. As with schizophrenia, studies using MRI have furthered knowledge already gained with CT and neuropathological techniques to investigate brain abnormalities in affective disorder. In particular, more specific quantitative evaluation of structural abnormalities and more sensitive detection of lesions have been possible with MRI. There are, however, difficulties in distinguishing findings from the effects of ageing in patients. This difficulty is compounded by the association between cerebrovascular disease and affective disorder (McDonald & Krishnan, 1992).

A number of MRI studies report ventricular enlargement and cortical atrophy, especially in elderly depressed patients. Reports of lateral- and third-ventricular enlargement in studies of patients with bipolar and unipolar illness have

been inconsistent (Coffey *et al.*, 1993). Temporal-lobe size reduction, reported in at least one study of patients with affective disorder (Altshuler *et al.*, 1991), was not confirmed in another (Johnstone *et al.*, 1989). Coffey *et al.* (1993) found reduced volume of cerebrum, frontal and temporal lobes, amygdala and hippocampus and an increase in lateral- and third-ventricle volume in depressed patients. However, only frontal-lobe volume was significantly decreased in depressed patients after adjustment for age, sex education and cranial size. Coffman *et al.* (1990) found no difference in sagittal frontal-lobe areas between young bipolar patients and controls.

It has been suggested that any reduction in brain tissue in depressed patients is progressive rather than arising out of a developmental change, as hypothesised for schizophrenia. It has been linked to hypercortisolaemia secondary to overactivity of corticotrophin-releasing factor from the pituitary. Pituitary enlargement, as demonstrated by MRI in depressed patients, is consistent with this hypothesis (McDonald & Krishnan, 1992).

Bilateral reduction of caudate volume has been demonstrated in a group of patients with major depression after considering the effects of age (Krishnan *et al.*, 1992). Degeneration of striatal neurons or terminals could lead to disrupted pathways involved in mood regulation. Alteration of other brain structures in patients with affective disorder include reports of a smaller brainstem and cerebellar vermis (Shah *et al.*, 1992).

T2-weighted MR images in older normal subjects often reveal clinically silent hyperintensities, also known as unknown bright objects (UBOs). These features sometimes correspond to hypodensities noted on CT scans. Hyperintensities are usually detected in periventricular or deep white matter (DWMHs) and in subcortical grey matter. Hyperintensities are thought to result from a variety of degenerative brain changes, including atherosclerosis, arteriolar hyalinisation, lacunar infarcts, atrophic demyelination and leakage of CSF into periventricular spaces. These supposed lesions are more prevalent in older depressed patients with risk of cardiovascular disease (Krishnan *et al.*, 1988). A number of studies have found increased frequency and size of DWMHs and hyperintensities in subcortical nuclei in elderly patients with depression and in patients with bipolar disorder (Coffey *et al.*, 1993). In a study of elderly depressed patients, 62% had periventricular hyperintensities, compared with 23% in controls, 55% had DWMHs compared with 14% of controls and basal-ganglia lesions were present in 51% of patients and only 5% of controls (Coffey *et al.*, 1990). The occurrence of these lesions was associated with risk of cerebrovascular disease. To take account of cardiovascular risk factors, Figiel *et al.* (1991) compared early- and late-onset depressed patients with a control group well matched for cardiovascular risk factors. Basal-ganglia lesions and large DWMHs were more commonly seen in late-onset depressives than in depressives of early onset.

The clinical significance of hyperintensities is unknown. Hyperintensities may be related to cognitive impairment, poorer response to treatment and increased sensitivity to medication and ECT (McDonald & Krishnan, 1992).

Conclusions and future directions

MRI has contributed a great deal to the evidence that structural brain abnormalities underlie the functional psychoses. This evidence is particularly strong in schizophrenia. Patterns of structural brain abnormalities that have emerged include modest enlargements of lateral and third ventricles and cortical sulci, generalised slight diminution in cerebral size and specific reduction in cerebral cortical grey matter volume. Whether regional volume loss in the temporal lobes and hippocampi occurs over and above general grey-matter reduction is still not clear. Recently, the iatrogenic enlargement of caudate nuclei with antipsychotic drugs has also been shown.

An important area of current and future research lies in linking structural and functional brain abnormalities. Already some links have been suggested between cerebral anatomy de-

tected by MRI and clinical symptoms, e.g. size of the superior temporal gyrus and auditory hallucinations in schizophrenia. Sciences concerned with brain function are increasingly being used in conjunction with structural MRI of the brain. These disciplines include neuropsychology, neurophysiology and functional neuroimaging. The newest technique of functional neuroimaging, functional MRI, now provides the first opportunity to perform structural and functional measures in the same subject at the same sitting.

Acknowledgement

We gratefully acknowledge the help of Dr Christine Heron, Consultant Radiologist, MRI Unit, St George's Hospital, London, and that of Catriona Woodruff for preparing the figures and for help with the manuscript.

References

Akbarian, S., Bunney, W.E., Potkin, S.G., Wigal, S.B., Hagman, J.O., Sandman, C.A. Jones, E.G. (1993a) Altered distribution of nicotinamide-adenosine dinucleotide phosphate-diaphorase cells in frontal lobe of schizophrenics implies disturbances of cortical development. *Arch. Gen. Psychiatry* 50, 169–77.

Akbarian, S., Vinuela A., Kim, J.J., Potkin S.G., Bunney W.E. Jones E.G. (1993b) Altered distribution of nicotinamide-adenosine dinucleotide phosphate-diaphorase cells in frontal lobe of schizophrenics implies disturbances of cortical development. *Arch. Gen. Psychiatry* 50, 178–87.

Altshuler, L.L., Conrad, A., Hauser, P. *et al.* (1991) Reduction of temporal lobe volume in bipolar disorder: a preliminary report of magnetic resonance imaging. *Arch. Gen. Psychiatry* 48, 482–3.

Andreasen, N.C., Nasrallah, H.A., Dunn, V. *et al.* (1986) Structural abnormalities in the frontal system in schizophrenia. *Arch. Gen. Psychiatry* 43, 137–44.

Andreasen, N.C., Erhardt, J.C., Swayze, V.W. *et al.* (1990) Magnetic resonance imaging of the brain in schizophrenia: the pathophysiologic significance of structural abnormalities. *Arch. Gen. Psychiatry* 47, 35–44.

Andreasen, N.C., Flaum, M., Swayze, V. *et al.* (1993) Intelligence and brain structure in normal individuals. *Am. J. Psychiatry* 150 (1), 130–4.

Arndt, S., Cohen, G., Alliger, R.J. *et al.* (1991) Problems with ratio and proportion measures of imaged cerebral structures. *J. Psychiatry Res. Neuroimaging* **40** (1), 79–89.

Barta, P.E., Pearlson, G.D., Powers, R.E., Richards, S.S. & Tune, L.E. (1990) Auditory hallucinations and smaller superior temporal gyral volume in schizophrenia. *Am. J. Psychiatry* **147**, 1457–62.

Bear, D., Schiff, D., Saver, J., Greenberg, M. & Freeman, R. (1986) Quantitative analysis of cerebral asymmetries. *Arch. Neurol.* **43**, 598–603.

Benes, F., McSparren, J., Bird, E.D., San Giovanni, J.P. & Vincent, S.L. (1991) Deficits in small interneurons in prefrontal and cingulate cortices of schizophrenic and schizoaffective patients. *Arch. Gen. Psychiatry* **48**, 996–1001.

Berman, K.F., Ostrem, J.L., Mattay, V.S., *et al.* (1994) The roles of the dorsolateral prefrontal cortex and hippocampus in working memory and schizophrenia (Society of Biological Psychiatry 1994 Annual Meeting, abstract). *Biol. Psychiatry* **35**, 27.

Bigelow, L.B., Nasrallah, H.A. & Rauscher, F.P. (1983) Corpus callosum thickness in chronic schizophrenia. *Br. J. Psychiatry* **142**, 284–7.

Bilder, R.M., Wu, H., Bogerts, B. *et al.* (1994) Absence of regional hemispheric volume asymmetries in first episode schizophrenia *Am. J. Psychiatry* **151**, 1437–47.

Blansjaar, B.A., Vielvoye, G.J., van Dijk, J.G. *et al.* (1992) Similar brain lesions in alcoholics and Korsakoff patients: MRI, psychometric and clinical findings. *Clin. Neurol. Neurosurg.* **24**, 197–203.

Bogerts, B., Ashtari, M., Degreef, G., Alvir, J.M.J., Bilder, R.M. & Lieberman, J.A. (1990) Reduced temporal limbic structure volumes on magnetic resonance images in first episode schizophrenia. *Psychiatry Res. Neuroimaging* **35**, 1–13.

Bornstein, R.A., Schwarzkopf, S.B., Olson, S.C. & Nasrallah, H.A. (1992) Third ventricle enlargement and neuropsychological deficit in schizophrenia. *Biol. Psychiatry* **31**, 954–61.

Breier, A., Buchanan, R.W., Elkashef, A., Munson, R.C., Kirkpatrick, B. & Gellad, F. (1992) A magnetic resonance imaging study of limbic, prefrontal cortex, and caudate structures. *Arch. Gen. Psychiatry* **49**, 921–5.

Brugha, T.S., Wing, J.K., Brewin, L.R. *et al.* (1988) The problems of people in long term psychiatric care. An introduction to the Camberwell High Contact Survey. *Psychol. Med.* **18**, 457–68.

Cannon, T.D., Mednick, S.A. & Parnos, J. (1989) Genetic and perinatal determinants of structural brain deficits in schizophrenia. *Arch. Gen. Psychiatry* **46**, 883–9.

Carlen, P.L., Wortzman, G., Holgate, R.C. *et al.* (1978) Reversible cerebral atrophy in recently abstinent chronic alcoholics measured by computed tomography scans. *Science* **200**, 1076–8.

Casanova, M.F., Sanders, R.D., Goldberg, T.E. *et al.* (1990) Morphometry of the corpus callosum in monozygotic twins discordant for schizophrenia: a magnetic resonance imaging study. *J. Neurol. Neurosurg. Psychiatry* **53**, 416–21.

Cazzullo, C.L., Sacchetti, E., Vita, A. *et al.* (1985) Cerebral ventricular size in schizophrenic spectrum disorders: relationship to clinical neuropsychological, and immunogenetic variables. In Shagass, C., Josiassen, R.C., Bridger, W.H. *et al.* (eds) *Biological Psychatry*. Elsevier Science Publishing, New York.

Chakos, M.H., Leiberman, J.A. & Bilder, R.M. (1994) Caudate volume increases in first episode schizophrenia after treatment. *Am. J. Psychiatry* **151**, 1430–6.

Chang, K.H., Cha, S.H., Han, M.H. *et al.* (1992) Marchiafava–Bignami disease: serial changes in corpus callosum on MRI. *Neuroradiology* **34**, 480–2.

Chick, J.D., Smith, M.A., Engleman, H.M. *et al.* (1989) Magnetic resonance imaging of the brain in alcoholics: cerebral atrophy, lifetime alcohol consumption, and cognitive defects. *Alcoholism Clin. Exp. Res.* **13**, 512–18.

Clarke, B., Arthur Wigan (1987) The duality of mind. *Psychol. Med.* Monograph supplement 11.

Coffey, C.E., Djang, W.T. & Weiner, R.D. (1990) Subcortical hyperintensities on MRI: a comparison of normal and depressed elderly subjects. *Am. J. Psychiatry* **147**, 187–9.

Coffey, C.E., Weiner, R.D., Djang, W.T. *et al.* (1991) Brain anatomic effects of electroconvulsive therapy: a prospective magnetic resonance imaging study. *Arch. Gen. Psyhiatry* **48**, 1013–21.

Coffey, C.E., Wilkinson, W.E., Weiner, R.D. *et al.* (1993) Quantitative cerebral anatomy in depression: a controlled magnetic resonance imaging study. *Arch. Gen. Psychiatry* **50**, 7–16.

Coffman, J.A., Bornstein, R.A., Olson, S.C., Schwarzkopf, S.B. & Nasrallah, H.A. (1990) Cognitive impairment and cerebral structure by MRI in bipolar disorder. *Biol. Psychiatry* **27**, 1188–96.

Coger, R.W. & Serafetinides, E.A. (1990) Schizophrenia, corpus callosum, and inter-hemispheric communication: a review. *Psychiatry Res.* **34**, 163–84.

Dauphinais, D., DeLisi, L.E., Crow, T.J. *et al.* (1990) Reduction in temporal lobe size in siblings with schizophrenia: a magnetic resonance imaging study. *Psychiatry Res.* **35**, 137–47.

David, A.S., Minne, C., Jones, P., Harvey, I. & Ron, M.A. (1995) Structure and function of the corpus callosum in schizophrenia: what's the connection? *Eur. Psychiatry* **10**, 28–35.

Degreef, G., Ashtari, M., Bogerts, B. *et al.* (1992) Volumes of ventricular system subdivisions measured from magnetic resonance images in first-episode schizophrenic patients. *Arch. Gen. Psychiatry* **49**, 531–7.

De Lacoste-Utamsing, C. & Holloway, R.L. (1982) Sexual dimorphism in the human corpus callosum. *Science* **216**, 1431–2.

DeLisi, L.E., Goldin, L.R., Harnovit, V.R. *et al.* (1986) A family study of the association of increased ventricular size with schizophrenia. *Arch. Gen. Psychiatry*, **43**, 48–53.

DeLisi, L.E., Hoff, A.L., Schwartz, J.E. *et al.* (1991) Brain morphology in first episode schizophrenia-like patients: a quantitative magnetic resonance imaging study. *Biol. Psychiatry* **29**, 159–75.

DeLisi, L.E., Stritzke, P., Riordan, H. *et al.* (1992) The timing of brain morphological changes in schizophrenia and their relationship to clinical outcome. *Biol. Psychiatry* **31**, 241–54.

DeMeyer, M.K., Gilmor, R.L., Hendrie, H.C. *et al.* (1988) Magnetic resonance brain images in schizophrenic and normal subjects: influence of diagnosis and education. *Schizophr. Bull.* **14**, 21–38.

Eagles, J.M., Gibson, I., Bremner, M.H. *et al.* (1990) Obstetric complications in DSM-3 schizophrenics and their siblings. *Lancet*, **335**, 1139–41.

Edwards, G., Chandler, J., Hensman, C. *et al.* (1972) Drinking in a London suburb. *Quart. J. Studies Alcoholism* Suppl. 6, 69–128.

Falkai, P., Bogerts, B., Kleinschmidt, A. *et al.* (1994) The planum temporale in schizophrenia. A comparison of post-mortem and MRI data. *Schizophr. Res.* **11** (2), 131.

Farmer, A., Jackson, R., McGuffin, P. *et al.* (1987) Cerebral ventricular enlargement in schizophrenia: consistencies and contradictions. *Br. J. Psychiatry*, **150**, 324–30.

Figiel, G.S., Krishnan, K.R.R., Doraiswamy, P.M., Rao, V.P., Nemeroff, C.B. & Boyko, O.B. (1991) Subcortical hyperintensities on brain magnetic resonance imaging: a comparison between late age onset and early onset elderly depressed subjects. *Neurobiol. Aging* **26**, 245–7.

Francis, A.F. (1979) Familial basal ganglia calcification and schizophreniform psychosis. *Br. J. Psychiatry* **133**, 360–2.

Goldberg, T.E., Raglan, J.D., Torrey, E.F., Gold, J.M., Bigelow, L.B. & Weinberger, D.R. (1990) Neuropsychological assessment of monozygotic twins discordant for schizophrenia. *Arch. Gen. Psychiatry* **47**, 1066–72.

Gunther, W., Petsch, R., Steinberg, R. *et al.* (1991) Brain dysfunction during motor activation and corpus callosum alterations in schizophrenia measured by cerebral blood flow and magnetic resonance imaging. *Biol. Psychiatry* **29**, 535–53.

Gur, R.E., Mozley, P.D., Resnick, S.M. *et al.* (1991) Magnetic resonance imaging in schizophrenia. *Arch. Gen. Psychiatry* **48**, 407–12.

Gur, R.E., Mozley, P.D., Shtasel, D.L. *et al.* (1994) Clinical subtypes of schizophrenia: differences in brain and csf volume. *Am. J. Psychiatry* **151** (3), 343–350.

Harper, C.G. & Kril, J.J. (1990) Neuropathology of alcoholism. *Alcohol Alcoholism* **25**, 207–16.

Harvey, I., Ron, M.A., DuBoulay, G., Wicks, D., Lewis, S.W. & Murray, R.M. (1993) Reduction of cortical volume in schizophrenia on magnetic resonance imaging. *Psychol. Med.* **23**, 591–604.

Harvey, I., Williams, M., Toone, B.K. *et al.* (1990) The ventricle-brain ratio (VBR) in functional psychoses: the relationship of lateral ventricular and total ventricular area. *Psychol. Med.* **20**, 55–62.

Haug, J.O. (1962) Pneumoencephalographic studies in mental disease. *Acta Psychiatr. Scand.* **38** (Suppl. 165), 1–104.

Hauser, P., Dauphinais, D., Berrettini, W., DeLisi, L.E., Gelernter, J., Post, R.M. (1989) Corpus callosum dimensions measured by magnetic resonance imaging in bipolar affective disorder and schizophrenia. *Biol. Psychiatry* **26**, 659–68.

Iacono, W.G., Smith, G.N., Morean, M. *et al.* (1988) Ventricular and sulcal size at the onset of psychosis. *Am. J. Psychiatry* **145**, 820–4.

Illowsky, B., Juliano, D.M., Bigelow, L.B. *et al.* (1988) Stability of CT scan findings in schizophrenia. *J. Neurol. Neurosurg. Psychiatry* **51**, 209–12.

Izquierdo, G., Quesada, M.A., Chacon, J. *et al.* (1992) Neuroradiologic abnormalities in Marchiafava–Bignami disease of benign evolution. *Eur. J. Radiol.* **15** (1), 71–4.

Jack, C.R., Gehring, D.G., Sharbrough, F.W. *et al.* (1988) Temporal lobe volume measurement from MR images: accuracy and left right asymmetry in normal persons. *J. Computer Assisted Tomogr.* **12**, 21–9.

Jacobson, R.R. & Lishman, W.A. (1990) Cortical and diencephalic lesions in Korsakoff's syndrome: a clinical and CT scan study. *Psychol. Med.* **20**, 63–75.

Jensen, G.B. & Pakkenberg, B. (1993) Do alcoholics drink their neurones away? *Lancet* **342**, 1201–4.

Jernigan, T.L., Press, G.A. & Hesselink, J.R. (1990) Methods for measuring brain morphologic features on magnetic resonance images, validation and normal aging. *Arch. Neurol.* **47**, 27–32.

Jernigan, T.L., Butters, N., DiTraglia, G. *et al.* (1991a) Reduced cerebral grey matter observed in alcoholics using magnetic resonance imaging. *Alcoholism Clin. Exp. Res.* **15** (3), 418–27.

Jernigan, T.L., Schafer, K., Butters, N. *et al.* (1991b) Magnetic resonance imaging of alcoholic Korsakoff patients. *Neuropsychopharmacology* **4**, 175–86.

Jernigan, T.L., Archibald, S.L., Berhow, M.T., Sowell, E.R., Foster, D.S. & Hesselink, J.R. (1991c) Cerebral structure on MRI, Part I: localization of age-related changes. *Biol. Psychiatry* **29**, 55–67.

Jernigan, T.L., Zisook, S., Heaton, R.K. *et al.* (1991d) Magnetic resonance imaging abnormalities in lenticular nuclei and cerebral cortex in schizophrenia. *Arch. Gen. Psychiatry* **48** (10), 881–90.

Johnstone, E.C., Owens, D.G.C., Crow, T.J. *et al.* (1989) Temporal lobe structure as determined by nuclear magnetic resonance in schizophrenia and bipolar affective disorder. *J. Neurosurg. Psychiatry* **52**, 736–41.

Jones, P & Murray, R.M. (1991) The genetics of schizophrenia is the genetics of neurodevelopment. *Br. J. Psychiatry* **158**, 615–23.

Jones, P.B., Harvey, I, Lewis, S.W. *et al.* (1994) Cerebral ventricle dimensions as risk factors for psychosis. An epidemiological approach to analysis. *Psychol. Med.* **24**, 995–1011.

Kaiya, H., Uematsu, M., Ofuji, M. *et al.* (1989) Computerised tomography in schizophrenia. Familial versus non-familial forms of illness. *Br. J. Psychiatry* **155**, 444–50.

Kelsoe, J.R., Cadet, J.L., Pickar, D. & Weinberger, D.R. (1988) Quantitative neuroanatomy in schizophrenia. *Arch. Gen. Psychiatry* **45**, 533–41.

Kemali, D., Maj, M., Galderini, S. *et al.* (1983) Clinical, biological and neuropsychological features associated with lateral ventricular enlargement in DSM-III schizophrenic disorder. *Psychiatry Res.* **21**, 137–49.

Kemali, D., Maj, M., Galderini, S., Milici, N. & Salvati, A. (1989) Ventricle to brain ratio in schizophrenia: a controlled follow-up study. *Biol. Psychiatry* **26**, 756–9.

Kleinschmidt, A., Falkai, P., Huang, Y., Schneider, T., Furst G. & Steinmetz, H. (1994) *In vivo* morphometry of planum temporale asymmetry in first-episode schizophrenia. *Schizophr. Res.* **12**, 9–18.

Krishnan, K.R.R., Goli, V., Ellinwood, E.H., France, R.K., Blazer, D.G. & Nemeroff, C.B. (1988) Leukoencephalopathy in patients diagnosed as major depressive. *Biol. Psychiatry* **23**, 519–22.

Krishnan, K.R.R., McDonald, W.M., Escalona, P.R. *et al.* (1992) Magnetic resonance imaging of the caudate nuclei in depression. *Arch. Gen. Psychiatry* **49**, 553–7.

Kroft, C.L., Gescuk, B., Woods, B.T. *et al.* (1991) Brain ventricular size in female alcoholics: an MRI study. *Alcohol* **8**, 31–4.

Kuhnley, E.J., White, D.H. & Granoff, A.L. (1981) Psychiatric presentation an arachnoid cyst. *J. Clin. Psychiatry*, **42**, 167–9.

Kulynych, J.J., Vladar, K., Jones, D.W. & Weinberger, D.R. (1994) Gender differences in the normal lateralization of the supratemporal cortex: MRI surface-rendering morphometry of Heschl's gyrus and the planum temporale. *Cereb. Cortex* **4**, 107–18.

Leira, H.L., Myhr, G., Nilsen, G. & Dale, L.G. (1992) Cerebral magnetic resonance imaging and cerebral computerized tomography for patients with solvent-induced encephalopathy. *Scand. J. Work Environment Health* **18** (2), 68–70.

Lewis, S. W. (1987) Schizophrenia with and without intracranial abnormalities on CT scan. Unpublished MPhil thesis, University of London.

Lewis (1989) Congenital risk factors for schizophrenia. *Psychol. Med.* **19**, 5–13.

Lewis, S.W. (1990) Computed tomography in schizophrenia, 15 years on. *Br. J. Psychiatry* **157** (Suppl 9) 16–24.

Lewis, S.W. & Mezey, G.C. (1985) Clinical correlates of septum pellucidum cavities: an unusual association with psychosis. *Psychol. Med.* **15**, 43–54.

Lewis, S.W., Reveley, M.A., David, A.S. & Ron, M.A. (1988) Agenesis of the corpus callosum and schizophre-

nia: a case report. *Psychol. Med.* **18**, 341–7.

McDonald, W.M. & Krishnan, K.R.R. (1992) Magnetic resonance in patients with affective illness. *Eur. Arch. Psychiatry Clin. Neurosci.* **241**, 283–90.

Mander, A.J., Whitfield, A., Kean, D.M. *et al.* (1987) Cerebral and brain stem changes after ECT revealed by nuclear magnetic resonance imaging. *Br. J. Psychiatry* **151**, 69–71.

Mann, K., Batra, A., Gunthner, A. & Schroth, G. (1992) Do women develop alcoholic brain damage more readily than men? *Alcoholism Clin. Exp. Res.* **16** (6), 1052–6.

Mann, K., Opitz, H., Petersen, D. *et al.* (1989) Intracranial CSF volumetry in alcoholics: studies with MRI and CT. *Psychiatry Res.* **29**, 277–9.

Matthew, R.J., Partain, C.L., Prakash, R., Kulkarni, M.V., Logan, T.P. & Wilson, W.H. (1985) A study of the septum pellucidum and corpus callosum in schizophrenia. *Acta Psychatr. Scand.* **72**, 414–21.

di Michele, V., Rossi, A., Stratta, P. *et al.* (1992) Neuropsychological and clinical correlates of temporal lobe anatomy in schizophrenia. *Acta Psychiatr. Scand.* **85**, 484–8.

Murphy, D.G.M., DeCarli, C., Schapiro, M.B., Rapoport, S.I. & Horwitz, B. (1992) Age-related differences in volumes of subcortical nuclei, brain matter, and cerebrospinal fluid in healthy men as measured with magnetic resonance imaging. *Arch. Neurol.* **49**, 839–45.

Murray, R.M., Lewis, S.W. & Reveley, A.M. (1985) Towards an aetiological classification of schizophrenia. *Lancet*, i, 1023–6.

Nasrallah, H.A., Andreasen, N.C., Coffman, J.A. *et al.* (1986) A controlled magnetic resonance imaging study of corpus callosum thickness in schizophrenia. *Biol. Psychiatry* **21**, 274–82

Nasrallah, H.A., Schwarzkopf, S.B., Olson, S.C. & Coffman, J.A. (1990) Gender differences in schizophrenia on MRI brain scans. *Schizophr. Bull.* **16** (2), 205–10.

Nimgaonkar, V.L., Wessley, S. & Murray, R. M. (1988) Prevalence of familiality, obstetric complications and structural brain damage in schizophrenic patients. *Br. J. Psychiatry*, **153**, 191–7.

O'Callaghan, E., Larkin, C. & Waddington, J.L. (1990) Obstetric complications in schizophrenia and the validity of maternal recall. *Psychol. Med.* **20**, 89–94.

Owens, D.G.C., Johnstone, E.C., Bydder, G.M. *et al.* (1980) Unsuspected organic disease in chronic schizophrenia demonstrated by computed tomography. *J. Neurol. Neurosurg. Psychiatry* **43**, 1065–9.

Owens, D.G.C., Lewis, S.W. & Murray, R.M. (1988) Obstetric complications and schizophrenia: a computed tomographic study. *Psychol. Med.* **18**, 332–40.

Owens, D.G.C., Lewis, S.W. & Murray, R.M. (1989) Family history and cerebral ventricular enlargement in schizophrenia: a case control study. *Br. J. Psychiatry* **154**, 629–34.

Pearlson, G.D., Garbacz, D.J., Moberg, P.J. *et al.* (1985) Symptomatic, familial, perinatal and social correlates of computerised axial tomography (CAT) changes in schizophrenics and bipolars. *J. Nerv. Ment. Dis.* **173**, 42–50.

Pearlson, G.D., Kim, W.S., Kubos, K.L. *et al.* (1989) Ventricle–brain ratio, computed tomographic density, and brain area in 50 schizophrenics. *Arch. Gen. Psychiatry* **46**, 690–7.

Penfield, W. & Perrot, P. (1963) The brain record of auditory and visual experience. *Brain* **86**, 595–6.

Pettergrew, J.W., Keshaven, M.S., Panchalingam, K.*et al.* (1991) Alterations in brain high-energy phosphate and membrane phospholipid metabolism in first episode, drug naive schizophrenics. *Arch. Gen. Psychiatry* **48**, 563–8.

Pfefferbaum, A., Lim, K.O., Zipursky, R.B. *et al.* (1992) Brain gray and white matter volume loss accelerates with aging in chronic alcoholics: a quantitative MRI study. *Alcoholism Clin. Exp. Res.* **16** (6), 1078–89.

Philpot, M. & Lewis, S.W. (1990) Psychopathology of basal ganglia calcification. *Behav. Neurol.* **2**, 227–34.

Raine, A., Harrison, G.N., Reynolds, G.P., Sheard, C., Cooper, J.E. & Medley, I. (1990) Structural and functional characteristics of the corpus callosum in schizophrenics, psychiatric controls, and normal controls. *Arch. Gen. Psychiatry* **47**, 1060–3.

Reveley, A.M. & Reveley, M.A. (1983) Aqueduct stenosis and schizophrenia. *J. Neurol. Neurosurg. Psychiatry,* **46**, 18–22.

Reveley, A.M., Chitkara, B. & Lewis, S.W. (1988) Ventricular and cranial size in schizophrenia: a 4 to 7 year follow-up. *Schizophr. Res.* **1**, 163.

Reveley, A.M., Reveley, M.A. & Murray, R.M. (1984) Cerebral ventricular enlargement in non-genetic schizophrenia: a controlled twin study. *Br. J. Psychiatry* **144**, 89–93.

Romani, A., Merrelo, S., Gozzoli, L. *et al.* (1987) P300 and CT scan in patients with chronic schizophrenia. *Br. J. Psychiatry* **151**, 506–13.

Ron, M.A. (1983) The alcoholic brain: CT scan and psychological findings. *Psychol. Med.* Suppl. 3, 1–32.

Rosenthal, R. & Bigelow, L.B. (1972) Quantitative brain measurements in chronic schizophrenia. *Br. J. Psychiatry* **121**, 259–64.

Rossi, A., Stratta, P., D'Albenzio, L. *et al.* (1990) Reduced temporal lobe areas in schizophrenia: preliminary evidence from a controlled multi-planar magnetic resonance imaging study. *Biol. Psychiatry* **27**, 61–8.

Rossi, A., Stratta, P., Gallucci, M., Passariello, R. & Casacchia, M. (1988) Brain morphology in schizophrenia by magnetic resonance imaging. *Acta Psychiatr. Scand.* **77**, 741–5.

Rossi, A., Stratta, P., Gallucci, M., Passariello, R. & Casacchia, M. (1989) Quantification of corpus callosum and ventricles in schizophrenia with nuclear magnetic resonance imaging: a pilot study. *Am. J. Psychiatry* **46**(1), 99–101.

Rossi, A., Stratta, P., Mattei, P. *et al.* (1992) Planum temporale in schizophrenia: a magnetic resonance study. *Schizophrenia Res.* **7**, 19–22.

Schlaepfer, T.E., Harris, G.J., Tien, A.Y. *et al.* (1994) Decreased rational cortical gray matter volume in first episode schizophrenia. *Am. J. Psychiatry* **151**, 842–8.

Schmauss, C. & Krieg, J.C. (1987) Enlargement of cerebrospinal fluid spaces in long-term benzodiazepine abusers. *Psychol. Med.* **17**, 869–73.

Seidman, L.J., Yurgelin-Todd, D., Kremen, W.S. *et al.* (1994) Relationship of prefrontal and temporal lobe MRI measures to neuropsychological performance in chronic schizophrenia. *Biol. Psychiatry* **35**, 235–46.

Shah, S.A., Doraiswamy, P.M., Husain, M. *et al.* (1992) Posterior fossa abnormalities in major depression: a controlled magnetic resonance imaging study. *Acta Psychiatr. Scand.* **85** (6), 474–9.

Shenton, M.E., Kikinis, R., Jolesz, F.A. *et al.* (1992) Left-lateralized temporal lobe abnormalities in schizophrenia and their relationship to thought disorder: a computerized, quantitative MRI study. *N. Engl. J. Med.* **327**, 604–12.

Smith, R.C., Baumgartner, R. & Calderon, M. (1987) Magnetic resonance imaging studies of the brains of schizophrenic patients. *Psychiatry Res.* **20**, 33–46.

Squire, L.R., Amaral, D.G., Press, G.A. *et al.* (1990) Magnetic resonance imaging of the hippocampal formation and mammillary nuclei distinguish medial temporal lobe and diencephalic amnesia. *J. Neurosci.* **10** (9), 3106–17.

Strang, J. & Gurling, H. (1989) Computerized tomography and neuropsychological assessment in long-term high-dose heroin addicts. *Br. J. Addiction* **84**, 1011–19.

Stratta, P., Rossi, A., Gallucci, M., Amicarelli, I., Passariello, R. & Casacchia, M. (1989) Hemispheric asymmetries and schizophrenia: A preliminary magnetic resonance imaging study. *Biol. Psychiatry* **25**, 275–84.

Suddath, R.L., Christison, G.W., Torrey, E.F., Casanova, M.F. & Weinberger, D.R. (1990) Anatomical abnormalities in the brains of monozygotic twins discordant for schizophrenia. *N. Engl. J. Med.* **322**, 789–94.

Swayze, W., Andreasen, N.C., Erhardt, J.C., Yuh, W.T.C., Allinger, R.J. & Cohen, G.A. (1990) Development abnormalities of the corpus callosum in schizophrenia: an MRI study. *Arch. Neurol.* **47**, 805–8.

Turner, S.W., Toone, B.K. & Brett-Jones, J.R. (1986) Computerised tomographic scan changes in early schizophrenia preliminary findings. *Psychol. Med.* **16**, 219–25.

Vita, A., Dieci, M., Giobbio, G.M. *et al.* (1994) A reconsideration of the relationship between cerebral structural abnormalities and family history of schizophrenia. *Psychiatry Res.* **53**, 41–55.

Weinberger, D.R., Berman, K.F., Suddath, R. & Torrey, E.F. (1992) Evidence of dysfunction of a pre-frontal–limbic network in schizophrenia: a magnetic resonance imaging and regional cerebral blood flow study of discordant monozygotic twins. *Am. J. Psychiatry* **149**, 880–97.

Williams, A.O., Reveley, M.A., Kolakowska, T. *et al.* (1985) Schizophrenia with good and poor outcome II: cerebral ventricular size and its clinical significance. *Br. J. Psychiatry* **146**, 239–46.

Williamson, P., Pelz, D., Merskey, H., Morrison, S. & Conlon, P. (1991) Correlation of negative symptoms in schizophrenia with frontal lobe parameters on magnetic resonance imaging. *Br. J. Psychiatry* **159**, 130–4.

Witelson, S.F. (1989) Hand and sex differences in the isthmus and genu of the human corpus callosum. *Brain* **112**, 799–833.

Witelson, S.F. & Goldsmith C.H. (1991) The relationship of hand preference to anatomy of the corpus callosum in men. *Brain Research* **545**, 175–82.

Woodruff, P.W.R. & Murray, R.M. (1994a) The aetiology of brain abnormalities in schizophrenia. In Ancill, R., Higenbottam, J. & Holliday, S. (eds) *Schizophrenia 1994: A State of the Art*. John Wiley & Sons, Chichester.

Woodruff, P.W.R., Howard, R., Rushe, T., Graves, M. Murray, R.M. (1994b) Frontal lobe volume and cognitive estimation in schizophrenia. *Schizophr. Res.* **11** (2), 133–4.

Woodruff, P.W.R., McMannus, I.C., David, A.S. (1995) A meta-analysis of corpus callosum size in schizophrenia. *J. Neurol. Neurosurg. Psychiatry*, **58**, 451–61.

Woodruff, P.W.R., Pearlson, G.D., Geer, M.J., Barta, P.E. & Chilcoat, H.D. (1993) A computerized magnetic resonance imaging study of corpus callosum morphology in schizophrenia. *Psychol. Med.* **23**, 45–56.

Young, A.H., Blackwood, D.H.R., Roxborough, H., McQueen, J.K., Martin, M.J. & Kean, D. (1991) A magnetic resonance imaging study of schizophrenia: brain structure and clinical symptoms. *Br. J. Psychiatry* **158**, 158–64.

Zipursky, R.B., Lim, K.C. & Pfefferbaum, A. (1989) MRI study of brain changes with short-term abstinence from alcohol. *Alcoholism* **13**, 664–6.

Zipursky, R.B., Lim, K.O. & Sullivan, E.V. (1992) Widespread cerebral grey matter volume in schizophrenia. *Arch. Gen. Psychiatry* **49** (3), 195–205.

11: Functional Imaging in Schizophrenia

P. F. Liddle

Concepts and techniques

Conceptual issues in imaging brain function

Functional imaging techniques generate quantitative images of the neural activity associated with a particular state of mental activity, and hence offer the prospect of delineating the links between mental disorder and brain disorder. A full description of the neural mechanisms of mental symptoms requires knowledge of many aspects of neuronal activity, including the anatomical location of the neurons involved; the way in which the activity of these neurons is related to activity of neurons elsewhere in the brain; pharmacological characteristics of the neurons implicated; and the time course of the neural events. Functional imaging techniques have the potential to provide information about all of these aspects of neural activity, as noted in Chapter 5.

The most firmly established techniques for identifying the anatomical location of relevant neurons are the techniques for imaging regional cerebral blood flow (rCBF). These techniques include the cortical-probe technique using the radioactive isotope of xenon, ^{133}Xe, as tracer; single-photon emission tomography (SPET) using the tracer hexamethylpropyleneaminoxine (HMPAO) labelled with the metastable isotope of technetium, ^{99m}Tc; and positron emission tomography (PET) using either CO_2 or H_2O labelled with an isotope of oxygen, ^{15}O. Functional magnetic resonance imaging (fMRI) generates images that reflect CBF, but this technique is still very new (see Chapter 6). Images of glucose or oxygen metabolism have also been used to demonstrate the location of active neurons, but metabolism is a less sensitive indicator of neural activity and images of metabolism take longer to acquire, making them less suitable for mapping neural activity associated with transient mental activity.

The most direct approach to exploring the relationship between neural activity in different regions is to obtain a series of images in an individual subject during which the subject is engaged to a varying degree in a particular type of mental process. The correlation between temporal variations in neural activity at any pair of brain sites represents the degree of functional connectivity between those two brain sites for the relevant type of mental processing. Such functional connections between brain sites might be mediated by either direct or indirect anatomical connections. The strength and sign of the functional connection between two brain sites can vary depending on the type of mental process. Using PET it is possible to obtain images embracing the entire brain sampled at 10 or more points in time. Such sets of rCBF images provide substantial information about functional connections between brain regions. fMRI allows sampling at a multitude of points in time, but current techniques cannot easily be employed to image the entire brain. Fast MRI techniques with the potential to achieve this are discussed in Chapter 6.

Identification of the pharmacological characteristics of the relevant neurons is even more difficult than measuring functional connections. The issue can be addressed indirectly by measuring the effect of pharmacological agents on rCBF, but the interpretation is complex because a localised change in CBF at a particular site does not necessarily indicate that the pharmacological agent acted at that site. It would perhaps be more informative to measure changes in level of occupation of receptors by endogenous neurotransmitters between different mental states. In principle, PET might be used to make such measurements, but it has yet to be established that naturally occurring changes in receptor occupancy are large enough to be measured with current techniques (see Chapter 7).

The techniques we have listed so far produce images of activity averaged over a period of several seconds or minutes. The events of neuronal firing occur on a time-scale of milliseconds. The only techniques that offer the ability to measure events on a time-scale measured in milliseconds are topographic electroencephalography (EEG) (see Chapter 8), recordings of event-related potentials (ERP) and magnetoencephalography (MEG) (see Chapter 9). Although these techniques offer high temporal resolution, they provide limited information about the spatial location of the neurons implicated.

Thus, a range of techniques are likely to be required to map the various aspects of brain function relevant to mental disorder, but at this stage rCBF techniques offer the most thoroughly established approach to dynamic measurement of the spatial distribution of neural activity. Therefore this chapter will build on Chapter 5 with techniques for imaging rCBF, and will illustrate the use of these techniques in the investigation of schizophrenia.

Because images of rCBF are sensitive to many different influences, we shall consider in some detail the ways in which the variations in rCBF which are informative can be distinguished from the various confounding sources of variance. We shall also consider the way in which imaging studies can be designed to reveal particular types of abnormality of mental function. For example, patterns of spontaneous aberrant mental activity corresponding to concurrent symptoms are likely to be most clearly demonstrated in images of

rCBF during a resting state or during performance of a simple routine task. On the other hand, comparisons of rCBF during the performance of a task which the patient has difficulty in performing with rCBF during an appropriate control condition might reveal difficulty in activating the relevant brain areas. Measurement of rCBF during a task in a domain of mental function relevant to the illness but which the patient can apparently perform adequately might reveal abnormal pattern of utilisation of different brain areas to perform the task, that is, aberrant patterns of functional connectivity.

Regional perfusion and metabolism as indicators of regional neuronal activity

Typically, a simple motor task, such as flexion and extension of a joint repeated approximately once per second, is associated with a change in rCBF in the relevant primary motor area of about 15%, while a regular sensory stimulus at a similar rate is associated with an increase in rCBF in the primary sensory cortex of similar magnitude. The changes in rCBF in association cortical areas during execution of higher mental processes tends to be somewhat less. For example, frontal changes during the generation of words at a rate of one every few seconds is about 5–10%. In general, the magnitude of the activation in association cortex is only weakly dependent on the rate at which the task is performed. Studies using fMRI with echo planar imaging, which allows very rapid image acquisition, indicate a lag of a few seconds between a change in brain activity and the associated change in cerebral perfusion. Thus, the temporal resolution of rCBF measurements is inevitably greater than a second or so.

The change in regional glucose metabolism (rCMRglu) during sensory activation is somewhat less than the corresponding change in rCBF. For example, Raichle *et al.* (1987) found an increase of glucose metabolism of 11% in sensorimotor cortex during somatosensory stimulation similar to that producing an increase of 26% in rCBF. Thus, rCBF provides a more sensitive measure of changes in local neuronal activity than rCMRglu. However, in the absence of gross disease, steady-state perfusion and metabolism are relatively tightly coupled, and it is probable that images of rCBF and rCMRglu provide a similar indication of steady-state neural activity.

Techniques for measuring regional perfusion and metabolism

Cortical-probe technique

This technique entails the use of an array of detectors attached to the scalp to detect the photons emitted by the decay of ^{133}Xe as it arrives in the brain after inhalation of air containing a trace of ^{133}Xe. Xenon is a freely diffusible tracer, and its rate of accumulation in a given area of the brain reflects the perfusion in that area. Because the photon emitted by the decay of the isotope has a relatively low energy and is strongly absorbed by cerebral tissue, only radioactive-decay events from near the brain surface are detected. Thus, the initial slope of the curve, representing count rate as a function of time, at each detector provides a measure of the perfusion in the cortex immediately beneath that detector. Data from an array of detectors provides a map of cortical activity. The advantages of this rCBF technique are low radiation exposure and rapid clearance of the isotope from the brain, allowing multiple scans of an individual subject during a single scanning session. The disadvantage is the lack of information about rCBF in deep brain structures. Despite its limitations, this technique has been used in some of the landmark studies of brain function in mental illness. In particular, it was the technique used by Ingvar and Franzen (1974) in the first demonstration of frontal underactivity in chronic schizophrenic patients. It was also the technique used by Weinberger and colleagues (1986) to demonstrate that schizophrenic patients have a diminished ability to activate prefrontal cortex during the Wisconsin Card Sorting Test (WCST).

Single-photon emission tomography (SPET)

SPET entails administration of a tracer substance labelled with a radioactive isotope that decays by emission of a single photon. Tomographic reconstruction is employed to generate a two-dimensional image of radioactive decay events in an axial slice of brain. Tomographic reconstruction requires knowledge of direction of travel of the detected photon. In SPET, lead collimators (tubes) are employed to define the direction of travel of photons reaching a specific detector. Consequently, SPET is an inherently inefficient technique (compared with PET) because a substantial proportion of the emitted photons are absorbed in the lead. Consequently, the technique requires relatively high radiation exposure to generate a single image, thereby limiting the possibility of performing repeated studies in the same individual. Furthermore, unlike the situation in PET, where the total distance traversed by each pair of photons is virtually the same irrespective of location of the decay event in the brain, in the case of SPET the photons from decay events deep in the brain are more likely to be absorbed than those from decay events nearer the surface, so the sensitivity of the technique varies throughout the brain, being less for deeper structures.

The tracer usually employed in SPET studies of rCBF is ^{99m}Tc-HMPAO. The tracer is virtually all fixed in tissue during the first pass through the brain, and hence the density of radioactive-decay events in a given area reflects the perfusion of that brain area in a period of a few seconds shortly after administration of the tracer. The dose of radiation required to generate an adequate image is approximately 5 millisieverts (mSv), which is similar in magnitude to the annual radiation dose from background sources. The long half-life of ^{99m}Tc makes it difficult to obtain separate images of two different brain states in a single scanning session. If comparison of a brain state of interest with a reference brain state is required, it is possible to perform a split-dose technique, in a which second dose of tracer is administered during a second brain state but while a substantial amount of tracer from the first dose remains in the brain, and the projected count rate from the radiation arising from the first dose of tracer is subtracted from that after the second dose.

Some SPET studies, such as the study by Andreasen *et al.* (1992) of cerebral activation in schizophrenic patients during the Tower of London task, have employed ^{133}Xe, which is cleared from the body rapidly, thus allowing repeated scans, but high absorption of the photons emitted by that isotope seriously limits the information available about deep brain structures.

Positron emission tomography (PET)

PET employs tracers that contain positron-emitting isotopes, such as ^{15}O, and exploits the fact that the annihilation of a positron by an electron generates two oppositely directed photons, each with an energy of 0.5 megaelectron-volts (MeV). An array of detectors around the head are connected to enable the identification of the coincident arrival of two photons at two different detectors, indicating the occurrence of a positron-annihilation event along the straight line joining the two detectors. Coincidence detection ensures that the direction of travel of the photons is known, and tomographic reconstruction is possible without the need for collimators. Because all pairs of photons traverse an approximately equal combined distance through brain tissue, there is relative uniformity of sampling within a brain slice. PET cameras employ a set of rings arranged so that contiguous slices spanning the entire brain can be imaged. If the detectors are connected not only within but also between rings, pairs of photons travelling obliquely to the longitudinal axis can be detected, allowing three-dimensional reconstruction, thus enhancing efficiency.

PET can be used to measure rCBF by imaging the distribution in the brain of H_2O labelled with ^{15}O. The half-life of ^{15}O is 2.1 min. The tracer is usually administered as a slow intravenous bolus, and an adequate image can be generated within approximately 1 min. If three-dimensional reconstruction is employed, an adequate image can be obtained with a radiation exposure of approximately 0.5 mSv. Since the radioactivity level falls to an insignificant level after 10 min, it is feasible to obtain up to 12 images of different brain states in a single imaging session.

The spatial resolution of PET measurements of rCBF is limited by the fact that a positron emitted by ^{15}O typically travels a distance of the order of 2 mm in brain tissue before an annihilating encounter with an electron. A serious practical limitation of PET is the necessity of having a nearby cyclotron to generate the short-lived ^{15}O.

Functional magnetic resonance imaging (fMRI)

When neurons are activated the local increase in perfusion exceeds that required to meet the increased metabolic requirements, resulting in an increase in the level of oxygenation of the blood. Since oxyhaemoglobin is less paramagnetic than deoxyhaemoglobin, the paramagnetism of the blood decreases, leading to a local change in the magnetic-spin relaxation time of protons in water molecules. This change can be detected by MRI, using a fast imaging sequence, such as echo planar imaging. The technique offers the advantages of high spatial resolution characteristic of proton MRI; time resolution limited by the time-scale of the intrinsic response of rCBF to neuronal activity; and no exposure to either radiochemicals or any other pharmacological agents, thereby removing restrictions on the number of scans that can be performed safely. However, it is a technique prone to artefactual influence, such as movement artefacts. It has been used to study changes in cerebral activity associated with various sensory, motor and mental tasks in normal individuals (Neil, 1993). fMRI is discussed fully in Chapter 6.

Sources of variance in rCBF

Because the changes in rCBF associated with local neuronal activity are typically in the range

5–15%, while, on the other hand, many factors contribute to variation in rCBF, both between individuals and within an individual over time, it is imperative to design studies in a way that addresses the multiple sources of variance if the observations are to be interpreted usefully. The major sources of variance are:

1 The type of mental activity performed during imaging;

2 individual differences in the way the brain is used to perform a particular activity;

3 differences in brain shape, size and orientation that result in differences in the location (with respect to external landmarks) of specific groups of neurons;

4 differences in global CBF which are unrelated to local neuronal activity.

The first two sources of variance are potentially informative about cerebral function, provided appropriate comparisons are performed, while the third and fourth sources of variance are usually confounding variables, for which allowance must be made if rCBF images are to be interpreted reliably.

Differences in current mental activity

The observation that rCBF varies with neuronal activity indicates that it is necessary to design studies in a way that allows either direct or indirect comparison in rCBF during a mental state of interest with that during some reference mental state. There are two major types of approach to study design in schizophrenia. One is to seek to identify cerebral activity associated with the expression of a particular type of symptom by comparing rCBF in the presence of a particular symptom with that in the absence of that symptom, exemplified in the study of auditory hallucinations by McGuire *et al.* (1993).

The other approach is to examine the pattern of activity associated with a specified task involving mental processes implicated in the pathophysiology of schizophrenia. This can be done by comparing rCBF during the performance of that task with rCBF during an appropriate reference activity. This type of approach was developed by Weinberger *et al.* (1986) in an influential series of studies of rCBF during performance of the WCST. However, interpretation of such neuropsychological activation studies is complex if the task is one which the schizophrenic patients perform poorly, because patients might differ from controls either because they are not achieving the same goal as the controls, or because they use their brains differently to achieve a particular goal. That is, the observed differences might reflect either different level of performance or different patterns of brain usage. Furthermore, it is important to recognise that the pattern of cerebral activity observed during neuropsychological activation reflects the experimentally imposed task, rather than the expression of symptoms, although, of course, it is possible that symptom profile might influence cerebral activity associated with task performance.

Individual differences in patterns of brain use

Although there has been little systematic investigation of individual differences between normal individuals in pattern of cerebral activity during the performance of a specified task, PET studies of rCBF patterns in a single subject reveal that there is a modest degree of variation in patterns of activity during tasks such as word generation or the Stroop colour-naming test in normal subjects. There are likely to be substantial differences between schizophrenic patients and normal individuals in the patterns of brain activity during a specified activity.

Ideally, such proposed differences in patterns of cerebral connectivity might be delineated by comparing images of cerebral activity in patients with those of normal individuals during the performance of a task which, on the one hand, is relevant to the types of mental processing implicated in schizophrenia, but which, on the other hand, is not too demanding, so that patients can achieve a level of performance similar to that of controls. This approach has been employed by the PET group at Hammersmith Hospital to compare rCBF during the paced generation of words, paced at a rate slow enough to ensure that patients and controls produce a similar number of words (Friston *et al.*, 1994; Liddle *et al.*, 1994). However, while pacing at a slow rate ensures similar observable performance in patients and controls, it does not eliminate differences in facility of task performance.

Differences in brain shape, size and orientation

Differences in brain shape, size and orientation can introduce two related types of problem. First, such differences make it difficult to perform between-subject comparisons of sites of focal activation associated with a specific mental activity. Secondly, structural differences between individual brains are likely to produce differences in partial-volume effects.

The difficulty in comparing sites of activation in different subjects can be minimised by reorientating and plastically transforming the shape of each brain image to produce the optimal match to a standard template. Such a transformation is known as *stereotactic renormalisation*. In principle, the mathematical parameters for such a transformation might best be estimated by determining the transformation necessary to produce the best match between an MRI structural image of the subject's brain and a standard MRI template derived from averaging MRI images from many subjects. The same transformation might then be applied to the functional image. Such an approach requires the ability to produce accurate coregistration of images across imaging modalities. Recent developments in cross-modality coregistration have made this approach feasible. It should be noted that there is not necessarily a one-to-one correspondence between brain structure and function even in normal individuals, so there is probably no ideal solution to the issue of mapping functional images of individual subjects on to a single template. Fortunately, the spatial smoothing of images that is usually employed to improve signal-to-noise ratio (at the price of reduced

spatial resolution) helps to minimise the importance of differences between subjects in location of a specific site of activation.

An alternative to the use of structural images to derive the optimum transformation parameters is to determine the transformation that produced the best match between the individual's functional image and a standard template derived by averaging functional images from many individuals (Friston *et al.*, 1991). Such an approach avoids the problem of inaccurate coregistration across modalities and also the issue of correspondence between brain structure and function. However, the process of transforming the image so as to match the standard template as closely as possible inevitably tends to reduce the apparent magnitude of the differences in function which are of interest.

The second problem is that of partial-volume effects. Because of limitations on spatial resolution, the apparent rCBF at a specific grey-matter site will be an average of rCBF values at adjacent sites, usually including white matter. Since perfusion of white matter is substantially lower than that of grey matter, such partial-volume effects decrease the magnitude of apparent rCBF at the grey-matter site of interest. This effect will be greater in an individual with reduced volume of grey matter in the vicinity of interest. Hence, apparent deficits in local grey-matter CBF in an individual might reflect a decrease in grey-matter volume rather than a decrease in activity per unit volume of tissue.

Differences in global perfusion

Global cerebral perfusion is influenced by a number of biochemical influences (such partial pressure of CO_2 in the blood) that are not a direct reflection of local neuronal activity. Such fluctuations in global flow tend to obscure changes in rCBF attributable to local neural activity. The potentially confounding contribution from variation in global CBF to variation in local CBF can be removed by analysis of covariance, treating the global flow as the covariate (Friston *et al.*, 1990).

This approach assumes that local flow consists of two independent contributors: a contribution from local neural activity and a contribution that is proportional to global flow (at least over a limited range of values of global flow). This assumption has reasonable face validity and is supported by empirical evidence (Friston *et al.*, 1990). Alternatively, some investigators (e.g. Early *et al.*, 1987) have corrected for variation in global flow by dividing local flow by global flow. Such a normalisation procedure implicitly assumes that the magnitude of changes in local flow due to neural activity is proportional to those of global flow, which is unlikely to be the case. However, the errors arising from such a normalisation procedure are usually small.

Studies of flow or metabolism in schizophrenia

Differences in resting cerebral activity between patients and normal controls

The earliest studies using the cortical-probe technique found that chronic schizophrenic patients tended to exhibit frontal hypoperfusion relative to normal controls (Ingvar & Franzen, 1974). In particular, the hypofrontality was most pronounced in socially withdrawn, catatonic patients, raising the possibility that this abnormality is not a feature of schizophrenia in general, but, rather, of the specific symptoms characteristic of this chronic patient group.

Eighteen of the 35 studies comparing resting-state rCBF or regional cerebral metabolism in schizophrenic patients and normal controls, published in the period 1975 to 1990, found evidence of significant either absolute or relative hypofrontality in the schizophrenic patients (Andreasen *et al.*, 1992). Only a minority of studies of acute, unmedicated patients reported hypofrontality. For example, in a carefully executed study of acute, never-medicated patients, taking account of potentially confounding factors such as variation in global flow and variation in brain size, Early *et al.* (1987) found no evidence

of hypofrontality. They found that the only significant difference between acute schizophrenic patients and normal controls was increased rCBF in the left globus pallidus. Overall, it can be concluded from the various studies of resting rCBF and metabolism that schizophrenic patients do exhibit abnormal patterns of resting cerebral activity, but these patterns depend on symptom profile and/or phase of illness.

Differences in cerebral activity associated with symptom expression

It is likely that each specific symptom is associated with a specific pattern of neural activity, but one problem in identifying such patterns of neural activity is the fact that symptoms tend to covary together. This problem can be addressed in one of two ways. The first approach is based on the observation that, at least in patients with persistent symptoms, three major syndromes can be identified (Liddle, 1987). The symptoms within each syndrome tend to covary together, while the correlations between symptoms from different syndromes are trivial. The fact that the symptoms within a syndrome tend to covary implies that they share substantial features of their underlying pathophysiology. The absence of correlation between the syndromes ensures that, provided a reasonably large cohort of subjects is studied, the correlation between cerebral activity and severity of any one syndrome will not be influenced by variance in either of the other two syndromes. The three distinguishable syndromes are *psychomotor poverty* (the core negative features: poverty of speech; blunted affect; decreased spontaneous movement); *disorganisation* (disorders of the form of thought, inappropriate affect); and *reality distortion* (delusions and hallucinations).

In a PET study of medicated patients with persistent, stable symptoms, Liddle *et al.* (1992a) found that each of the three syndromes was associated with a specific pattern of CBF. Psychomotor poverty was associated with decreased perfusion in the prefrontal cortex and left parietal cortex and with increased perfusion in the caudate nuclei. Disorganisation was associated with decreased perfusion in the right ventral prefrontal cortex and adjacent insula and with increased perfusion in the right anterior cingulate cortex and in the thalamus. Reality distortion was associated with increased perfusion in left medial-temporal lobe and with decreased perfusion in right posterior-cingulate cortex and left lateral-temporal cortex.

Each of the syndromes was associated with areas of increased perfusion and areas of decreased perfusion, implying a dynamic imbalance between different cerebral areas, rather than a fixed loss of function at a specific locus. Furthermore, for each syndrome, the associated pattern of rCBF involved the site maximally activated in normal individuals during performance of the type of mental processing implicated in that syndrome (Liddle *et al.*, 1992b).

In a SPET study of acute, unmedicated patients, Ebmeier *et al.* (1993) replicated the finding of a negative correlation between psychomotor and prefrontal rCBF, the positive correlation between disorganisation and rCBF in the right anterior cingulate and the negative correlation between reality distortion and left lateral-temporal lobe perfusion. They did not find evidence of the various correlations between syndromes and deep brain structures reported by Liddle *et al.* (1992a), possibly reflecting the reduced sensitivity of SPET to regions deeper within the brain. It is of interest to note that, when Ebmeier *et al.* (1993) compared their acute, unmedicated patients with normal controls the major finding was of increased frontal rCBF in the schizophrenic patients as a group, despite the reported negative correlation between psychomotor poverty and prefrontal flow. This observation implies that some other aspect of acute schizophrenia, perhaps psychomotor excitation, is associated with hyperfrontality.

The association between negative symptoms and resting-state hypofrontality has been reported in studies using the cortical-probe technique with ^{133}Xe (Suzuki *et al.*, 1992), and has also been demonstrated in PET studies of glucose metabolism in unmedicated patients (Tamminga *et al.*, 1992; Wolkin *et al.*, 1992). Thus, the association between the core negative symptoms that constitute the psychomotor-poverty syndrome and underactivity of the frontal cortex in the resting state, originally foreshadowed by the findings of Ingvar and Franzen (1974) in the first functional imaging study of schizophrenia, appears to be a very robust finding.

The second approach to establishing the relationship between symptoms and cerebral activity is to perform a longitudinal study, in which patients are studied while exhibiting the symptom of interest and again after resolution of that symptom. Because of the tendency of different symptoms to covary, it is necessary to perform an analysis of covariance, treating other symptoms as covariates. This is the approach employed by McGuire *et al.* (1993) in their SPET study of the rCBF pattern associated with auditory hallucinations. The most significant change between the hallucinating and non-hallucinating state was an excess rCBF in Broca's area while hallucinations were present. They also found increased rCBF in the left medial-temporal lobe, consistent with a similar finding in a SPET study by Musalek *et al.* (1989), and also with the observation by Liddle *et al.* (1992a) that reality distortion is associated with increased left medial-temporal rCBF. Matsuda *et al.* (1989) and Suzuki *et al.* (1993) have reported an association between hallucinations and increased left lateral-temporal rCBF, measured using SPET.

Impaired cerebral activation during neuropsychological challenge

Weinberger *et al.* (1986) introduced a fruitful approach to functional imaging in schizophrenia with a series of studies of rCBF measured using the cortical-probe technique, during performance of the WCST. This task is associated with activation of the frontal lobes in normal individuals. An important feature of the experimental design was comparison of the rCBF during the WCST with that during rest, and also with that during a number-matching task not expected to engage the frontal cortex. By measuring change in rCBF in comparison with the resting state, they were able to detect differences between patients and normal subjects in the cerebral activity associated with the task. They found that schizophrenic patients exhibit a lesser degree of activation of lateral prefrontal cortex than normal subjects during the WCST. They demonstrated that this finding could not be accounted for by non-specific factors, such as level of arousal, mental effort or attention, and, furthermore, that similar findings were observed in medicated and unmedicated patients.

The finding of diminished activation of prefrontal cortex in schizophrenic patients during the WCST has been replicated by Weinberger's group (Weinberger *et al.*, 1988) and by others (Rubin *et al.*, 1991). In view of the probable importance of interactions between frontal cortex and the corpus striatum, it is of special interest to note that Rubin *et al.* (1991) found that the diminished prefrontal activation in schizophrenic patients was accompanied by impaired suppression of striatal rCBF during the WCST.

Weinberger *et al.* (1986) reported a significant negative correlation between performance of the WCST and degree of prefrontal activation in the schizophrenic patients, but not in normal individuals, implying that the function of the prefrontal cortex is the limiting factor in WCST performance in schizophrenia. In contrast, they reported that in patients with Huntington's chorea, who also exhibit impaired WCST performance, there was no diminution of prefrontal activation. These observations imply that abnormal prefrontal function is specifically implicated in the impairment of WCST performance in schizophrenic patients. However, in their later replication study in schizophrenic patients, Weinberger *et al.* (1988) did not find a negative correlation between WCST performance and prefrontal activation, so the interpretation of the finding remains uncertain.

Although Weinberger and colleagues have not reported a correlation between diminished pre-

frontal activation during the WCST and any specific group of schizophrenic symptoms, they have reported that the degree of diminution of prefrontal activation is correlated with low cerebrospinal fluid (CSF) levels of the dopamine metabolite homovanillic acid (HVA) (Weinberger *et al.*, 1988). Investigation of twins discordant for schizophrenia indicates that prefrontal impairment is not confined to a subgroup of patients. In a study of 14 discordant twin pairs, Berman *et al.* (1992b) found that the twin with schizophrenia exhibited lesser activation of the prefrontal cortex in every twin pair, even though in some of the affected cases the degree of prefrontal activation was not outside the normal range. This implies not only that the schizophrenic disease process is associated with diminished prefrontal function compared with that which might have been expected in the absence of schizophrenia, but also that this diminution of prefrontal function is not determined genetically. In the same study, Berman *et al.* (1992b) found that, in twin pairs concordant for schizophrenia, the twin with the greater diminution of prefrontal function tended to have received less antipsychotic medication, confirming the conclusion that the relevant prefrontal impairment is not due to treatment with antipsychotic medication.

Andreasen *et al.* (1992) reported that medial prefrontal activation occurring in normal individuals during the Tower of London test, a planning task designed to test frontal activity, was diminished in never-medicated schizophrenic patients. Furthermore, the degree of diminution of prefrontal activation was correlated with severity of negative symptoms.

Patterns of cerebral activity during a specific task

While there is convincing evidence that schizophrenic patients, especially those with negative symptoms, have diminished ability to activate the prefrontal cortex during tasks in which the patients perform poorly, activation studies employing such tasks do not address the question of whether or not schizophrenic patients activate prefrontal cortex less than normal individuals while achieving a similar level of performance in a frontal task. This question can be addressed by measuring rCBF during paced word generation, paced at a rate which is within the capacity of schizophrenic patients, and comparing with normal individuals performing the same task at the same rate. Using such a strategy, Liddle *et al.* (1994) demonstrated that in schizophrenic patients, even those with marked poverty of speech, the prefrontal activation is equal in magnitude to that occurring in normal individuals. Thus, the resting hypofrontality associated with psychomotor poverty (core negative symptoms) is not an irreversible loss of function. Furthermore, during the paced word-generation task, the patients exhibited a different pattern of functional connectivity between frontal cortex and other brain regions, especially the temporal lobe. In normal individuals, prefrontal activation during word generation is accompanied by suppression of cortical activity in the lateral aspect of the left temporal lobe, but, in schizophrenic patients, this normal temporal suppression is replaced by a temporal activation, implying a different working relationship between frontal and temporal cortex.

The demonstration of an abnormal relationship between frontal and temporal activation in schizophrenic subjects during a word-generation task raises the question of whether or not there is a more widespread disorder of functional connectivity between brain areas in schizophrenia. The overall pattern of relationships between brain areas during a particular type of mental processing can be summarised succinctly in terms of the magnitude of the principal components of the covariance matrix describing the covariance of rCBF between all pairs of pixels in a series of the brain images recorded when the subject is engaged in tasks that include the relevant type of mental processing. In normal individuals performing tasks that entail word generation, the first principal component has strong positive loadings on left lateral-frontal cortex, medial-frontal cortex and thalamus and negative loadings on left lateral-temporal lobe and posterior cingulate (Friston *et al.*, 1994). These are the brain areas in which there is a significant difference when rCBF during articulation of internally generated words is compared with that during articulation of an externally provided list of words. In particular, the areas having greater rCBF during *internal* generation have positive loadings of the first principal component and the areas with lower rCBF have negative loadings, and the magnitude of the loadings approximately reflects the magnitude of the difference in rCBF between internal and external generation conditions (Frith *et al.*, 1991). Thus, the first principal component appears to be an appropriately weighted distribution of functionally connected brain areas specifically engaged in internal generation of words.

The degree to which the pattern of functional connectivity seen in any specific individual during word-generation tasks includes the pattern of rCBF occurring in normal individuals during the internal generation of words can be quantified by calculating the relevant 2-norm (that is, the length of the vector derived by forming the product of the matrix representing the patterns of cerebral activity in the index individual while engaged in a series of word-generation tasks, with the vector representing the first principal component accounting for the variance during word-generation tasks in normal individuals). Using such an approach, Friston *et al.* (1994) found a marked difference between the values of the 2-norm in a group of 18 schizophrenic patients and the range of values of the 2-norm in normal subjects. This indicates that schizophrenia is characterised by an abnormal pattern of functional connectivity between brain areas during the internal generation of words.

Neuropharmacological challenge

The earliest neuropharmacological challenge study using PET in human subjects was a study by Cleghorn *et al.* (1991) examining the effects of the dopamine agonist apomorphine on regional glucose metabolism in normal individuals and in schizophrenic patients. They found that apomorphine challenge produced a decrease in metabolism in the corpus striatum in schizophrenic subjects, but no change in striatal metabolism in normal controls. This observation is consistent with the evidence that prolonged dopaminergic blockade can increase striatal metabolism in schizophrenic patients.

However, the effects of dopaminergic blockade on striatal metabolism appear to depend on whether or not the patient shows a therapeutic response to dopamine-blocking medication. For example, in a study using PET to compare regional glucose metabolism after a 5-week period of placebo treatment with that after a 5-week period of treatment with haloperidol, Buchsbaum *et al.* (1992) demonstrated that those schizophrenic patients who exhibited a reduction in symptoms during treatment had exhibited low striatal metabolism while treated with placebo and that this deficit in striatal metabolism had been alleviated by treatment with haloperidol. Patients who did not respond to haloperidol did not exhibit increase in striatal metabolism after treatment.

In view of the fact that monoamine neurotransmitters such as dopamine act as neuromodulators which regulate the tone of the concurrent brain activity, perhaps the most meaningful questions to ask about the effect of dopaminergic agonists or antagonists are what effects they have on the patterns of cerebral activity associated with specific mental processes. Such questions can be addressed by combining neuropharmacological with neuropsychological challenge. The first studies of this type were performed by Weinberger and colleagues, using the cortical-probe technique to examine the effect of the indirect dopaminergic agonist, amphetamine, on the prefrontal activation during the WCST. They found that amphetamine produced an increase in prefrontal activation during the WCST in the schizophrenic patients and, furthermore, produced a slight alleviation of the WCST performance deficit

(Daniel *et al.* (1991).

Thus, imaging rCBF during pharmacological challenge, either alone or in combination with neuropsychological challenge, demonstrates that dopaminergic agonists produce changes in the cerebral activity in those brain regions implicated in the pathophysiology of schizophrenia, especially the frontal cortex and basal ganglia. The effects are consistent with the hypothesis that the pathophysiology of schizophrenia entails abnormal dopaminergic influence at these brain sites. In particular, the evidence is consistent with proposal that the pathophysiology of schizophrenia entails underactivity of prefrontal dopaminergic projections and hyperactivity of subcortical dopaminergic projections. While it is necessary to be cautious in interpreting the findings until the techniques of pharmacological-challenge studies in human subjects are more firmly established, the available evidence indicates the potential value of these techniques for exploring the pathophysiology of schizophrenia and for the development of improved treatments.

References

Andreasen, N.C., Rezai, K., Alliger, R. *et al.* (1992) Hypofrontality in neuroleptic-naive patients and in patients with chronic schizophrenia: assessment with xenon 133 single-photon emission computed tomography and the Tower of London. *Arch. Gen. Psychiatry* **49**, 943–58.

Berman, K.F., Zec, R.F. & Weinberger, D.R. (1992a) Physiologic dysfunction of dorsolateral prefrontal cortex in schizophrenia. II: Role of neuroleptic treatment, attention, and mental effort. *Arch. Gen. Psychiatry* **43**, 126–35.

Berman, K.F., Torrey, E.F., Daniel, D.G. & Weinberger, D.R. (1992b) Regional cerebral blood flow in monozygotic twins discordant and concordant for schizophrenia. *Arch. Gen. Psychiatry* **49**, 927–35.

Buchsbaum, M.S., Potkin, S.G., Siegel, B.V. *et al.* (1992) Striatal metabolic rate and clinical response to neuroleptics in schizophrenia. *Arch. Gen. Psychiatry* **49**, 966–74.

Cleghorn, J.M., Szechtman, H., Garnett, E. *et al.* (1991) Apomorphine effects on brain metabolism in neuroleptic-naive schizophrenic patients. *Psychiatry Res. Neuroimaging* **40**, 135–53.

Daniel, D.G., Weinberger, D.R., Jones, D.W. *et al.* (1991) The effect of amphetamine on regional cerebral blood flow during cognitive activation in schizophrenia. *J. Neurosci.* **11**, 1907–17.

Early, T.S., Reiman, E.R., Raichle, M.E. & Spitznagel, E.L. (1987) Left globus pallidus abnormality in never-medicated patients with schizophrenia. *Proc. Nat. Acad. Sci. USA* **84**, 561–3.

Ebmeier, K.P., Blackwood, D.H.R., Murray, C. *et al.* (1993) Single photon emission tomography with ^{99m}Tc-exametazime in unmedicated schizophrenic patients. *Biol. Psychiatry* **33**, 487–95.

Friston, K.J., Frith, C.D., Liddle, P.F., Lammertsma, A.A., Dolan, R.D. & Frackowiak, R.S.J. (1990) The relationship between global and local changes in PET scans. *J. Cerebr. Blood Flow Metab.* **10**, 458–66.

Friston, K.J., Frith, C.D., Liddle, P.F. & Frackowiak, R.S.J. (1991) Plastic transformation of PET images. *J. Comput. Assist. Tomogr.* **15**, 634–9.

Friston, K.J., Herold, S., Fletcher, P. *et al.* (1994) Abnormal fronto-temporal interaction in schizophrenia. In Watson, S.J. (ed.) *Biology of Schizophrenia and Affective Disorders*. Raven Press, New York.

Frith, C.D. Friston, K.J., Liddle, P.F. & Frackowiak, R.S.J. (1991) Willed action and the prefrontal cortex in man: a study with PET. *Proc. Roy. Soc. (London) B* **244**, 241–6.

Ingvar, D.H. & Franzen, G. (1974) Abnormalities of cerebral blood flow distribution in patients with chronic schizophrenia. *Acta Psychiatr. Scand.* **50**, 425–62.

Liddle, P.F. (1987) The symptoms of chronic schizophrenia: a re-examination of the positive–negative dichotomy. *Br. J. Psychiatry* **151**, 145–51.

Liddle, P.F., Friston, K.J., Frith, C.D., Jones, T., Hirsch, S.R. & Frackowiak, R.S.J. (1992a) Patterns of cerebral blood flow in schizophrenia. *Br. J. Psychiatry* **160**, 179–86.

Liddle, P.F., Friston, K.J., Frith, C.D. & Frackowiak, R.S.J. (1992b) Cerebral blood flow and mental processes in schizophrenia. *J. Roy. Soc. Med.* **85**, 224–7.

Liddle, P.F., Herold, S., Fletcher, P., Friston, K.J., Silbersweig, D. & Frith, C.D. (1994) A PET study of word generation in schizophrenia. *Schizophrenia Res.* **11**, 168.

McGuire, P.K., Shah, G.M.S. & Murray, R.M. (1993) Increased blood flow in Broca's area during auditory hallucinations in schizophrenia. *Lancet* **342**, 703–6.

Matsuda, H., Gyobu, T., Hisada, K. & Ii, M. (1989) SPECT imaging of auditory hallucination using ^{123}I-IMP. *Adv. Functional Neuroimaging* **2**, 9–16.

Musalek, M., Podreka, I., Walter, H. *et al.* (1989) Regional brain function in hallucinations: a study of regional cerebral blood flow with ^{99m}-Tc-HMPAO-SPECT in patients with auditory hallucinations, tactile hallucinations and normal controls. *Comprehens. Psychiatry* **30**, 99–108.

Neil, J.J. (1993) Functional imaging of the central nervous system using magnetic resonance imaging and positron emission tomography. *Curr. Opin. Neurol.* **6**, 927–33.

Raichle, M.E., Fox, P.T., Mintun, M.A. & Dense, C. (1987) Cerebral blood flow and oxidative glycolysis are uncoupled by neuronal activity. *J. Cerebr. Blood Flow Metab.* **7** (Suppl. 1), S300.

Rubin, P., Holm, S., Friberg, L. *et al.* (1991) Altered modulation of prefrontal and subcortical activity in newly diagnosed schizophrenia and schizophreniform disorder. *Arch. Gen. Psychiatry* **48**, 987–95.

Suzuki, M., Kurachi, M., Kawasaki, Y., Kiba, K. & Yamaguchi, N. (1992) Left hypofrontality correlates with blunted affect in schizophrenia. *Japan. J. Psychiatry Neurol.* **46**, 653–7.

Suzuki, M., Yuasa, S., Minabi, Y., Murata, M. & Kurachi, M. (1993) Left superior temporal blood flow increases in schizophrenic and schizophreniform patients with auditory hallucinations: a longitudinal case study using ^{131}IMP SPECT. *Eur. Arch. Psychiatry Clin. Neurosci.* **242**, 257–61.

Tamminga, C.A., Thaker, G.K., Buchanan, R. *et al.* (1992) Limbic system abnormalites identified in Schizophrenia using positron emission tomography with fluorodeoxyglucose and neocortical alterations with deficit syndrome. *Arch. Gen. Psychiatry* **49**, 522–30.

Weinberger, D.R., Berman, K.F. & Zec, R.F. (1986) Physiologic dysfunction of dorsolateral prefrontal cortex in schizophrenia. 1. Regional cerebral blood flow evidence. *Arch. Gen. Psychiatry* **43**, 114–24.

Weinberger, D.R., Berman, K.F. & Illowsky, B.P. (1988) Physiological dysfunction of the dorsolateral prefrontal cortex in schizophrenia. III. A new cohort and evidence for a monoaminergic mechanisms. *Arch. Gen. Psychiatry* **45**, 609–15.

Wolkin, A., Sanfilipo, M., Wolf, A.P., Angrist, B., Brodie, J.D. & Rotrosen, J. (1992) Negative symptoms and hypofrontality in chronic schizophrenia. *Arch. Gen. Psychiatry* **49**, 959–65.

12: Brain Imaging in Affective Disorders

R. J. Dolan and G. M. Goodwin

Introduction

Understanding how pathological brain structure and function determine abnormal mental states is essential to progress in biological psychiatry. The place of brain imaging in promoting an understanding of the nature, prognosis and treatment of depressive illness is, in our view, likely to be of increasing theoretical and practical importance over the next decade. The direct measurement of cerebral neurophysiology appears to validate neuropsychological constructs accounting for components of normal cognition and can reasonably be assumed to hold out similar possibilities for psychiatric diagnostic constructs. The potential reversibility of the depressed state provides a unique model for the testing of specific hypotheses about its functional anatomy and psychopharmacology.

In the absence of direct measures of *in vivo* brain function, the neurobiology of affective disorders has remained, hitherto, largely a matter of speculation. Traditional neurological approaches to localisation of function have relied upon the interpretation of the effects of critical brain lesions; the apparent absence of a singular locus that can be implicated in mood disorder has, therefore, required a methodology that can implicate multiple or distributed neuronal systems. Further, while pursuing the neurobiology of affective illness is a goal in itself, this enquiry relates to the broader issues encompassed within the regulation of human emotion. An essential starting-point is the definition of an underlying functional anatomy of affective states, by which we mean the organised brain systems that provide the neural substrate for both the behavioural and the conscious components of emotional experience, including morbid mental states.

The requirement for a theory of the emotions

It will be obvious that, in offering a functional map of the brain areas involved in emotion, we are attempting to bridge the traditional divide between mind and body at a single, perhaps overambitious, stroke. What precisely should we be expecting of such a map? Psychological theories have had a dominant role in the study of human emotion. However, they have had a diversity and an absence of consensus that are daunting (e.g. Robbins, 1983). Thus emotion can be seen as a state of pure feeling, as a secondary sensory consequence of visceral responses or as a 'context' strongly influenced by thoughts and memories. Traditional distinctions between emotion and cognition have been undermined by the application of the term cognitive variously to sensory processing, to thinking in general and to the acquisition of knowledge (Moroz, 1972). Given this broader definition, it has been argued that emotions can be conferred the legitimacy of cognitive status (Armon-Jones, 1991). The presence of emotional disturbance in patients following damage to cortical association areas, typically associated with higher cognitive functions (Damasio & Van Hoesen, 1983), and conversely, the presence of cognitive impairment in patients with primary depression (e.g. Austin *et al.*, 1992a) support the view that emotion and cognitive function are non-independent. Emotion and more classical cognitive constructs, such as attention and memory, may not require uniquely separate brain systems but, rather, different modes of mental processing, perhaps within a related functional anatomy. Indeed, it has been hypothesised that such modes might be computational, resulting in conceptual elaboration, in the case of cognition and evaluative, determining value or significance, in the case of emotion (Parrott & Schulkin, 1993).

It is our view that cognitive neuroscience will increasingly demand that the relative merits of competing psychological theories be gauged by biological measures (Sherer, 1993), provided primarily by functional brain imaging. Thus, the general acceptance of the premise that emotional experience is realised through activity in central neural systems has paralleled an increasing emphasis on the direct investigation of brain function in patients with affective disorders. Structural imaging can address whether there are trait differences between the brains of patients with major depression and controls, in the form of either unique focal pathologies or non-specific structural deficits. Functional imaging techniques based on regional perfusion address the relationship between mental states and brain states in terms of functional anatomy. In its current application, it can also address questions such as the relationship between illness manifestations and regional brain function, as well as the critical issue of how brain neurophysiology covaries with recovery. It can be anticipated that future developments may enable the examination of specific neurochemical questions concerning fundamental mechanisms of disease.

This chapter will review and anticipate developments in the following areas: the structural and functional brain abnormalities associated with affective illness; the anatomy of brain systems underlying the phenomena and component symptoms of affective illness; and the neuropsychological mechanisms that account for component symptoms and their relationship to functional anatomy.

Structural imaging in affective disorders

X-ray computed tomography (CT) provided the first non-invasive approach to the study of *in vivo* brain morphology in the functional psychiatric disorders. The technique provides relatively low anatomical resolution of brain structure but a good resolution of brain from surrounding cerebrospinal fluid (CSF), particularly for the ventricular system. This has enabled quantitative measurements of ventricular size and estimates of sulcal width within patient populations, from which alterations in underlying brain morphology can be inferred. The limited ability to differentiate grey and white matter has not allowed quantitative measurements of component brain structures.

As described in Chapter 10, the earliest application of CT in psychiatry was in the study of schizophrenia, where lateral ventricular enlargement has been described in a significant proportion of patients; the distribution across many studies is compatible with an effect on patients in general rather than upon an aberrant subgroup (Daniel *et al.*, 1991). The first study of this kind (Johnstone *et al.*, 1976) provided a modern landmark in the adoption of a more biologically based approach to the functional psychoses. It thus provided the impetus for similar studies in the affective disorders.

The first study employing CT was of a cohort of elderly depressed patients, where a small but significant minority exhibited enlarged ventricles. These patients appeared clinically distinct in that they had a later age of onset and a high endogenous-symptom profile (Jacoby & Levy, 1980). On follow-up, they also had a higher mortality compared with patients with normal ventricles, although the sample size was small (Jacoby *et al.*, 1981). An initial report in a younger sample of patients with bipolar disorder indicated the presence of ventricular enlargement in younger patients (Pearlson & Veroff, 1981), as did a comparative study of consecutive admissions with mania and schizophrenia (Nasrallah *et al.*, 1982). The latter study provided preliminary evidence that morphological brain changes were a feature of both affective disorder and schizophrenia. Other comparative studies of affective cohorts, primarily bipolar patients, and schizophrenic samples provided similar evidence (Rieder *et al.*, 1983).

One of largest controlled CT studies showed that ventricular size and sulcal width was a feature of patients spanning all age ranges (Dolan *et al.*, 1986) and occurred in both bipolar and unipolar depression. Patients exhibited significantly larger ventricles and greater sulcal width, particularly in the frontal and parietal regions, compared with controls. No relationship emerged between morphological brain changes and illness characteristics, such as age of onset, illness duration or course. It was concluded that morphological changes acted as vulnerability factors for depression and the findings were broadly in keeping with another large study of unipolar patients (Shima *et al.*, 1984), although in this study enlarged ventricles were associated with a latter age of onset and a more chronic illness course. A minority of studies have examined other parameters, particularly the size of the third ventricle. The findings are broadly similar to studies of lateral ventricular size, with some, but not all, reporting differences with respect to controls (Tanaka *et al.*, 1982; Schlegel & Kretzschmar, 1987).

Although a majority of studies have reported morphological brain changes in patients with affective disorders, a significant proportion of investigations have failed to replicate these findings (Schlegel & Kretzschmar, 1987; Dewan *et al.*, 1988; Iacono *et al.*, 1988). This failure has also been a feature of similar studies in schizophrenia and may be expected for small studies pursuing relatively modestly sized effects (Chapter 10).

Magnetic resonance imaging (MRI) has an improved potential for the acquisition and quantitative analysis of structural images because of its superior spatial resolution. This may have important implications for our better understanding of psychiatric disorder if some of the problems of quantification can be solved. The required techniques are only now beginning to be applied to schizophrenia (e.g. Bartzokis *et al.*, 1993). The potential in affective illness where outcome is equally variable, but treatment more effective, remains largely unexplored. As already implied, the evidence from CT for structural brain abnormality in major depression has been largely non-specific. A distinct topographical focus of brain impairment was achieved with the finding of Coffey *et al.* (1993), suggesting a small but selective reduction in frontal-lobe volume in depressive illness. Findings in elderly volunteers also suggest that preferential involvement of frontal cortex may be a feature of age-related change in brain structure (Jernigan *et al.*, 1991; Coffey *et al.*, 1992). Reduced size of subcortical nuclei has also been reported in depression with MRI (Krishnan *et al.*, 1992).

In addition to abnormal brain dimensions, there have been consistent reports of increased rates of white-matter lesions in affective disorder. The best known clinicopathological entity characterised by related white-matter change is otherwise known as Binswanger's disease (Kinkel *et al.*, 1985) (see Chapter 13). It is held to be a consequence of diffuse arteriosclerosis in white-matter vessels, itself a vague and still unsatisfactory description (Hachinski, 1991). *In vivo* white-matter changes have attracted similarly imprecise descriptive terms such as 'leucoaraiosis' on CT (Kinkel *et al.*, 1985). White-matter lesions in T2-weighted images are seen even more commonly with MRI (Coffey *et al.*, 1990; Mirsen *et al.*, 1991). They also occur in asymptomatic elderly subjects, so the choice of controls is critical (Guze & Szuba, 1992). Rate and severity of white-matter lesions are less in controls than in depressed patients (Coffey *et al.*, 1990, 1993). In elderly controls, they did not appear to predict neuropsychological impairment on a measure such as the digit symbol-substitution test (Tupler *et al.*, 1992). In depressive illness, the matter remains to be properly addressed. White-matter changes are also common in Alzheimer dementia, where they are commonest in women and may be associated with more extreme cognitive impairment and perhaps premature death (Steingart *et al.*, 1987; Diaz *et al.*, 1991). Neuropathologically, white-matter pallor is the clearest correlate of leucoaraiosis (Janota *et al.*, 1989).

Accepting that a proportion of patients with affective disorder display morphological brain changes does not establish their biological significance. There is uncertainty as to whether structural change occurs only in a subgroup or simply represents the tail of a shifted normal distribution. The absence of any consistent relationship with clinical or phenomenological features suggests that morphological changes act at the level of vulnerability. The aetiology of these structural changes remains unknown. Perhaps the most interesting implication is that the change may reflect accelerated ageing. Independent family studies suggest that the fathers of individuals with major depression show premature death due to non-psychiatric causes (Vaillant *et al.*, 1992). In contrast, in schizophrenia structural abnormality appears more likely to arise through failure in brain development, without evidence of subsequent progressive loss of brain volume. This may explain why similar-looking brain changes may lead to schizophrenia on the one hand and affective disorder on the other. However, it underlines the relatively crude nature of current morphological methods for *in vivo* imaging. Whether superior measures of tissue integrity will be discernible with new methods based on MRI, such as proton spectroscopy will be of considerable interest (see Chapter 6).

The relationship between structural abnormality, vulnerability and cognitive impairment

It remains uncertain whether vulnerability and poor outcome in affective disorder can be related to the degree of structural brain change. The necessary outcome studies have not been done with modern MRI methods. The mediating mechanisms for the vulnerability that the brain changes may imply are similarly uncertain. One

possibility is that a general impairment of cognitive processing contributes, at least in the elderly. This is compatible with the findings of Abas *et al.* (1990). Depression may then arise for a host of reasons, including precipitant life circumstances, which may be mediated, in part, by a reduced capacity for effective information processing. However, we can be much less certain of the most likely basis of the corresponding vulnerability and variation in outcome in younger patients, including those with a strongly familial pattern of affective disorder (often bipolar). There are reports of white-matter and basal-nuclear lesions in young patients with bipolar illness (e.g. Dupont *et al.*, 1990; Botteron *et al.*, 1992), but most of the existing studies are in older subjects and have employed limited imaging methods. The development of contrast enhancement of white-matter lesions with MRI will facilitate a more systematic investigation of this phenomenon than has been possible hitherto.

The link between the old and the young with depressive illness remains tenuous for explanations of vulnerability based on structural brain abnormality. However, preliminary but related neuropsychological findings may justify a similar approach in young and old. Abas *et al.* (1990) described impaired recognition memory function after recovery from depressive illness in elderly patients. More curiously, in young patients with seasonal affective disorder (O'Brien *et al.*, 1993), an enduring impairment of the performance of the same recognition-memory task was also reported. However, the effect was confined to response latency rather than accuracy. This evidence of slowed performance has echoes of the more general psychomotor slowing seen in the depressed state. It is possible that impairment in the efficiency of cognitive processing may contribute to the vulnerability to depression, even in young subjects. This view is given circumstantial support by Wolfe *et al.* (1987), who reported that bipolar patients, who are more likely to have early-onset disease with a genetic loading, presented even greater cognitive impairment than unipolars, and that their memory

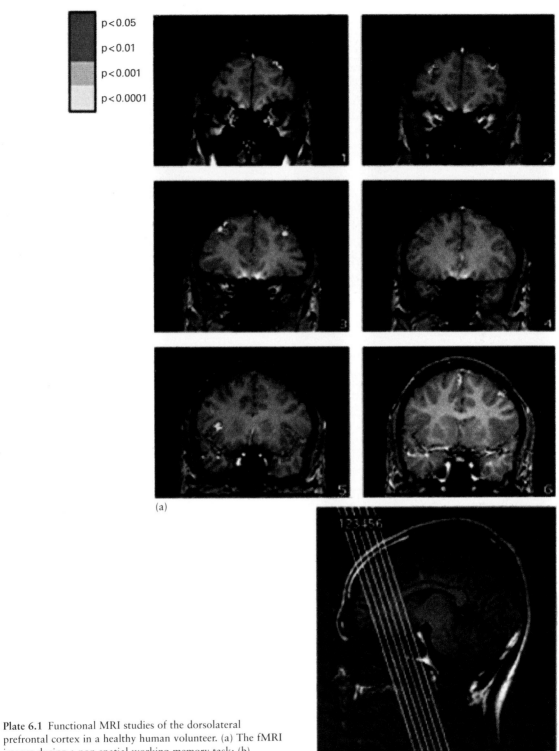

p < 0.05
p < 0.01
p < 0.001
p < 0.0001

(a)

(b)

Plate 6.1 Functional MRI studies of the dorsolateral prefrontal cortex in a healthy human volunteer. (a) The fMRI images during a non-spatial working-memory task; (b) sagittal view showing slice selection.

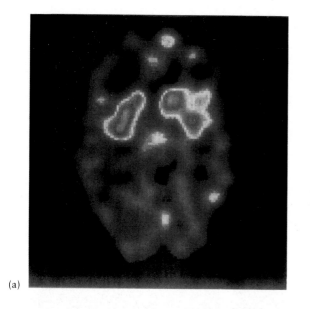

(a)

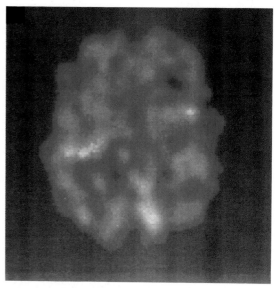

(b)

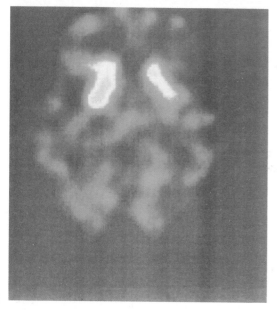

(c)

Plate 7.1 (a) ^{123}I-IBZM SPET scan from an untreated schizophrenic patient. The basal ganglia are clearly seen in the image as two central red areas. (b) A patient on typical antipsychotic drugs. No basal ganglia signal is visible. The cold drug prevents ^{123}I-IBZM binding to D2 receptors by occupying these sites. (c) A patient treated with clozapine. Occupancy is 50% lower than that of typical antipsychotic drugs and the basal ganglia are visible.

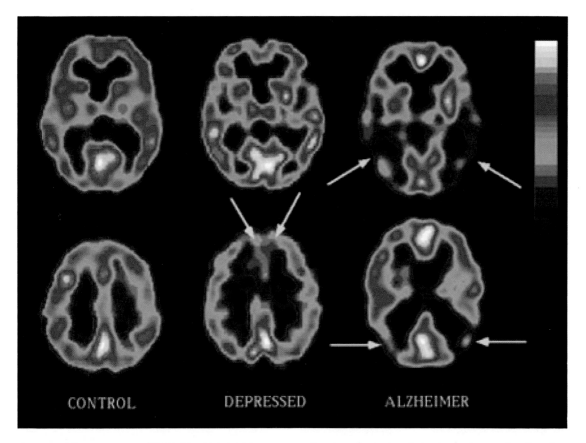

Plate 12.1 The appearance of ^{99m}Tc-HMPAO SPET scans in normal elderly, elderly depressed and patient with Alzheimer dementia. Note (indicated by arrows) the frontal reductions in the upper scan and the preservation of parietotemporal perfusion in the depressed patient. In contrast, there is a classic posterior perfusion deficit in the Alzheimer patient.

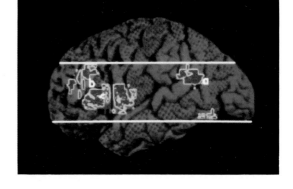

Plate 12.2 A statistical parametric map (SPM) of the correlation between a behavioural dimension of psychomotor retardation and rCBF. The area of greatest correlation, in terms of spatial extent, is in the left dorsolateral prefrontal cortex. These findings are comparable with the findings illustrated by SPET data in Fig. 12.1 b. a = angular gyrus, b = dorsolateral prefrontal cortex.

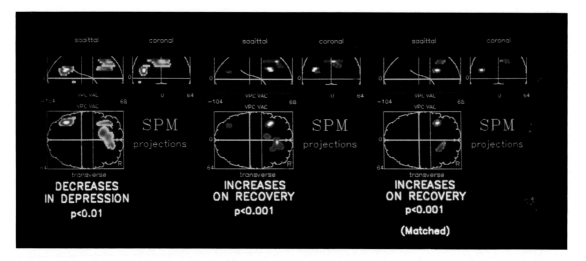

Plate 12.3 Statistical parametric map (SPM), displayed as orthogonal projections, of adjusted regional cerebral blood flow (rCBF) differences in (left) 25 depressed patients at index assessment, compared with 23 controls; (centre) 25 depressed patients at index compared with same patients on recovery (non-matched for medication); and (right) 15 depressed patients at index compared with recovery (matched for medication). Two of the regions that show maximal decreases at index assessment, the left dorsolateral prefrontal cortex and the anterior cingulate cortex, are the areas that show maximal increases with recovery. In contrast, the left angular gyrus shows relatively little change on recovery.

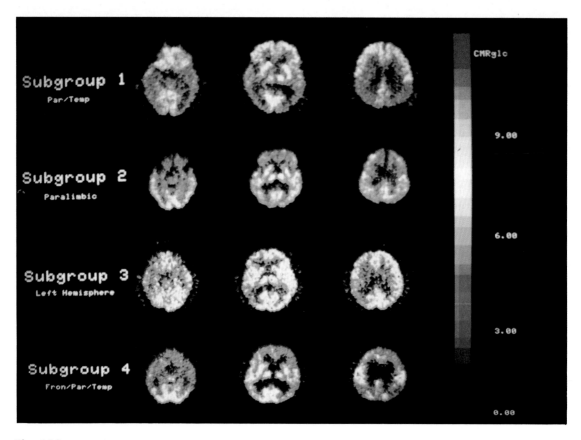

Plate 14.1

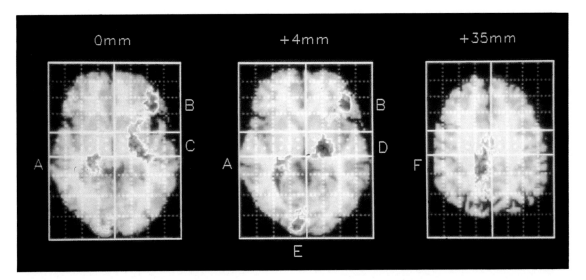

Plate 15.1 Three transverse planes demonstrating areas where there were significant positive correlations between symptom intensity and rCBF in a group of patients with OCD (McGuire *et al*, 1994). The PET data have been superimposed on a magnetic resonance (MR) image from one of the patients, which has been transformed into the stereotactic space of the Talairach and Tournoux atlas, to serve as an anatomical reference. The level of each plane relative to the anterior commissure–posterior commissure (AC–PC) line is shown above each slice. The right side of the brain is seen on the viewer's right. In the 0 mm plane, positive correlations are evident in the left hippocampus (A), right inferior frontal gyrus (B) and right putamen and globus pallidus (C). At +4 mm, positive correlations can be seen in the left hippocampus (A), right inferior frontal gyrus (B), right thalamus (D) and left cuneus (E). In the 35 mm plane there are positive correlations in the left posterior cingulate gyrus (F).

Plate 14.1 (*opposite*) PET scan images from four AD patients that characterise four metabolic subgroups identified with principal-component analysis. Three planes are shown for each subject: left, at the level of the orbitofrontal cortex (30 mm above the inferior orbitomeatal (IOM) line); middle, at the level of the basal ganglia (45 mm above IOM line); and right, at the level of the centrum semiovale (70 mm above IOM line). The subgroup numbers correspond to the subgroups described in the text. Metabolic rate is shown in mg/100 g brain/min (scale is on the right of the figure, CMRglc = cerebral metabolic rate for glucose). Data were obtained using a Scanditronix PC1024-7B tomograph.

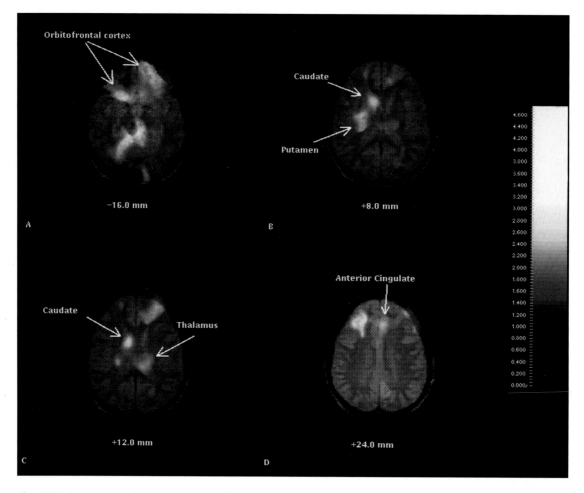

Plate 15.2 Areas activated in association with the evocation of symptoms in a group of patients with OCD are shown on a series of transverse slices (Rauch *et al.* 1994). The PET data have been superimposed on a nomal magnetic resonance (MR) image, which has been transformed into the stereotactic space of the Talairach and Szikla atlas, to serve as an anatomical reference. The height of each slice relative to the AC–PC line is shown in millimetres. The right side of the brain is seen on the viewer's left. Significant increases in rCBF are evident in the orbitofrontal cortex (A), the striatum (B and C) and the anterior cingulate (D).

Plate 15.4 (*opposite*) Transverse PET images (upper row) showing the distribution of rCBF during anticipatory anxiety, panic and teeth clenching. All these conditions are associated with increasing rCBF in the region of the temporal poles, but coregistration with MR images (lower row) demonstrates that these functional changes are localised to the overlying extracranial musculature (bottom, right) (Drevets *et al*, 1992).

Plate 15.3 Asymmetry of resting parahippocampal blood flow, as measured by PET, in a patient with a predisposition to lactate-induced panic (Reiman *et al*, 1984). Resting rCBF in a transverse slice including the parahippocampal gyri. The left half of this figure illustrates left-hemispheric blood flow, while the right half shows the differences between rCBF in the right and left hemispheres, expressed as a percentage of the left-hemisphere blood flow. There is a region of asymmetry in the right parahippocampal gyrus, which was not evident in controls.

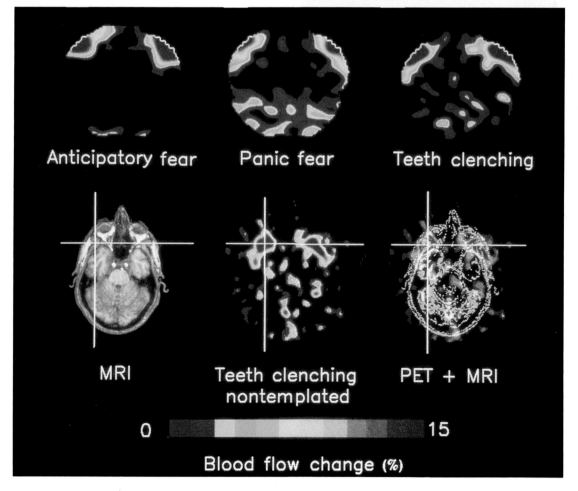

Plate 15.4

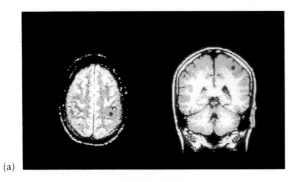

(a)

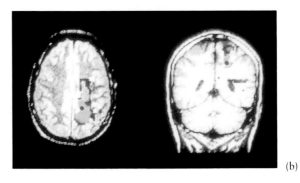

(b)

Plate 16.1 Colour-coded representation of the instantaneous distribution of electrical activity at the level of the sensory motor strip during a left index-finger movement obtained from magnetic-field tomography analysis of MEG. Activity is shown (a) 240 ms and (b) 280 ms after the stimulus to move the finger. The red dot marks the maximum current. The activation appears over the central sulcus on the contralateral side. Courtesy of Dr A.A. Ioannides, Open University, UK.

profiles when depressed closely resembled those of patients with Huntington's disease.

However, impairment of cognitive function has been a neglected feature of depressive illness. In patients under 65 with major depression, worsening depressive illness was associated with increasing cognitive impairment; episodic-memory tasks and visuomotor speed were particularly affected (Austin *et al.*, 1992a). This is unlike schizophrenia, where symptom severity and cognitive impairment do not appear to be correlated (Goldberg *et al.*, 1993). In the elderly, the overlap in memory dysfunction between major depression and Alzheimer-type dementia was so large that 25% of depressed patients could have been misclassified as demented on the basis of their memory deficit (O'Carroll *et al.*, 1994). These findings are not explained by a global attentional difficulty, since performance on measures of attention (e.g. digit span) was virtually unaffected (Austin *et al.*, 1992a).

Most studies of cognitive dysfunction in depression have focused on traditional episodic-memory tests such as word-list learning and story recall (see review by Robbins *et al.*, 1992). However, studies of amnesic patients clearly show that 'memory' is not a unitary function (Parkin & Leng, 1993) and may be fractionated into different components which have dissociable functional neuroanatomies. A detailed analysis of memory dysfunction is now required in major depression, employing currently accepted divisions into short-term and long-term, episodic and semantic, explicit and implicit, and positive and negative hedonic bias. A selective effect on memory performance would favour a localising mechanism underlying the depressive illness, whereas generalised cognitive impairment would not.

Functional imaging in affective disorders

In the functional imaging literature, employing either single-photon emission tomography (SPET) or positron emission tomography (PET), it is possible to identify three methodological approaches in the affective disorders, all based on analyses of subjects studied under resting, non-activated, conditions and each addressing distinct issues. Firstly, there are *case–control* experiments, whereby a depressed subject group is compared with a control group. This has been the most widely adopted approach and essentially provides information on the common sites of neural dysfunction within the population of patients under investigation. It also risks confounding reduced perfusion with reduced brain mass. This would be especially difficult if brain volume showed localised change, although, until Coffey *et al.* (1993), there was little evidence that reduced brain volume was markedly localised in depression. A generalised loss of brain volume of the sort most commonly described would be largely corrected for by normalisation within individual subjects. A second group of experimental studies, using *correlational* analyses, provides information on the relationship between particular behavioural impairments and regional brain function. This type of approach may identify brain areas not revealed in case–control experiments, where the averaging of data from behaviourally heterogeneous patients samples tends to highlight shared deficits. The third approach is that based on longitudinal assessments of patients studied on more than one occasion, usually when ill and on recovery. This approach addresses the question of how regional deficits, identified at an index assessment, covary with recovery or alteration of a behavioural state and can determine whether deficits represent trait or state markers. It is unlikely to be confounded by regional reductions in brain mass.

An approach based on activation, using either psychological, pharmacological or conjoint activation techniques remains the most intriguing, but undeniably the most difficult to design. In principle, activation studies can provide more sophisticated information on brain function, such as the patterns of connectivity, both functional and effective, between regional brain systems (Friston *et al.*, 1993a,b). The theoretical promise of formulating psychiatric disorder in terms of disordered functional networks subserving relevant neuropsychological mechanisms is an appealing one. It offers to transcend the mere phenomenology of symptoms and to offer predictive models of the disease process. It remains limited, nevertheless, by the difficulty of measuring connectivity within the nervous system using methods that measure neuronal function on the basis of vascular change and by our current ability to conceptualise the necessary neuropsychology.

Single-photon emission tomography (SPET)

Perfusion imaging with SPET employs the widely available ligand ^{99m}Tc-hexamethylpropyleneaminoxime (HMPAO; Exametazime). This is injected intravenously, taken up into brain tissue in proportion to regional perfusion and trapped in the brain (Neirinckx *et al.*, 1987). Because of the perceived limitations of SPET reconstruction algorithms, the low resolution of many rotating camera systems, and the poor stability of the ^{99m}Tc-HMPAO complex in plasma, there were early reservations about the quantitation of ^{99m}Tc-HMPAO uptake. Certainly, it has not been possible with SPET to obtain absolute values for brain perfusion: the 'gold standard' for tomographic studies of aggregate brain function is, therefore, provided by ^{15}O-PET. However, the high variance of global flow seen across conditions in a single subject, or between subjects for a single condition, makes it necessary to normalise PET perfusion data before its analysis. Normalised SPET data can, unequivocally, be treated similarly. The critical difference from ^{99m}Tc-HMPAO SPET is that modification of PET cameras and acquisition software has improved sensitivity to a point where it is possible to study whole-brain perfusion for 12–18 conditions (30 s sampling windows) on the same subject for a radiation exposure comparable to that of a single ^{99m}Tc-HMPAO SPET scan (Silbersweig *et al.*, 1993). These developments mean that ^{99m}Tc-HMPAO SPET is best employed experimentally for simple comparisons within or between patient

groups. However, it is feasible to employ SPET in large and fully representative clinical studies and it is likely to be the only isotope-based technique widely available for clinical use. The adaptation of pixel-by-pixel analysis to SPET data has been slow but is entirely feasible. However, all the analyses to be described below have employed data derived from region-of-interest analysis (see Chapter 5).

Cross-sectional studies with ^{99m}Tc-HMPAO SPET

In patients under 65 with major depression, reduced brain perfusion was found in the majority of cortical and subcortical regions examined, most significantly in temporal and inferior frontal areas and in the caudate area bilaterally (Austin *et al.*, 1992b). Unlike most of the structural findings, the SPET data suggested an effect predominantly in anterior brain structures. This also resembled functional findings with non-tomographic techniques, usually based on ^{133}Xe (Mathew *et al.*, 1980; Warren *et al.*, 1984; Schlegel *et al.*, 1989; Sackeim *et al.*, 1990) and tomographic tracer techniques using PET (Buchsbaum *et al.*, 1986; Post *et al.*, 1987; Baxter *et al.*, 1989; Hurwitz *et al.*, 1990; Martinot *et al.*, 1990; Bench *et al.*, 1992). Subsequently, Yazici *et al.* (1992) have also reported similar decrements with ^{99m}Tc-HMPAO SPET; negative results have been reported by Maes *et al.* (1993). Group effects were generally small and, in some studies, strongly influenced by patient age (Austin *et al.*, 1992b); there was relatively higher uptake in younger patients and lower uptake in the older members of the sample. Perfusion of neocortex was not age-related for controls with ^{99m}Tc-HMPAO SPET or ^{15}O PET (Martin *et al.*, 1991).

The interpretation of correlations with a 'trait' variable (age) is not straightforward. The finding could imply that relatively diffuse cross-sectional differences from controls in functional scans are potentially trait-related. They may even be related to structural abnormalities since white-matter abnormalities are primarily placed anteriorly. In contrast, as will be explained below, there is good evidence for some of the variation in anterior brain perfusion being attributable to patterns of symptoms. The present findings underline that cross-sectional designs are inadequate in themselves to answer the range of questions that fall within the scope of a functional imaging study.

The impact of increasing patient age was further examined by comparing uptake of ^{99m}Tc-HMPAO at rest for subjects over 60 with major depressive disorder or Alzheimer-type dementia with normal volunteers (Curran *et al.*, 1993). Cross-sectional differences between the three groups were highly statistically significant but primarily reflected the reductions in cortical uptake in the Alzheimer group (cf. Upadhyaya *et al.*, 1990). A detailed comparison of depressed patients and controls identified decrements in anterior cingulate, temporal and frontal cortex and in caudate and thalamus in male patients only (Fig. 12.1a). These decrements were correlated with impairment of performance on the trail-making task (Fig. 12.1b), but were also associated with continuing treatment with antidepressants and/or benzodiazepines. There was a weak association between good outcome at 6–18 months and increased tracer uptake in subcortical areas.

Since parietotemporal uptake of tracer in elderly depressed patients and age-matched controls was similar, it is highly significant that marked bilateral reductions in this area are characteristic in Alzheimer-type dementia (Holman *et al.*, 1992). Our results therefore imply that by focusing on these areas ^{99m}Tc-HMPAO SPET can contribute to the differential diagnosis of depression and dementia. Quantitative analysis with a standard template shows, in Fig. 12.2, the overlap between depressed and control groups for anterior cingulate (partial) and parietal cortex (complete except for one outlier). In contrast, the Alzheimer patients show lower uptake in both regions. The qualitative differences are illustrated for individual cases in Plate 12.1 (facing p. 230). Any diagnostic decision is likely to be between dementia and depression, so this contrast is, of

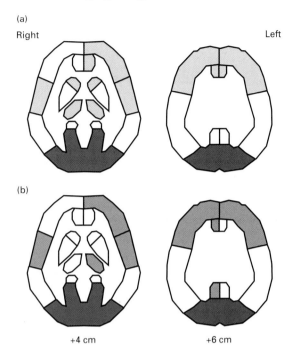

Fig. 12.1 (a) The relationship between decrements in the uptake of ^{99m}Tc-HMPAO in depressed male patients and male controls (upper) and (b) correlations between tracer uptake and trail-making test B (lower) in same male patients. Uptake was expressed relative to posterior visual sensory areas (dark grey). Decrements and correlations (all negative) are shown by light grey and dark grey shading respectively of regions of interest in which reductions were individually statistically significant ($P <$ 0.05). The brain regions are reproduced as they appear in the templates fitted to scan data. The relationship to a standard brain atlas is shown in Fig. 1 of Austin *et al.* (1992b). Slices at 4 cm and 6 cm above the orbitomeatal line.

course, much more relevant than a comparison between demented patients and normal controls. However, post-mortem-confirmed Alzheimer-type dementia can be most reliably distinguished from controls when both structural and SPET findings are combined (Jobst *et al.*, 1992). The clinical potential of combining images from both modalities has yet to be established.

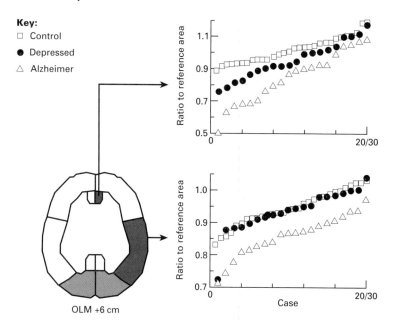

Key:
□ Control
● Depressed
△ Alzheimer

OLM +6 cm

Fig. 12.2 The attenuation of uptake of ^{99m}Tc-HMPAO in anterior cingulate and its preservation in posterior parietal cortex in elderly depressed patients. The ratio between uptake of ^{99m}Tc-HMPAO into the two brain areas (shown drak grey) and a reference sensory area (light grey) for the controls (open squares), depressed patients (filled circles) and Alzheimer patients (open triangles). The data for each group were ordered and plotted by ascending magnitude across the sample. For further discussion, see text. OLM, Orbitomeatal line.

The functional topography of depressive symptoms with SPET

Once age had been controlled for, the SPET study of Austin *et al.* (1992b) showed evidence of state-related correlations within the patient group. However, instead of the expected negative association between brain perfusion and symptom severity, there was a strong positive association between uptake and scores on the Newcastle scale, an arbitrary estimate of 'endogenicity', especially in cingulate areas, frontal cortex and caudate nuclei. The Newcastle scale is itself correlated with a more valid sign-based measure of motor abnormalities in major depression (Parker *et al.*, 1993). The involvement of frontal and caudate areas would seem to make sense in relation to motor symptoms. However, the 'sign' of the effect was the opposite of that seen in older patients and described in detail below for ^{15}O studies using pixel-by-pixel analysis. This may not matter for where correlations are found, but it implies that correlations with state variables must be highly influenced by patient selection as well as

being confounded in part by global severity (Austin *et al.*, 1992b; Bench *et al.*, 1993). The potential for more detailed cross-sectional correlational analysis relating symptoms to brain topography will be explored below in relation to PET data.

Changes in regional brain function on recovery from depression

Measurements made by tomographic functional-imaging techniques are potentially confounded in brains with reduced tissue mass. In depressed patients the evidence for increased ventricular–brain ratios, cerebral atrophy and diminished caudate nucleus volume, particularly in older patients, has been noted above. These difficulties may be overcome for SPET or ^{15}O PET in a test–retest design. Longitudinal studies thus enable some constraints to be placed on the range of exploratory analyses with findings from index assessments serving as the hypotheses to be tested. It is therefore surprising that there have been few longitudinal studies in depression, given its suitability to such approaches. The most important limitations of longitudinal studies are the potential confounding effects of order, the related problem of interpretation if changes in an index group are used to 'validate' maxima or minima at index examination and the bias introduced by patients dropping out.

State effects were determined in the Edinburgh SPET sample by comparing brain topography when ill and after recovery. In this sample, 28 patients previously investigated when ill were followed up at an interval of 9–28 months, after full recovery (Goodwin *et al.*, 1993). Significant bilateral increases in tracer uptake were confined to inferior anterior cingulate cortex and basal ganglia in those matched for drug treatment (4) or on both occasions drug-free (12); there were no statistically discernible changes in the neocortex. The remainder of the sample yielded inconclusive evidence of increased tracer uptake in left temporal cortex. This represents change within a far more restricted anatomical network than had been implied by cross-sectional comparisons. It occurred within a patient group showing little clinical evidence of motor retardation and a particularly good clinical outcome.

Since recovery from a major depressive episode was associated with functional changes within a restricted anatomical network, it appeared possible that the acute effects of electroconvulsive treatment (ECT) might be localised within the same areas. Fifteen patients with major depression being treated with ECT were investigated before and 45 min after a single ECT, using split-dose SPET. Significant decreases in tracer uptake were confined to the inferior anterior cingulate cortex (Scott *et al.*, 1994). These changes were correlated with the current severity of depressive symptoms and more weakly with decrements of memory function produced by ECT; there was no significant correlation with stimulus intensity or electroencephalographic measures of seizure duration. The results implied that ECT did indeed produce changes within the same restricted network, which changed following recovery. This is comparable with the locus of change in other

studies of short-term intervention with sleep deprivation, which modulated symptom severity (Wu *et al.*, 1992). Together or separately, these findings are all highly indicative of the anterior cingulate as a central locus of state change in depressive illness.

Positron emission tomography

PET is the most sophisticated technique available for the investigation of the functional anatomy of the living human brain. The most widely utilised technique involves perfusion mapping, using radioactive oxygen-15-labelled water (^{15}O-H$_2$O) or metabolic mapping using fluorine-18-labelled deoxyglucose (FDG). The basic principle in both techniques is that increases or decreases in synaptic activity are reflected in changes in local perfusion or energy consumption. The net magnitude of the effect observed is necessarily ambiguous, because it must reflect the combination of excitation, active inhibition, deactivation, etc. occurring within a particular region. However, where an effect is observed is much less ambiguous and it is for this reason that these methods are said to generate a functional anatomy. As there has been only preliminary work using PET to measure receptor density or neurotransmitter turnover in depression, this review will confine itself to perfusion and metabolic mapping studies.

Cross-sectional studies with ^{15}O PET

Early PET studies of depressed patients reported disparate findings, including decreased metabolism in the inferior frontal lobe (Buchsbaum *et al.*, 1984), lower hemispheric metabolic rates in bipolar patients (Baxter *et al.*, 1985), relative caudate hypometabolism in unipolar patients (Schwartz *et al.*, 1987) and impaired left dorsolateral prefrontal cortex (DLPFC) metabolism in both subgroups (Baxter *et al.*, 1989). These early studies were based on relatively small sample sizes and have not been consistently replicated. Perhaps the most robust finding from these early studies has been decreased metabolism in the left DLPFC (Martinot *et al.*, 1990; Bench *et al.*, 1992).

Bench *et al.* (1992) have reported the largest PET study of affective disorders to date, involving 40 patients with moderate to severe depression. This study, in contrast to previous work, which was based on region-of-interest analyses, used a pixel-by-pixel approach, sampling all brain regions, within a stereotactic coordinate framework. It was thus possible to identify three sites of maximal regional brain dysfunction: the left DLPFC, the left anterior cingulate cortex and the left angular gyrus. In other words, the depressed state was associated with a dysfunction in a neural system that involved paralimbic and association cortex. The findings were not an artefact of medication, being present in both medicated and non-medicated patients, and were not related to age, being present in both younger and older patients. In our view, it is likely to be significant that the regions identified are interconnected by reciprocal corticocortical connections (Goldman-Rakic, 1987).

A study, using very similar techniques of perfusion and parametric statistical mapping, has reported the apparently contradictory findings of *increased* regional cerebral blood flow (rCBF) in the left ventrolateral prefrontal and medial prefrontal cortices and the amygdala (Drevets & Raichle, 1992; Drevets *et al.*, 1992). This study confined itself to patients meeting criteria for familial pure depressive disorder (FPDD) and involved a small sample of 13 subjects of relatively young age (mean age 37). This study is therefore at odds with previous investigations reporting decrements in regional perfusion. An obvious explanation for this discrepant finding rates to the patient population studied. The SPET study by Austin *et al.* (1992b) also found relatively higher frontal perfusion in younger patients. Alternatively, the FPDD subtype may be unusual since it is most closely related to bipolar illness (Winokur, 1980). The majority of studies in the literature have been confined principally to unipolar patients. However, the areas implicated

overlap to some extent, at least in regard to left DLPFC. As noted previously, the magnitude and perhaps even the sign of metabolic or perfusion effects may be less critical than their anatomy. The potential for identifying different cross-sectional abnormalities when different diagnostic groups are employed within the very wide umbrella of major depression deserves further attention and perhaps the addition of information from structural scanning.

The functional topography of depressive symptoms with PET

A further approach to understanding the phenomenological heterogeneity of major depression lies in relating brain perfusion to symptoms or mental-state constructs rather than to diagnosis. Depression involves not only mood disturbance but also changes in psychomotor speed, attention and memory (Silfverskiöld *et al.*, 1987). The lack of consistency in findings from functional imaging studies in depression could be the consequence of clinical heterogeneity in the expression of these mental-state abnormalities. If there is a measurable relationship between brain and behaviour, how could the range of behavioural abnormalities encompassed within what are termed affective illnesses be attributable to a single pattern of regional brain dysfunction? It follows that specific syndromes of depression might be related to unique patterns of neurophysiological dysfunction. This can be explored in cross-sectional studies by relating regional deficits to phenomenological and neuropsychological profiles, using correlational analyses. The cross-sectional correlation structure of subjects scanned in the same behavioural state is dependent on variance experimentally introduced by subject selection. The basic assumption of this approach is that, if subjects exhibit variability in a single behavioural score, for example a psychopathological rating, then brain systems underlying that behaviour can be expected to exhibit neuronal activity which correlates with the behavioural score. The particular advantage of using pixel-by-pixel analysis is that this maximises the use of the available data set for detecting patterns of correlations.

In fact, it has been demonstrated that specific clinical components of affective disorder can be associated with individual patterns of rCBF, using pixel-by-pixel analysis (Bench *et al.*, 1993). Specifically, increased blood flow in the posterior cingulate cortex and inferior parietal lobule correlated with increased loading on a score for a clinical dimension of psychomotor agitation/anxiety, and decreased rCBF in the left DLPFC and the left angular gyrus was highly correlated with a dimension of psychomotor retardation and mood disturbance. In the left anterior medial prefrontal cortex, decreased rCBF was correlated with increasing cognitive impairment.

Such correlational studies are hypothesis-generating. It is important to establish their behavioural generality by confirmatory studies in other patient groupings or by modelling the behavioural deficit in terms of the neuropsychological process involved. The latter approach has the advantage of enabling predictions to be made as to the neural basis of particular neuropsychological processes in normal subjects. For example, a striking finding in the study of Bench *et al.* (1993) was the emergence of a relationship between psychomotor retardation and hypoperfusion in the left DLPFC (Plate 12.2, facing p. 230). Psychomotor retardation is characterised by difficulties in the initiation of action, with a restriction of both verbal and motor expression. Depressed patients will give normal but delayed and slowed responses to questions but generate little in the way of propositional speech. In schizophrenia, the presence of psychomotor poverty, is likewise highly correlated with an area of decreased rCBF in the left DLPFC. The PET finding is an important stimulus to understanding the common cognitive deficit underlying poverty of speech in the two conditions. A key hypothetical component of both conditions may be an impairment of intentional or willed behaviour. Intentional behaviours are those in which we must generate and consciously select between alternatives rather than be subject to external guidance. If the DLPFC is critical in the expression of intentional or willed behaviours, it should be activated in intentional action. This has been shown to be the case in separate studies of self-generated words and movements in normal subjects (Frith *et al.*, 1991). It follows that DLPFC hypoperfusion is associated more with a behavioural deficit than with a diagnosis. By pooling data from two cohorts of patients with depression and schizophrenia, poverty of speech, but not diagnosis, predicted hypoperfusion in the left DLPFC (Dolan *et al.*, 1993). Significant correlations between patterns of rCBF and other behavioural measures should cross diagnostic boundaries. Equally, the critical differences between poverty of speech in depression and schizophrenia, assuming they are not actually identical, may be interpretable once a more refined understanding of the spontaneous generation of words has been obtained. Functional-imaging studies thereby reinforce the potential interest of neuropsychological constructs. Neuropsychological deficits that are common to different diagnostic categories should be accounted for by similar sites of neurophysiological deficit.

Cognitive performance and regional brain function

Neuropsychological deficits are an invariable component of depression. These deficits range from mild subclinical impairments to a pervasive state of clinical dementia, the dementia of depression. The neuropsychological deficits have been characterised as involving attentional and mnemonic function. The neural basis of cognitive deficits in depression has been the subject of a number of studies. In a comparison of depressed patients with and without global cognitive deficits, determined on the Mini-Mental State Examination (MMSE), a decrease in rCBF in the medial prefrontal cortex was reported in patients with global cognitive impairments (Dolan *et al.*, 1992). This was extended to a series containing more patients with milder impairment, using a correlational approach with the same result (Bench *et al.*, 1993).

The previous findings left open the question of whether specific components of cognitive impairment in depression might be associated with separable patterns of regional neuronal dysfunction. This possibility was explored in a neuropsychological study of a representative subsample of the same patients. Two factors, one related to episodic memory function and the other related to attention, explained most of the variance in the cognitive impairment (Bench *et al.*, 1993). Both these factors demonstrated significant correlations with rCBF in the medial prefrontal cortex and frontal polar cortex (Dolan *et al.*, 1994). For posterior brain regions, the memory factor correlated with areas such as the retrosplenial cingulate cortex and precuneus; a similar association was reported by Austin *et al.* (1992b). These posterior brain areas have been previously identified as part of a neuronal network involved in auditory-verbal memory (Grasby *et al.*, 1993). For the attentional component, there were significant posterior correlations that encompassed the inferior parietal lobule and inferior postcentral gyrus.

Changes in regional brain function on recovery from depression

As with the SPET study of Goodwin *et al.* (1993), the study of the same patients when ill and, again, when recovered with ^{15}O PET provided a method of bolstering findings from cross-sectional studies. The expectation was that some, or all, the brain regions identified as dysfunctional during an illness episode should show maximal change, towards normalisation, with recovery.

To date the longitudinal studies reported with PET have been, in most cases, small in scale and limited to region-of-interest methodology. Hurwitz *et al.* (1990) found no differences in rCBF in patients after 5–7 weeks of imipramine treatment whereas Kanaya and Yonekawa (1990) found a trend for cortical rCBF to increase to normal values after treatment. Wu *et al.* (1992) reported

a decrease, from index assessment, in cingulate and amygdala metabolism post-treatment in a subgroup of patients who responded to sleep deprivation. Drevets and Raichle (1992) found that in three patients recovery was associated with decreased activity in the DLPFC and a non-significant increase in the left caudate. Other studies have described a relative normalisation of left DLPFC hypometabolism with recovery (Baxter *et al.*, 1989; Martinot *et al.*, 1990). No firm conclusions can be drawn from these studies in view of small sample sizes and varying medication status between pre- and post-treatment assessments.

Bench *et al.* (1995) have reported the largest longitudinal study to date employing PET. The study involved 25 patients, who were scanned when ill and on recovery. The methodology again involved a pixel-by-pixel analysis in conjunction with an image-realignment algorithm (Woods, R.P. *et al.*, 1992). Compared with normal controls, patients displayed persisting decreases in rCBF in the DLPFC, anterior cingulate and angular gyrus, despite clinical remission. The critical comparison involved a paired comparison of the same patients when ill and following recovery. It was evident that remission was associated with significant increases in rCBF in the left DLPFC and medial prefrontal cortex, including the anterior cingulate. The change in anterior cingulate at least is comparable with that described in a similarly designed SPET study by Goodwin *et al.* (1993). There was no significant change in rCBF in the angular gyrus. Thus the greatest regional variation occurred in areas previously identified as maximally dysfunctional during illness episodes (Plate 12.3, facing p. 230). Persistent decreases in rCBF in all three brain regions, of lesser magnitude than when subjects were ill, could represent either state abnormalities that had not fully normalised or, alternatively, trait abnormalities. The disadvantage of this study design is that the interpretation of changes in areas originally identified as areas of extreme relative increases or decreases in perfusion is difficult. Obviously an area identified because it shows extreme values will tend to show some normalisation on rescanning, an effect usually referred to as regression to the mean. This issue can only be resolved by scanning a cohort of stable recovered patients. Such an approach could also tackle the issue of the clinical significance, in terms of prognosis and clinical course, of persistent deficits in regional brain function.

The induction of low mood in volunteers has been investigated in a single ^{15}O PET study by Pardo *et al.* (1993). Increases in perfusion occurred in inferior frontal/orbital cortex, most prominently on the left side. The interpretation of these findings is complicated by the absence of an adequate control condition. Thus the increases could have been due to the recall or ruminatory processes required for the induction of a negative mood state rather than the mood itself. Nevertheless, the experimental manipulation of human emotion in normal subjects during imaging paradigms may yet prove of interest.

Conclusions from functional-imaging studies

The major limitations of the majority of functional-imaging studies in affective disorders have been the small sample sizes and the use of relatively unsophisticated modes of data analysis based on regions of interest. A consensus has now emerged in the functional-imaging literature that strongly favours pixel-by-pixel data-analysis techniques, in conjunction, for group studies, with the use of stereotaxis. Despite this, the majority of studies have demonstrated widespread reduction in anterior brain function in affective disorder. This has been more consistent than the 'hypofrontality' sometimes claimed in schizophrenia (see Chapter 11). The most frequent localising finding from cross-sectional studies has been decreased function in the left DLPFC in depression. Other important brain regions that have been highlighted in more recent studies, using both correlational and longitudinal designs, which have related local perfusion to symptoms, include the anterior and posterior cingulate and medial prefrontal cortices. The existence of a relationship between patterns of symptoms and regional perfusion may account for the apparent lack of consistency of detail in the literature, because symptom heterogeneity will necessarily introduce variation. The fact that specific symptomatic manifestations, including cognitive deficits, are related to regional brain neurophysiology indicates that the principal-symptom profile of any patient grouping can bias findings in an averaged data set. The more widespread use of a symptomatic approach to the analysis of functional-imaging data might provide one way forward and explain the often discrepant findings in the literature.

Specific ligands for SPET and PET: uses in affective disorder

There are two potential uses for such ligands, which are discussed in detail in Chapter 7. High-affinity compounds will indicate the density of receptors and will be highly resistant to displacement by agonists of lower affinity. For example, ^{123}I-iomazenil binding may provide an assay of gamma-aminobutyric acid (GABA) receptor numbers. It is highly specific for the benzodiazepine site and has an affinity 10-fold higher than that of the corresponding PET ligand ^{11}C-flumazenil (Innis *et al.*, 1991; Woods, S.W. *et al.*, 1992). It will, therefore, provide a good measure of receptor density in neocortical areas. This is of interest in several contexts. For example, loss of GABAergic interneurons would be expected to produce increases in postsynaptic GABA receptors, as described in cingulate cortex post-mortem in schizophrenia by Benes *et al.* (1992). Alternatively, the loss of pyramidal cells which normally express the receptor should produce decrements, and would be expected in Alzheimer-type dementia and perhaps also in elderly depressed patients.

Lower-affinity compounds can be used to indicate displacement from a specific receptor by competing agonists or antagonists. In principle, ligands that bind selectively to receptors for serotonin (5-hydroxytryptamine (5-HT)) would be of interest in understanding the effects of drug treatment and in the investigation of reported abnormalities from post-mortem brain studies. In practice, the use of the available selective SPET and PET ligands in depressive illness has, thus far, been minimal.

Future directions with functional imaging

The studies in affective disorder reviewed here have been based primarily on investigations carried out in the resting state. This has long seemed unsatisfactory. Pertubation of a complex system either with a suitably designed cognitive task or a selective drug offers a potential way of understanding the underlying dynamics. How to achieve an unambiguous advance by this means has, however, proved elusive. At a simple level, challenges determine the functional integrity of particular brain systems. Thus, Andreasen *et al.* (1992) showed that only half of the studies carried out in schizophrenia during the resting state found reduced frontal perfusion, whereas three-quarters of studies using an activation task did. The difficulty is that activation requires performance and patients with schizophrenia perform all cognitive tasks relatively poorly (Saykin *et al.*, 1991). Reduced prefrontal activation is thus regularly associated with poor task performance in schizophrenia. This echoes a recent finding in demented patients performing a verbal-memory task (Riddle *et al.*, 1993). In our view, such an 'abnormality' tells us less about the illness in question than about the particular task. The only outcome of such a study which might be interesting would be where, under conditions of matched performance, the pattern of brain activity was qualitatively different in patients compared with controls. To our knowledge, no such outcome has yet been observed. The worst outcome from activation studies is that activation obliterates differences quite easily detected at rest: this appeared to be the result in a pilot SPET study of verbal fluency in elderly depressed patients (Philpot *et al.*, 1993).

Where a drug acutely influences the symptoms

that define a condition, such pharmacological analysis has obvious meaning. However, the pharmacological theories invoking 5-HT and nor adrenaline in depression derive from drug actions that are delayed. This is unfavourable for imaging studies and means that drug challenge with selective agonists, such as clonidine or apomorphine, appear preferable. Neither has prominent effects on mood so it may be necessary to define their action on brain perfusion in relation to target cognitive tasks rather than the baseline (Grasby *et al.*, 1992a,b). However, the interpretation of the resulting effects is complicated. In addition, many psychotropic drugs act as direct pressor agents, and may change CBF independently of metabolism. Although it is global rather than regional changes that would be expected to result from alteration of blood-vessel innervation and it is regional changes in perfusion that are detected, it is seldom possible to refute the objection experimentally.

Non-human primate studies have begun to establish the role of neurotransmitter systems in the regulation of the neural systems subserving specific psychological states (Goldman-Rakic, 1988). Conjoint activation paradigms, involving cognitive and pharmacological challenges in the same scanning session, can therefore theoretically link psychology and pharmacology by specifying the neuroanatomical locus of interactions between neural systems subserving specific psychological processes and neurotransmitter inputs (Friston *et al.*, 1991). The potential of such an approach in the study of functional disorders, such as affective illness, is undeniable if it can be deployed to test theories of monoaminergic neurotransmitter dysregulation in depression within a systems framework.

As already indicated there are still unsolved conceptual difficulties in the use and interpretation of challenge studies, particularly psychological challenges, in patients with pathology. The critical issues involve the choice of psychological challenge and the nature of the experimental question. It is usually assumed that the psychological task should target a specific brain region or system that has been shown to be dysfunctional or engage a psychological process that is impaired in the patients under investigation. The difficulties in the interpretation of findings from these types of approach have been outlined already for hypofrontality in schizophrenia. One solution appears to be to constrain the performance of controls so as to match that of the patients. The probability is then that task difficulty will be quite different for the two groups. How should we conceptualise difficulty? If we attempt to escape the dilemma of task difficulty, we can instead use simple challenge paradigms which require minimal cognitive processing, tasks of trivial difficulty. Then, the assumption that the pheno-menon under investigation can be related to the dysregulation in the brain system of interest may be questionable.

Even if the choice of task can be made confidently, there remains the perennial problem, as in most areas of psychiatry, of behavioural heterogeneity within diagnostic categories. This poses formidable problems for any study of brain–behavioural relationships that involves averaging of data across subjects. It is a difficulty that can only be surmounted by selection of homogeneous patients within a diagnostic category, for example showing psychomotor retardation, or by resorting to single case-studies. While a surprising conclusion, the use of single case-studies has proved a resounding success within neuropsychology and an analogous approach is now feasible in conjunction with functional imaging, especially ^{15}O PET.

The advances to date in understanding the neurobiology of affective disorders have been modest. The central clinical issue is whether it is possible to identify brain abnormalities that are in any way predictive of vulnerability, treatment response, refractoriness or poor outcome: this has not yet been achieved. Nevertheless, we believe the current advances are of significance. Imaging studies strongly suggest that there is structural abnormality in the brains of patients with severe depressive illness: this is as important as the corresponding findings in schizophrenia. Brain

areas and systems that have been highlighted by functional imaging as the mediating structures for the disorder should now serve as target areas for investigation by other disciplines, such as neuro-pathology and neuropharmacology. Predictions based on functional deficits can be tested by hypothesis-led clinical studies. Methods to determine neurotransmitter mechanisms are likely to be implemented in the near future. It now seems likely that brain imaging advances will lead to a reconceptualisation of the nature of affective disorder which can incorporate both its psycho-social and its biological origins.

References

Abas, M.A., Sahakian, B.J. & Levy, R. (1990) Neuropsy-chological deficits and CT scan changes in elderly depressives. *Psychol. Med.* 20, 507–20.

Andreasen, N.C., Rezai, K., Alliger, R. *et al.* (1992) Hypofrontality in neuroleptic-naive patients and in patients with chronic schizophrenia. *Arch. Gen. Psychiatry* 49, 943–58.

Armon-Jones, C. (1991) *Varieties of Affect.* Harvester Wheatsheaf, London.

Austin, M.-P., Ross, M., Murray, C., O'Carroll, R.E., Ebmeier, K.P. & Goodwin, GM. (1992a) Cognitive function in major depression. *J. Affective Disorders* 25, 21–30.

Austin, M.-P., Dougall, N., Ross, M. *et al.* (1992b) Single photon emission tomography with ^{99m}Tc-Exametazime in major depression and the pattern of brain activity underlying the psychotic/neurotic continuum. *J. Affective Disorders* 26, 31–44.

Bartzokis, G., Mintz, J., Marx, P. *et al.* (1993) Reliability of *in vivo* volume measures of hippocampus and other brain structures using MRI. *Magnetic Resonance Imaging* 11, 993–1006.

Baxter, L.R., Phelps, M.E., Mazziotta, J.C. *et al.* (1985) Cerebral metabolic rates for glucose in mood disorders: studies with positron emission tomography and fluorodeoxyglucose F18. *Arch. Gen. Psychiatry* 42, 441–7.

Baxter, L.R., Schwartz, J.M., Phelps, M.E. *et al.* (1989) Reduc-tion of prefrontal cortex glucose metabolism common to three types of depression. *Arch. Gen. Psychiatry* 46, 243–50.

Bench, C.J., Friston, K.J., Brown, R.G., Scott, L.C., Frackowiak, S.J. & Dolan, R.J. (1992) The anatomy of melancholia – focal abnormalities of cerebral blood flow in major depression. *Psychol. Med.* 22, 607–15.

Bench, C.J., Friston, L.K.J., Brown, R.G., Frackowiak, R.S.J. & Dolan, R.J. (1993) Regional cerebral blood flow in depression measured by positron emission tomography: the relationship with clinical dimensions. *Psychol. Med.* **23**, 579–90.

Bench, C.J., Frackowiak, R.S.J. & Dolan, R.J. (1995) Changes in regional cerebral blood flow on recovery from depression. *Psychol. Med.* **25**, 247–61.

Benes, F.M., Vincent, S.L., Alsterberg, G., Bird, E.D. & SanGiovanni, J.P. (1992) Increased GABA$_A$ receptor binding in superficial layers of cingulate cortex in schizophrenics. *J. Neurosci.* **12**, 924–9.

Botteron, K.N., Figiel, G.S., Wetzel, M.W., Hudziak, J. & Van Eerdewegh, M. (1992) MRI abnormalities in adolescent bipolar affective disorder. *J. Am. Acad. Child Adolescent Psychiatry* **31**, 258–61.

Buchsbaum, M.S., DeLisi, L.E., Holcomb, H.H. *et al.* (1984) Anteroposterior gradients in cerebral gucose use in schizophrenia and affective disorders. *Arch. Gen. Psychiatry* **41**, 1159–66.

Buchsbaum, M.S., Wu, J., DeLisi, L.E. *et al.* (1986) Frontal cortex and basal ganglia metabolic rates assessed by positron emission tomography with [^{18}F]2-deoxyglucose in affective illness. *J. Affective Disorders* **10**, 137–52.

Coffey, C.E., Figiel, G.S., Djang, W.T. & Weiner, R.D. (1990) Subcortical hyperintensity on magnetic resonance imaging: a comparison of normal and depressed elderly subjects. *Am. J. Psychiatry* **147**, 187–9.

Coffey, C.E., Wilkinson, W.E., Parashos, I.A. *et al.* (1992) Quantitative cerebral anatomy of the aging human brain: a cross-sectional study using magnetic resonance imaging. *Neurology* **42**, 527–36.

Coffey, C.E., Wilkinson, W.E., Weiner, R.D. *et al.* (1993) Quantitative cerebral anatomy in depression. *Arch. Gen. Psychiatry* **50**, 7–16.

Curran, S.M., Murray, C.M., Van Beck, M. *et al.* (1993) A single photon emission computerised tomography study of regional brain function in elderly patients with major depression and with Alzheimer-type dementia. *Br. J. Psychiatry* **163**, 155–65.

Damasio, A.R. & Van Hoesen, G.W. (1983) Emotional disturbances associated with focal lesions of the limbic frontal lobes. In Heilma, K.M. & Satz, P. (eds) *Neuropsychology of Emotion*. Guilford Press, Guilford.

Daniel, D.G., Goldberg, T.E., Gibbons, R.D. & Weinberger, D.R. (1991) Lack of a bimodal distribution of ventricular size in schizophrenia: a Gaussian mixture analysis of 1056 cases and controls. *Biol. Psychiatry* **30**, 887–903.

Dewan, M.J., Haldipur, C.V., Lane, E.E., Ispahani, A., Boucher, M.F. & Major, L.F. (1988) Bipolar affective disorder I: comprehensive quantitative computed tomography. *Acta Psychiatr. Scand.* **77**, 670–6.

Diaz, J.F., Merskey, H., Hachinski, V.C. *et al.* (1991) Improved recognition of leukoaraiosis and cognitive impairment in Alzheimer's disease. *Arch. Neurol.* **48**, 1022–25.

Dolan, R.J., Calloway, S.P., Thacker, P.F. & Mann, A.H. (1986) The cerebral cortical appearance in depressed subjects. *Psychol. Med.* **16**, 775–9.

Dolan, R.J., Bench, C.J.B., Friston, K.J., Brown, R., Scott, L. & Frackowiak, R.S.J. (1992) Regional cerebral blood flow abnormalities in depressed patients with cognitive impairment. *J. Neurol. Neurosurg. Psychiatry* **55**, 768–73.

Dolan, R.J., Bench, C.J., Liddle, P.F. *et al.* (1993) Dorsolateral prefrontal cortex dysfunction in the major psychoses; symptom or disease specificity. *J. Neurol. Neurosurg. Psychiatry* **56**, 1292–8.

Dolan, R.J., Bench, C.J., Brown, R., Scott, L.C. & Frackowiak, R.S.J. (1994) Neuropsychological dysfunction in depression: its relationship to regional cerebral blood flow. *Psychol. Med.* **24**, 849–57.

Drevets, W.C. & Raichle, M.E. (1992) Neuroanatomical circuits in depression: implications for treatment mechanisms. *Psychopharmacol. Bull.* **28**, 261–74.

Drevets, W.C., Videen, T.O., Price, J.L., Preskorn, S.H., Carmichael, T. & Raichle, M.E. (1992) A functional anatomical study of unipolar depression. *J. Neurosci.* **12**, 3628–41.

Dupont, R.M., Jernigan, T.L., Butters, N. *et al.* (1990) Subcortical abnormalities detected in bipolar affective disorder using magnetic resonance imaging: clinical and neuropsychological significance. *Arch. Gen. Psychiatry* **47**, 55–9.

Friston, K.J., Grasby, P.M., Frith, C.D. *et al.* (1991) The neurotransmitter basis of cognition: psychopharmacological activation studies using positron emission tomography. In Foundation, C. (ed.) *Exploring Brain Functional Anatomy with Positron Tomography*. John Wiley & Sons, Chichester, pp. 76–92.

Friston, K.J., Frith, C.D. & Frackowiak, R.S.J. (1993a) Principal component analysis learning algorithms: a neurobiological analysis. *Proc. Roy. Soc. London Ser. B Biol. Sci.* **1**, 69–79.

Friston, K.J., Frith, C.D. & Frackowiak, R.S.J. (1993b) Time-dependent changes in effective connectivity measured with PET. *Hum. Brain Mapping* **1**, 69–79.

Frith, C.D., Friston, K.J., Liddle, P.F. & Frackowiak, R.S.J. (1991) Willed action and the prefrontal cortex in man: a study with PET. *Proc. Roy. Soc. London Ser. B Biol. Sci.* **244**, 241–6.

Goldberg, T.E., Gold, J.M., Greenberg, R. *et al.* (1993) Contrasts between patients with affective disorders and patients with schizophrenia on a neuropsychological test battery. *Am. J. Psychiatry* **150**, 1355–62.

Goldman-Rakic, P.S. (1987) Circuitry of primate prefrontal cortex and regulation of behaviour by representational memory. In Mountcastle, V.B., Bloom, F.E. & Geiger, S.R. (eds) *Handbook of Physiology—The Nervous*

System. Williams and Wilkins, Baltimore, pp. 373–417.

Goldman-Rakic, P.S. (1988) Topography of cognition: parallel distributed networks in primate association cortex. *Ann. Rev. Neurosci* **11**, 137–56.

Goodwin, G.M., Austin, M.-P., Dougall, N. *et al.* (1993) State changes in brain activity shown by the uptake of ^{99m}Tc-Exametazime with single photon emission tomography in major depression before and after treatment. *J. Affective Disorders* **29**, 243–53.

Grasby, P.M., Friston, K.J., Bench, C.J. *et al.* (1992a) The effect of apomorphine and buspirone on regional cerebral blood flow during the performance of a cognitive task—measuring neuromodulatory effects of psychotropic drugs in man. *Eur. J. Neurosci.* **4**, 1203–12.

Grasby, P.M., Friston, K.J., Bench, C. *et al.* (1992b) The effect of the $5HT_{1A}$ partial agonist buspirone on regional cerebral blood flow in man. *Psychopharmacology* **108**, 380–6.

Grasby, P.M., Frith, C.D., Friston, K.J., Bench, C.J., Frackowiak, R.S.J. & Dolan, R.J. (1993) Functional mapping of brain areas implicated in auditory-verbal memory function. *Brain* **116**, 1–20.

Guze, B.H. & Szuba, M.P. (1992) Leukoencephalopathy and major depression: a preliminary report. *Psychiatry Res. Neuroimaging* **45**, 169–75.

Hachinski, V.C. (1991) Multi-infarct dementia: a reappraisal. *Alzheimer Dis. Assoc. Disorders* **5**, 64–8.

Holman, B.L., Johnson, K.A., Gerada, B., Carvalho, P.A. & Satlin, A. (1992) The scintigraphic appearance of Alzheimer's disease: a prospective study using technetium-99m-HMPAO SPECT. *J. Nucl. Med.* **33**, 181–5.

Hurwitz, T.A., Clark, C., Murphy, E., Klonoff, H., Martin, W.R.W. & Pate, B.D. (1990) Regional cerebral glucose metabolism in major depressive disorder. *Can. J. Psychiatry* **35**, 684–8.

Iacono, W.G., Smith, G.N., Moreau, M. *et al.* (1988) Ventricular and sulcal size at the onset of psychosis. *Am. J. Psychiatry* **145**, 820–4.

Innis, R., Zoghbi, S., Johnston, E. *et al.* (1991) SPECT imaging of the benzodiazepine receptor in non-human primate brain with (I-123) RO 16-0154. *Eur. J. Pharmacol.* **193**, 249–52.

Jacoby, R.J. & Levy, R. (1980) Computed tomography in the elderly. 3. Affective disorder. *Br. J. Psychiatry* **136**, 270–5.

Jacoby, R.J., Levy, R. & Bird, J.M. (1981) Computed tomography and the outcome of affective disorder: a follow-up study of elderly patients. *Br. J. Psychiatry* **139**, 288–92.

Janota, I., Mirsen, T.R., Hachinski, V.C., Lee, D.H. & Merskey, H. (1989) Neuropathologic correlates of leuko-araiosis. *Arch. Neurol.* **46**, 1124–8.

Jernigan, T.L., Archibald, S.L., Berhow, M.T., Sowell, E.R. & Foster, D.S. (1991) Cerebral structure on MRI Part I:

Localization of age-related changes. *Biol. Psychiatry* **29**, 55–67.

Jobst, K.A., Smith, A.D., Barker, C.S. *et al.* (1992) Association of atrophy of the medial temporal-lobe with reduced blood flow in the posterior parietotemporal cortex in patients with a clinical and pathological diagnosis of Alzheimer's disease. *J. Neurol. Neurosurg. Psychiatry* **55**, 190–4.

Johnstone, E.C., Crow, T.J., Frith, C.D., Husband, J. & Kreel, L. (1976) Cerebral ventricular size and cognitive impairment in chronic schizophrenia. *Lancet* **ii**, 924–6.

Kanaya, T. & Yonekawa, M. (1990) Regional cerebral blood flow in depression. *Japan. J. Psychiatry Neurol* **44**, 571–6.

Kinkel, W.R., Jacobs, L., Polachini, I., Bates, V. & Heffner, R.R. (1985) Subcortical arteriosclerotic encephalopathy (Binswanger's disease): computed tomographic, nuclear magnetic resonance, and clinical correlations. *Arch. Neurol.* **42**, 951–9.

Krishnan, K.R.R., McDonald, W.M., Escalona, P.R., Doraiswamy, P.M. & Na, C. (1992) Magnetic resonance imaging of the caudate nuclei in depression: preliminary observations. *Arch. Gen. Psychiatry* **49**, 553–7.

Maes, M., Dierckx, R., Meltzer, H.Y. *et al.* (1993) Regional cerebral blood flow in unipolar depression measured with Tc-99m-HMPAO single photon emission computed tomography: negative findings. *Psychiatry Res. Neuroimaging* **50**, 77–88.

Martin, A.J., Friston, K.J., Colebatch, J.G. & Frackowiak, R.S.J. (1991) Decreases in regional cerebral blood flow with normal aging. *J. Cerebr. Blood Flow Metab.* **11**, 684–9.

Martinot, J.-L., Hardy, P., Feline, A. *et al.* (1990) Left prefrontal glucose hypometabolism in the depressed state: a confirmation. *Am. J. Psychiatry* **147**, 1313–17.

Mathew, R.J., Meyer, J.S., Francis, D.J., Semchuk, K.M., Mortel, K. & Claghorn, J.L. (1980) Cerebral blood flow in depression. *Am. J. Psychiatry* **137**, 1449–50.

Mirsen, T.R., Lee, D.H., Wong, C.J. *et al.* (1991) Clinical correlates of white matter changes on magnetic resonance imaging scans of the brain. *Arch. Neurol.* **48**, 1015–21.

Moroz, M. (1972) The concept of cognition in contemporary psychology. In Royce, J. & Rozeboom W. (eds) *The Psychology of Knowing*. Gordon & Breach, London.

Nasrallah, H.A., MacCalley-Whitters, M. & Jacoby, C.G. (1982) Cortical atrophy in schizophrenia and mania: a comparative study. *J. Clin. Psychology* **43**, 439–41.

Neirinckx, R.D., Canning, L.R., Piper, I.M. *et al.* (1987) Technetium-99m D, 1-HMPAO: a new radiopharmaceutical for SPECT imaging of regional cerebral blood perfusion. *J. Nucl. Med.* **28**, 191–202.

O'Brien J.T., Sahakian, B.J. & Checkley, S.A. (1993) Cognitive impairments in patients with seasonal affective disorder. *Br. J. Psychiatry* **163**, 338–43.

O'Carroll, R.E., Curran, S.M., Ross, M. *et al.* (1994) The differentiation of major depression from dementia of the Alzheimer type using within-subject neuropsychological discrepancy analysis. *Br. J. Clin. Psychology* **33**, 23–32.

Pardo, J.V., Pardo, P.J. & Raichle, M.E. (1993) Neural correlates of self-induced dysphoria. *Am. J. Psychiatry* **150**, 713–19.

Parker, G., Hadzi-Pavlovic, D., Brodaty, H. *et al.* (1993) Psychomotor disturbances in depression: defining the constructs. *J. Affective Disorders* **27**, 255–65.

Parkin, A.J. & Leng, N.R.C. (1993) *Neuropsychology of the Amnesic Syndrome.* Lawrence Erlbaum Associates, Hove, UK.

Parrott, W.G. & Schulkin, J. (1993) Neuropsychology and the cognitive nature of the emotions. In Watts, F. (ed.) *Neuropsychological Perspectives on Emotion.* Lawrence Erlbaum Associates, Hove, UK, pp. 43–60.

Pearlson, G.D. & Veroff, A.E. (1981) Computerised tomographic scan changes in manic-depressive illness. *Lancet* **ii**, 470.

Philpot, M.P., Banerjee, S., Needham-Bennett, H., Costa, D.C. & Ell, P.J. (1993) ^{99m}Tc-HMPAO single photon emission tomography in late life depression: a pilot study of regional cerebral blood flow at rest and during a verbal fluency task. *J. Affective Disorders* **28**, 233–40.

Post, R.M., De Lisi, L.E., Holcomb, H.H., Uhde, T.W., Cohen, R. & Buchsbaum, M.S. (1987) Glucose utilization in the temporal cortex of affectively ill patients: positron emission tomography. *Biol. Psychiatry* **22**, 545–53.

Riddle, W., O'Carroll, R.E., Dougall, N. *et al.* (1993) A single photon emission computerised tomography study of regional brain function underlying verbal memory in patients with Alzheimer-type dementia. *Br. J. Psychiatry* **163**, 166–72.

Rieder, R., Mann, L.S., Weinberger, D.R., van Kammen, D.P. & Post, R.M. (1983) Computed tomographic scans in patients with schizophrenia, schizo-affective disorder and bipolar affective disorder. *Arch. Gen. Psychiatry* **40**, 735–9.

Robbins, T.W. (1983) The neuropsychology of emotion. In Shepherd, M. & Zangwill, O.L. (eds). *Handbook of Psychiatry 1.* Press Syndicate of the University of Cambridge, Cambridge, pp. 123–45.

Robbins, T.W., Joyce, E.M. & Sahakian, B.J. (1992) Neuropsychology and imaging. In Paykel, E. (ed.) *Handbook of Affective Disorders.* Churchill Livingstone, Edinburgh.

Sackeim, H.A., Prohovnik, I., Moeller, J.R. *et al.* (1990) Regional cerebral blood flow in mood disorders. I. Comparison of major depressives and normal controls at rest. *Arch. Gen. Psychiatry* **47**, 60–70.

Saykin, A.J., Gur, R.C., Gur, R.E. *et al.* (1991) Neuropsychological function in schizophrenia. *Arch.*

Gen. Psychiatry **48**, 618–24.

Schlegel, S. & Kretzschmar, K. (1987) Computed tomography in affective disorders, part I: ventricular and sulcal measurements. *Biol. Psychiatry* **22**, 4–14.

Schlegel, S., Aldenhoff, J.B., Eissner, D., Lindner, P. & Nickel, O. (1989) Regional cerebral blood flow in depression: associations with psychopathology. *J. Affective Disorders* **17**, 211–18.

Schwartz, J.M., Baxter, L.R., Mazziotta, J.C., Gerner, R.H. & Phelps, M.E. (1987) The differential diagnosis of depression: relevance of positron emission tomography studies of cerebral glucose metabolism to the bipolar–unipolar dichotomy. *JAMA* **258**, 1368–74.

Scott, A.I.F., Dougall, N., Ross, M. *et al.* (1994) Short term effects of electroconvulsive treatment on the uptake of ^{99m}Tc-Exametazime into brain in major depression shown with single photon emission tomography. *J. Affective Disorders* **30**, 27–34.

Sherer, K.S. (1993) Neuroscience projections to current debates in emotion psychology. In Watts, F. (ed.) *Neuropsychological Perspectives on Emotion.* Lawrence Erlbaum Associates, Hove, UK, pp. 1–42.

Shima, S., Shikano, T., Kitamura, T. *et al.* (1984) Depression and ventricular enlargement. *Acta Psychiatr. Scand.* **70**, 275–7.

Silberswieg, D.A., Stern, E., Frith, C.D. *et al.* (1993) Detection of thirty second cognitive activations in single subjects with positron emission tomography: a new low-dose $H_2{}^{15}O$ regional cerebral blood flow three dimensional imaging technique. *J. Cerebr. Blood Flow Metab.* **13**, 617–29.

Silfverskiöld, P., Rosen, I., Risberg, J. & Gustafson, L. (1987) Changes in psychiatric symptoms related to EEG and cerebral blood flow following electroconvulsive therapy in depression. *Eur. Arch. Psychiatry Neurol. Sci.* **36**, 195–201.

Steingart, A., Hachinski, V.C., Lau, C. *et al.* (1987) Cognitive and neurologic findings in demented patients with diffuse white mater lucencies on computed tomographic scan (leukoaraiosis). *Arch. Neurol.* **44**, 36–9.

Tanaka, Y., Hazama, H., Fukuhara, T. & Tstsui, T. (1982) Computerised tomography of the brain in manic-depressive patients – a controlled study. *Fol. Psychiatr. Neurol. Japan* **36**, 137–44.

Tupler, L.A., Coffey, C.E., Logue, P.E., Djang, W.T. & Fagan, S.M. (1992) Neuropsychological importance of subcortical white matter hyperintensity. *Arch. Neurol.* **49**, 1248–52.

Upadhyaya, A.K., Abou-Saleh, M.T., Wilson, K., Grime, S.J. & Critchley, M. (1990) A study of depression in old age using single-photon emission computerised tomography. *Br. J. Psychiatry* **157**, 76–81.

Vaillant, G.E., Roston, E. & McHugo, G.J. (1992) An intriguing association between ancestral mortality and male affective disorder. *Arch. Gen. Psychiatry* **49**, 709–15.

Warren, L.R., Butler, R.W., Katholi, C.R., McFarland, C.E., Crews, E.L. & Halsey Jr, J.H. (1984) Focal changes in cerebral blood flow produced by monetary incentive during a mental mathematics task in normal and depressed subjects. *Brain Cognition* **3**, 71–85.

Winokur, G. (1980) Is there a common genetic factor in bipolar and unipolar affective disorder? *Comprehens. Psychiatry* **21**, 460–8.

Wolfe, J., Granholm, E., Butters, N., Saunders, E. & Janowski, D. (1987) Verbal memory deficits associated with major affective disorders: a comparison of unipolar and bipolar patients. *J. Affective Disorders* **13**, 83–92.

Woods, R.P., Cherry, S.R. & Mazziotta, J.C. (1992) A rapid automated algorithm for accurately aligning and reslicing positron emission tomography images. *J. Comput. Assist. Tomogr.* **16**, 620–33.

Woods, S.W., Seibyl, J.P., Goddart, A.W. *et al.* (1992) Dynamic SPECT imaging after injection of the benzodiazepine receptor ligand ^{123}I-iomazenil in healthy human subjects. *Psychiatry Res. Neuroimaging* **45**, 67–77.

Wu, J.C., Gillin, J.C, Buchsbaum, M.S., Hershey, T., Johnson, J.C. & Bunney Jr, W.E. (1992) Effect of sleep deprivation on brain metabolism of depressed patients. *Am. J. Psychiatry* **149**, 538–43.

Yazici, K.M., Kapucu, O., Erbas, B., Varoglu, E., Gulec, C. & Bekdik, C.F. (1992) Assessment of changes in regional cerebral blood flow in patients with major depression using the ^{99m}Tc-HMPAO single photon emission tomography method. *Eur. J. Nucl. Med.* **19**, 1038–43.

13: Structural Brain Imaging in Neuropsychiatry

G. D. Pearlson

Introduction

Space and reference constraints set reasonable limits on concise coverage of structural neuro-imaging in neuropsychiatric diseases. This chapter therefore confines itself to an examination of normal ageing and some of the commoner aetiopathological conditions resulting in adult dementia Alzheimer's disease (AD) vascular dementia, Huntington's chorea and acquired immune deficiency syndrome (AIDS)-associated dementia. This chapter will first review general issues, such as comparison of the use of computed tomography (CT) and magnetic resonance imaging (MRI), clinical and research assessment of structural scans, and issues of sensitivity and specificity. A discussion of specific diseases will then follow.

Structural neuroimaging currently does not meet criteria for an ideal diagnostic method in suspected dementia syndromes. This is because in most cases, it is not a sufficiently sensitive and specific tool to yield definitive cross-sectional diagnosis early in the course of the disease (or in presymptomatic genetically at-risk individuals). For *diagnostic* purposes, additional laboratory studies and follow-up neuroimaging are generally required. Therefore the appropriate current use of structural scans in neuropsychiatric illnesses is supportive, to aid diagnostic assessment in conjunction with other tests (such as blood tests, electroencephalography (EEG), functional imaging measures, etc.), and a careful history and clinical examination. This, however, is a distinct advance over the initial use of structural scans, which was mainly to rule out potentially treatable causes of dementia (e.g. tumours, subdurals). Additionally, structural neuroimaging has an important role in understanding and charac-terising the location and evolution of brain abnormalities associated with a particular disorder.

General issues

CT vs. MRI

As reviewed by Pearlson and Marsh (1993), MRI has superior anatomical resolution and, with volume image-acquisition sequences such as spoiled gradient recall acquisition in the steady state (GRASS), one can obtain anatomically useful artefact-free slices through virtually any structure of interest in any chosen plane, including regions poorly visualised on most CT scans (e.g. hippocampus and amygdala). MRI also boasts the advantage of improved grey/white contrast and is more sensitive to parenchymal changes. MRI has no bone-associated artefact and involves no exposure to ionising radiation. However, for many diagnostic purposes, CT is perfectly adequate and is also both less expensive and more widely available than MRI.

Clinical vs. research measures

Clinical scan interpretation by a skilled neuro-radiologist is helpful in the detection of some types of changes, while scan analysis using quantitative research methods is employed in others. As previously reviewed by Burns and Pearlson (1994), in addition to standard clinical ratings, structural brain scans are most often evaluated using the following means.

1 Visual qualitative ratings by trained observers (e.g. using standardised visual analogue or categorical scales).

2 Linear and area measures, including planimetric assessments.

3 Volumetric measures.

4 Tissue-density and thresholding methods to assess either volumes of cerebral components or their relative opacity to X-rays.

In general, reliability of ratings within one rater and between several raters needs to be high for meaningful conclusions to be drawn from scan analyses. Validity measurements employing *phantoms*, inert blocks of known physical characteristics or volumes, have been included as part of some studies.

Neuropathological validation

One ultimate goal of all neuroimaging methods is to reveal, during life, the extent of even subtle pathological brain changes, in a non-invasive manner. Because no single imaging method, or even combination of methods, can yet approach this aim, due to the non-specificity of many neuroimaging changes and the ever-present possibility of false positives or negatives, in many cases the neuropathological examination of the brain remains tremendously important as the ultimate validating procedure. Thus, for example, studies attempting to show the diagnostic specificity of a particular neuroradiological procedure in separating AD from multi-infarct dementia (MID) must rely for their validation on post-mortem examination, because of the considerable clinical overlap between the two conditions and the statistical likelihood of 'mixed' cases sharing pathological changes of both processes.

Sensitivity and specificity of changes

Ideally neuroimaging allows one to assess regionally specific abnormalities in brain locations most affected by the pathology of a particular syndrome, in preference to generalised and non-specific indices of cerebral atrophy. With newer methods, this is often feasible.

Generalised structural changes, such as lateral-ventricular enlargement, tend to be rather non-specific when a particular pathological group is compared with healthy controls. Not only do such changes not reveal the location of the primary neuropathology of the illness, but they are not specific to particular diseases. For example, lateral-ventricular enlargement (often measured as ventricular:brain ratio (VBR)), occurs both in putatively neurodevelopmental diseases, such as schizophrenia, and neurodegenerative conditions, such as AD. Measures such as VBR may be only weakly correlated with the severity of the pathological process and associated clinical measures. Even for more regionally specific structural radiological changes (e.g. amygdala volume in early AD measured from MRI scans), there can be 'floor' effects, i.e. lack of progression of atrophy beyond a certain level of severity. Thus measures which are relatively sensitive at the start of the illness may not evolve in a linear manner with disease severity.

Gene markers and presymptomatic diagnosis

In the last few years there has been an explosion in the identification of genetic markers for specific neuropsychiatric disorders, a trend which is likely to continue. Neuroimaging research is likely to evolve in response to the acquisition of this new genetic information. In particular, individuals are being studied who are gene-marker-positive for a neurodegenerative condition such as Huntington's chorea, but do not yet express any clinical symptoms. In such individuals, one can ask such questions as the following. At what stage and under what circumstances do the first cerebral changes occur? Can a putative treatment delay the onset of such changes? Are there neurodevelopmental as well as neurodegerative changes that affect the brains of individuals with a disease gene, which precede the neurodegenerative changes?

With the recent discovery of disease-related markers for AD and the characterisation of Alzheimer-like changes commonly found in ageing individuals with Down's syndrome, another condition of known genetic aetiology, opportunities for the marriage between neuro-imaging and genetics are expanding rapidly.

Normal ageing

Characteristic anatomical changes

As summarised by Coffey (1993), increasing age is associated with: (i) non-linear increases in lateral- and third-ventricular volume; (ii) increasing sulcal cerebrospinal fluid (CSF) volume; (iii) decreasing brain volume, especially of frontal lobes and cortical and subcortical grey matter; (iv) increasing variability in measures of brain size; and (v) increasing frequency and severity of subcortical hyperintensity of MRI. Many such changes appear to affect different brain systems to varied degrees, and to display a wide degree of normal variability.

Neuropathology

As reviewed by Jernigan *et al.* (1990, 1991a), studies of structural age-related cerebral changes in non-demented older persons document decreases in brain weight or volume, and in volume or cell density of cerebral cortex. Age-related decreases in cortical volume are especially marked in frontal and superior temporal regions. Haug (1977) examined cortical regions of human brains up to 90 years old, and found the average 75-year-old brain was 6% lighter than the average 25-year-old brain. Frontal cortex and basal ganglia were characterised by disproportionate volume loss relative to the parietal and entire cortex.

Neuroimaging: generalised age relationships

A large degree of variability in age-associated changes is observed for structural-neuroimaging volume measures, as also reported in neuropathological studies. CT studies of cerebral atrophy,

mostly cross-sectional in nature, show gradual age-related increases in sulcal and ventricular sizes until around 60 years of age, followed subsequently by more rapid increases. We documented similar changes in a cross-sectional CT study (Pearlson *et al.*, 1990). Several longitudinal studies assessing CSF volume demonstrated increases on reassessment of normal elderly subjects (e.g. Gado *et al.*, 1983), although not all such studies have demonstrated similar changes (e.g. Bird *et al.*, 1986). Jernigan *et al.* (1990), using MRI, studied cross-sectionally 58 normal volunteers with a mean age of 45 years (range 8–79) and described linear age-related decreases in the volume of the cerebrum and linear increases of ventricular and sulcal fluid. Curvilinear decreases in cortical volume related to age were demonstrable even in young adults.

Neuroimaging: regional changes

Jernigan *et al.* (1991a) measured individual cerebral grey-matter structures. In subjects between the ages of 30 and 79 years, significant age-related decreases occurred in the volume of the caudate and anterior diencephalic structures and in the grey matter of many cortical regions. Decreases in caudate volume with age on MRI are consistent with prior neuropathological data. Volumes of thalamus and anterior cingulate cortex showed no apparent age-related declines. Losses in association cortex and mesial temporal-lobe structures appeared to be relatively greater than for other cortical regions, again in agreement with neuropathological data. This has important implications for cognition. Lim *et al.* (1990) compared small samples of young and old healthy community-dwelling men on MRI, and demonstrated significant age-related increases in temporal-horn volume and a trend towards decreases in hippocampal volume.

White-matter changes

CT white-matter attenuation values have been demonstrated to decline with normal ageing in several studies (e.g. Zatz *et al.*, 1982b; Pearlson *et al.*, 1990), and multifocal periventricular areas of decreased attenuation on CT are reported in about 25% of AD patients and 10% of normal elderly (Faulstich, 1991). MRI has very high sensitivity to white-matter alterations, diffuse periventricular lucencies and *white-matter hyperintensities* (WMH). These areas of increased signal intensity, which are well visualised on T2-weighed (more specifically, long time to repetition (TR) with long or short time to echo (TE)) scans, have been reported in variable, although significant, proportions of MRI studies of normal elderly subjects (e.g. Awad *et al.*, 1986a,b; Agnoli & Feliciani, 1987; Hachinski *et al.*, 1987; Inzitari *et al.*, 1987). Such hyperintensities show no mass effect or contrast enhancement. These changes have been described in relation to increasing age, as well as vascular risk factors, such as hypertension, and may be associated with both sub-clinical functional (including cognitive) impairment and 'soft' neurological signs.

In healthy controls, highly non-linear age-related increases in the volume of signal hyperintensities were observed by Jernigan *et al.* (1990) in both cortical and subcortical regions. Significant age-related changes in white matter (increased T2 values) were also reported in a later study by Jernigan *et al.* (1991a). Elevations of T2 white-matter values in the elderly due to such hyperintensities could theoretically lead to misclassification of grey- and white-matter pixels.

The pathological status of these MRI features commonly seen in the elderly and their unitary nature remain to be clarified. Initial suggestions are that, pathologically, subcortical white-matter alterations may consist of dilated perivascular spaces, vascular ectasia and gliosis (Awad *et al.*, 1986b). Radiological periventricular changes, commonly found surrounding the frontal and occipital ventricular horns, may consist pathologically of astrocytic gliosis, possibly due to passage of CSF into parenchyma.

The terminology relating to various appearances of WMH is confusing because of the multiple descriptive terms used. These include '*unknown bright objects*' (UBOs), '*leucoencephalopathy*' and *leucoaraiosis*'. These latter two terms refer to non-specific radiological white-matter alterations seen on CT or MRI. These can be seen in, but are by no means synonymous with, diagnoses such as MID and 'Binswanger's disease', which are ultimately pathological rather than neuroradiological terms. White-matter changes, as noted, can be associated with a great variety of neuropathological states as well as normal ageing and are probably of multifactoral aetiology.

Sullivan *et al.* (1990) found both increased age and evidence of stroke to be significant independent multivariate predictors of the presence and severity of leucoencephalopathy on MRI scans, suggesting that subcortical ischaemia as well as non-vascular age-related changes contribute to the emergence of periventricular and other deep WMH in the elderly. Sullivan *et al.* (1990) developed scores for quantifying putative risk factors for leucoencephalopathy, such as age, a 13-item ischaemia scale, stroke and history of transient ischaemic attack, hypertension, cardiac disease and diabetes. The many reports documenting subcortical hyperintensities on MRI scans in the elderly are difficult to compare, however, because of differences in subject populations, scanning techniques and lesion definition.

Duara *et al.* (1989) investigated MRI abnormalities of periventricular white matter and in subcortical locations in 36 elderly normals, 87 AD patients, 12 patients with MID and 14 patients with mixed MID/AD. Mild degrees of periventricular signal enhancement were non-specific, as three-quarters of young normals and two-thirds of elderly normals had such findings. Higher degrees of periventricular abnormalities were found with increasing frequency in the various patient groups but not in the young normals (approximately one-fifth of elderly normals, two-thirds of AD patients and nine-tenths of MID patients). Subcortical hyperintensities of a mild nature were rare in young normals but found in one-third of elderly normals. No young and few elderly normals showed evidence of more marked subcortical changes, but approximately one-third of AD and half of the MID patients had scores in this range. No particular severity score for any of the MRI hyperintensities usefully separated AD from MID, however. Thus, both periventricular and sub-cortical lesions on MRI increase with age and further increase significantly in AD and MID.

Sensitivity and specificity

Many age-related neuroimaging changes, so far as is known, tend to be rather non-specific, with much overlap between changes that can occur in dementing illnesses effecting the elderly. The very variable effects of normal ageing on the brain confound structural assessment of dementia in the elderly; it is usually difficult to remove these confounds, since baseline premorbid scan measures are unavailable for most individuals. Thus, to help address these issues quantitatively, there is still a great need for more large-scale epidemiologically based studies of normal varia-tions in brain structures in randomly selected representative populations, in order to yield statistical information on sex, age and ethnically related variation.

Neuroimaging findings: relationship to cognition

As reviewed by Coffey (1993), relatively few studies of healthy volunteers have examined relationships between neuropsychological task performance and age-related changes in brain structures, and few clear results have emerged. Not all studies have agreed on the best statistical approach to examining simultaneous age effects on both brain structure and cognitive measures and effective means to exclude mildly demented subjects. Earnest *et al.* (1979) found significant correlations between scores on the digit symbol test and both linear and planimetric measures of lateral ventricular size on CT. Soinine *et al.* (1982) reported significant correlations between cognitive functioning and linear ventricular measures in both normal and demented elderly adults. It is has also been shown that fluid-volume

measures of the ventricles and the sulci correlated highly with memory-test scores, confrontation naming, visuospatial abilities and abstract reasoning, with maximal correlations found on the CT slice that contained primarily temporal and frontal lobes. In contrast, Jacoby *et al.* (1980) found no significant correlations, after age adjustment, between cortical-atrophy or ventricular-enlargement ratings and a test of memory and orientation. Matsubayashi (1992) found no significant relationship between VBR on CT scans and neuropsychological-test performance.

Now that more sophisticated anatomical assessment is possible, clarification of age-related cognitive–structural relations is increasingly feasible. Attempts to study these phenomena re-emphasise methodological issues related both to defining the population to be studied and to the means of recruitment.

Longitudinal changes

Preliminary evidence suggests that structural age-related changes are discontinuous in nature. This is probably true, as myelination and pruning processes are completed in early adult life. Pearlson *et al.* (1990) and others suggest that, after these normal changes occur, many age-related measures seem stable through adult life until approximately the age of 60. As mentioned earlier, regional atrophic changes may then begin, proceeding at different rates in different regions.

Alzheimer's disease

Characteristic changes

AD is the commonest aetiology of dementia in late life, and its prevalence rises with increasing age, affecting approximately 10% of individuals over the age of 65. AD is a familial progressive neurodegenerative disorder with age-dependent manifestation and is of unknown aetiology, although recently several gene markers have been identified. Certainly some forms of the illness have autosomal dominant inheritance. Interestingly, individuals with Down's syndrome have a very high risk of developing AD in midlife. Classically, AD presents with gradual impairment of short-term memory and higher-order cognitive functions, and is characterised by progressive, steady cognitive deterioration to apraxia, agnosia, acalculia, agraphia, disorientation and incontinence. Currently the disorder has no definitive biological markers, so that clinical diagnosis is made during life by exclusion of other causes of late-life dementia and ultimately validated by either biopsy (rarely) or neuropathological diagnosis. Thus, during life, clinical diagnosis depends on a combination of careful family history, history of present illness, pattern of cognitive loss, blood tests and brain-imaging investigations.

In AD, gross anatomical brain changes include reduced frontal and temporal gyral volumes, with sparing of primary somatosensory and motor cortices. The characteristic neuropathology consists of senile plaques, neurofibrillary tangles, granulovacuolar degeneration, amyloid deposits and neuronal loss. Changes in the nucleus basalis are inaccessible to structural neuroimaging, but the marked and early abnormalities seen in mesial temporal structures (limbic cortex) and the lateral temporal–parietal–occipital cerebral-cortical junction region are accessible to neuroimaging measurements.

Both regional and generalised cerebral atrophy has been reported in CT studies comparing AD patients with normal matched controls. Such reports have generally documented a fairly high degree of overlap between patients and controls, due to the previously mentioned issue of variability of brain atrophy associated with normal ageing.

MRI hyperintensities in Alzheimer's disease
(Fig. 13.1)

MRI hyperintensities are probably found in excess in the MRIs of patients with AD compared with those of normal elderly controls. Within AD they

may be associated with additional cognitive impairment, although this is not certain (Erkinjuntti *et al.*, 1989; Bowen *et al.*, 1990). This neuroradiological appearance could represent a subtype of AD, the superimposition of MID on AD (so called 'mixed dementia') or merely AD with more marked age-associated white-matter changes. Such white-matter changes, when present, do not usefully distinguish AD from MID.

Rusinek *et al.* (1991) used a segmentation algorithm to explore distributions of cerebral grey and white matter and intracranial CSF in 14 patients with AD compared with an equal number of healthy control subjects. The percentage of grey matter in the AD patients was significantly lower than in controls, with the most significant reduction occurring in temporal lobes and a central cerebral region.

Sensitivity and specificity

DeCarli *et al.* (1990) gives an excellent, concise review of the usefulness of CT measures in separating Alzheimer's patients from controls. As reviewed by Burns and Pearlson (1994), specificity is generally little altered by choice of analysis method, while sensitivity increases with increasing detail of analysis. To illustrate, the mean sensitivity of qualitative ratings is approximately 56%, while the mean sensitivity for volumetric ventricular ratings approaches 90%. Using measures of longitudinal change provides superior sensitivity. Sensitivity/specificity methods are dependent to some extent on the range of pathological severity of the patient population under examination. A review of the use of discriminant function methods in this context appears in Burns and Pearlson (1994). For clinically less advanced cases, temporal-lobe measures have attracted particular emphasis for CT studies. DeLeon *et al.* (1989) have reviewed such approaches. Since these methods may involve complex image reformatting, LeMay *et al.* (1986) documented that simpler suprasellar-cistern measures be used as a straightforward and reliable CT measure of medial-temporal atrophy

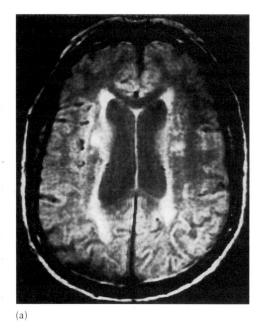

(a)

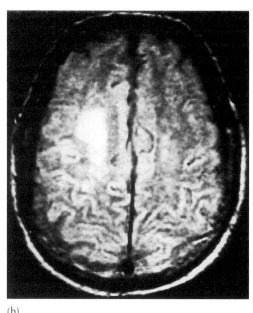

(b)

Fig. 13.1 (a) MRI scan of an 84-year-old male with mild Alzheimer's disease. Periventricular white-matter hyperintensities of a modest degree can be seen surrounding the bodies of the lateral ventricles, as can anterior periventricular 'caps'. TR = 2500, TE = 20, slice thickness = 5 mm, field of view = 24 cm, matrix = 256 × 256, field = 1.5 T. (b) Same individual as depicted in (a) with identical MRI scan parameters. An apical extension of the periventricular white-matter hyperintensities can be seen, 20 mm superior to the slice seen in (a).

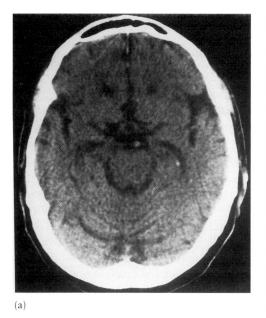

(a)

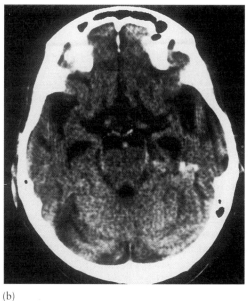

(b)

Fig. 13.2 (a) Suprasellar cistern in CT scan of a normal 80-year-old male (Mini-Mental State Examination = 27/30). Figure courtesy of Dr Elizabeth Aylward. (b) Suprasellar cistern in CT scan of an 84-year-old woman with Alzheimer's disease. Expansion of the cistern, accompanied by generalised cortical and subcortical atrophy, can be seen. CT parameters are identical to those in (a). Note that prominent Sylvian fissures and temporal ventricular-horn enlargement are visible.

(Fig. 13.2). Such an approach was taken by Pearlson *et al.* (1990), who demonstrated that suprasellar measures showed good discrimination both between Alzheimer's patients and appropriate controls and for demented versus non-demented Down's-syndrome adults. Few CT or MRI studies have yet attempted to discriminate Alzheimer's from MID.

Seab *et al.* (1988) and Pearlson *et al.* (1992) demonstrated that medial-temporal regions were severely structurally affected in AD subjects. The latter study demonstrated that these reduced volumes exceeded changes due to generalised atrophy (Figs 13.3–13.6). Amygdala and entorhinal cortical changes in the Pearlson *et al.* (1992) study best distinguished patients from controls, even after correction for global atrophy. Measures of global atrophy (e.g. CSF percentage) fared more poorly in a diagnostic discriminant-function analysis. This compares interestingly with other dementias. In the rare Creutzfeld – Jakob disease, altered signal in basal ganglia on MRI is an early finding (Barboriak *et al.*, 1994).

Clinical – cerebral associations

As reviewed by Burns and Pearlson (1994), a number of CT studies have studied the relationship between various atrophy measures in AD and degree of intellectual impairment. Earlier studies tended to look for such associations by combining populations of normal and demented subjects. Such CT studies tended to show correlational relationships between ventricular enlargement (measured by VBR) and cognitive loss, with weaker or no findings for cerebral-cortical atrophy. As pointed out by Burns and Pearlson (1994), however, ventricular measures are more reliably assessed as continuous variables than are cortical ones.

With reference to MRI, Pearlson *et al.* (1992) found superior temporal-gyral atrophy on MRI to be related to severity of language disorder, measured by the Boston naming test and category-naming test scores. Left-sided atrophy in this region tended to be most highly correlated

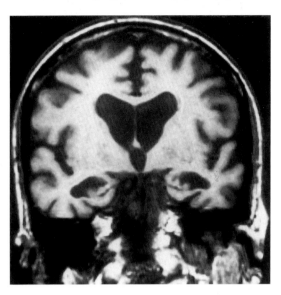

Fig. 13.3 An 81-year-old male with early Alzheimer's disease. Both cortical and subcortical atrophy are visible in this coronal MRI scan. Shrinkage of both temporal lobes and expansion of the Sylvian and interhemispheric fissures, as well as generalised cortical atrophy, are visible. Enlargement of both temporal horns can be seen, secondary to hippocampal shrinkage bilaterally. Field strength = 1.5 T, TR = 800, TE = 20, matrix = 256 × 256, field of view (FOV) = 24 cm, slice thickness = 5 mm.

with language disorder, consistent with its location close to lateralised language areas, including the dominant planum temporale. Seab *et al.* (1988) reported a significant relationship between overall brain atrophy and severity of cognitive impairment in AD, while Pearlson *et al.* (1992) did not. The latter study found no relationship between hippocampal and amygdala volumes and performance on a memory test, which they hypothesised was attributable to anatomical floor effects.

As noted earlier, the very variable effects of normal cerebral ageing complicate diagnostic assessment of dementia in the elderly, and baseline premorbid scan measures are usually unavailable.

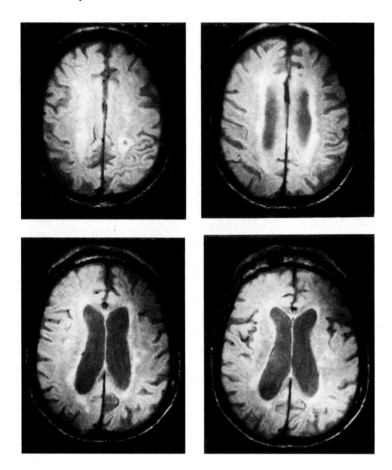

Fig. 13.4 Four non-consecutive axial MRI cuts through the brain of a normal 88-year-old individual, illustrating mild periventricular white-matter changes and lateral-ventricular enlargement. Field = 1.5 T, TR = 2500, TE = 20, matrix = 256 × 256, field of view (FOV) = 24 cm, slice thickness = 5 mm.

Longitudinal changes

Several studies in the 1980s showed that the rate of ventricular size increase at follow-up achieved excellent success in separating AD patients from normal controls. The largest published series, that of Burns *et al.* (1991), showed that several atrophy measures significantly increased in patients compared with controls over a 1-year period, and that increased ventricular size was associated with deterioration of memory scores. Difficulties associated with design and implementation of such longitudinal studies are reviewed by Burns *et al.* (1991). These include representativeness of subjects chosen, repositioning difficulties in the scanner and changes in scanner hardware and software. Another difficulty with longitudinal studies is that detectable neuroimaging changes take place over relatively prolonged periods of time. By the time they are conclusively demonstrable, diagnosis may well be obvious from clinical examination.

Few if any, longitudinal MRI studies in AD are currently published.

Presymptomatic diagnosis

Relatively recently, various putative markers for AD have become available. Presymptomatic diagnostic studies in individuals with and without AD gene markers and in at-risk individuals (i.e. with affected first-degree family members, in-

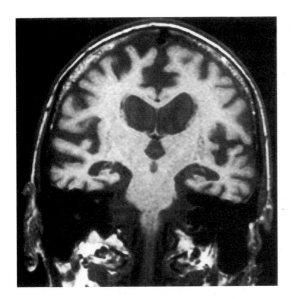

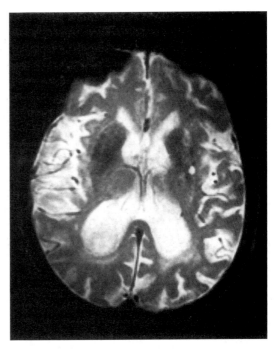

Fig. 13.5 Coronal MRI cut, illustrating hippocampal atrophy in Alzheimer's disease. Field = 1.5 T, TR = 800, TE = 20, matrix = 256 × 256, field of view (FOV) = 24 cm, slice thickness = 3 mm. This 88-year-old male, with both diabetes and Alzheimer's disease, demonstrates cortical and subcortical atrophy as well as hippocampal shrinkage.

Fig. 13.6 An 88-year-old male with moderately advanced Alzheimer's disease. Axial MRI cut shows ventricular enlargement and modest cortical atrophy, with pronounced Sylvian-fissure enlargement and a single left-sided punctuate white-matter hyperintensity. Periventricular white-matter changes are also visible surrounding the ventricular occipital horns. Field = 1.5 T, TR = 2500, TE = 80, matrix = 256 × 256, field of view (FOV) = 24 cm, slice thickness = 5 mm.

cluding twins, with the disorder) will undoubtedly take place over the next few years.

Vascular dementias (including multi-infarct disease)

Characteristic changes

After AD, vascular dementias are the commonest aetiology of cognitive loss in late life. They probably represent a family of disorders of varied aetiology, pathology, clinical expression and radiological appearance. As discussed by Tien *et al.* (1993), vascular dementias are probably associated with a variety of pathological entities, including multiple infarcts (both cortical and subcortical), strategically placed single strokes, ischaemic states (not necessarily resulting in infarction) and posthaemorrhagic and postanoxic states. Some of the variety of neuropathologies relating to these multiple causative factors have

been discussed in recent reviews, including those of Coffey (1993), Verny *et al.* (1991) and Starkstein and Robinson (1993).

It should thus be borne in mind that MID is only one form of vascular dementia and that multi-infarct *disease* can occur in the absence of cognitive changes. In fact, multi-infarct *disease* may be a general risk factor for several major mental illnesses with late-life onset (see Pearlson & Petty, 1993; Pearlson *et al.*, 1993). Clinically, vascular dementias are classically said to be distinguished by abrupt onset, history of stroke, stepwise, fluctuating course, focal neurological symptoms and/or signs, multiple vascular risk factors (e.g. hypertension, hyperlipidaemias) and emotional liability. Neuroimaging changes associated with vascular dementia can co-occur with those of AD, since both are common causes of late-life dementia, an occurrence often referred to as 'mixed dementia'. Finally, many elderly individuals have white-matter changes on both CT and MRI without clear-cut cognitive abnormalities. Useful work needs to be carried out comparing quantitative estimates of cerebral blood flow with structural measures of white-matter change, both in elderly normals and in patients with vascular dementia.

Much of the current terminology surrounding vascular dementia is inexact and in need of revision. Terms in current use tend to conflate *clinical states* (e.g. dementia), *aetiologies* (e.g. stroke), *neuropathological descriptions* (e.g. lacunar infarcts), *eponymous entities* (e.g. 'Binswanger's disease'), *neuroradiological findings* (e.g. subcortical MRI hyperintensities) and appearances on *different imaging methods* (e.g. MRI and CT). Neuroradiologically, given this clinical and pathological complexity, the most straightforward approach in examining a scan is to describe simply *which* changes are visualised, *where* the changes are occurring and their *severity*. The Consortium to Establish a Registry for Alzheimer's Disease (CERAD) scale (Davis *et al.*, 1989) is an illustrated MRI visual-analogue assessment scale based on these principles.

There has been much recent debate on the clinical diagnosis of vascular dementia and its relationship to neuropathology, clinical history and vascular risk factors. For these issues, the reader is referred to Salerno *et al.* (1992), Chui *et al.* (1992) and Erkinjuntti *et al.* (1987). Generally, the opinion expressed in recent reviews (e.g. Cummings & Benson, 1992; Tien *et al.*, 1993) is that MID is associated with cortical infarcts in approximately 20% of cases, lacunar infarcts in approximately 70% of cases, small-vessel ischaemia in 60–100% and a mixture of various pathologies in approximately 30%. 'Binswanger's disease' or 'subcortical arteriosclerotic encephalopathy' is best viewed as a subtype of vascular dementia disproportionately affecting subcortical white matter, relative to cortical grey matter. It should not be diagnosed on the basis of scan appearance alone.

On CT, diffuse cortical and subcortical changes in vascular dementias can be seen, as well as cerebral and subcortical infarctions and focal or widespread areas of reduced white-matter density (see Erkinjuntti *et al.*, 1986; Powell & Benson, 1990). The major types of changes that have been reported to occur on MRI in cases of vascular dementia are the following.

1 Smooth-appearing periventricular changes such as 'caps' and 'rims', best visualised on T2-weighted acquisition sequences and similar to those shown in Figs 13.1(a,b) and 13.7. These changes are common and, when less extensive and more regularly shaped, may have no pathological significance. They are also least clearly related to vascular aetiology. Irregular and more extensive periventricular changes, especially in association with ventricular enlargement, may be more associated with clinical cognitive change.

2 Non-periventricular deep subcortical WMH, sometimes termed 'leucoaraiosis', best seen on T2-weighted images, which are commonly attributed to chronic ischaemia but of unclear aetiology. Ischaemia can occur with or without parenchymal infarction. WMH may be a mixture of small or lacunar infarcts, focal demyelination and dilated perivascular spaces.

3 Cortical strokes and small deep infarcts ('lacunae') in deep grey matter and internal capsule.

Sensitivity and specificity

Pertinent remarks have been made earlier in the section on white-matter changes in normal ageing. In general, MRI is more sensitive but less specific than CT in the diagnosis of vascular dementia. Chui *et al.* (1992) addressed the need to distinguish MID from AD. Their study of ischaemia scales showed reasonable sensitivity and specificity for pure forms of AD or MID, but relative insensitivity to the presence of mixed disease. Since mixed disease is probably as common as pure MID, Chui *et al.* (1992) felt that a

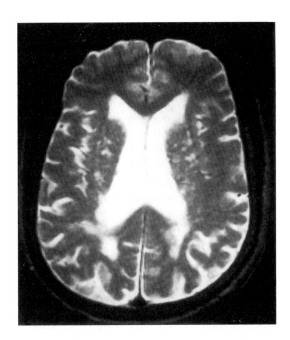

Fig. 13.7 An 84-year-old male with moderately advanced 'mixed dementia' (i.e. evidence for both Alzheimer's disease and vascular dementia). This T2-weighted axial MRI scan illustrates periventricular 'caps' and 'rims'. Both anterior and posterior 'caps' are visible. Field = 1.5 T, TR = 2500, TE = 80, matrix = 256 × 256, field of view (FOV) = 24 cm, slice thickness = 5 mm.

combination of clinical plus radiological criteria presented the optimum diagnostic approach, as reflected in their subsequent recommendations to the State of California criteria for ischaemic vascular dementia.

MRI changes resemble those seen on CT, but MRI is more sensitive to white-matter hypodensities. Erkinjuntti *et al.* (1986) compared large series of patients with AD, MID and probable vascular dementia (PVD), using CT. In this series, 89% of MID, 41% of PVD and 2% of AD had cerebral infarcts. Areas of low white-matter attenuation, especially in patients aged <75 years and without severe dementia, were associated with vascular aetiology.

Erkinjuntti *et al.* (1988) examined post-mortem neuropathology in a subset of 233 demented patients. Of these, 27 patients were studied who had met clinical criteria for vascular dementia during life and who had been previously studied with CT; this accounted for approximately 50% of all such patients. Of the 27 individuals studied, 23 met neuropathological criteria for MID and three for mixed AD/MID. Of the latter 23, 22 had bilateral infarcts and none met the criteria for 'Binswanger's disease'. While the presence of infarcts or reduced areas of white-matter attenuation on CT helped distinguish MID from AD, the degree of cortical or central atrophy did not.

Clinical–cerebral associations

Boone *et al.* (1992) studied 100 healthy, elderly individuals with MRI. Approximately 50% had no white-matter lesions, 25% had minimal or moderate lesions and 6% had large areas of MRI hyperintensities greater than 10 cm² total. Such large areas were associated with disturbances in basic attention and selected frontal-lobe skills, suggesting that a 'threshold' of white-matter lesions must be present before clear cognitive deficits become demonstrable. Similar suggestions have been made for the genesis of classic vascular dementias.

Erkinjuntti *et al.* (1986) found brain atrophy on CT to be positively correlated with degree of dementia in MID and PVD. Others have argued that, in vascular dementia, the Hachinski ischaemia score predicts CT findings less well than the CT scan appearance allows the prediction of the ischaemia score.

Liu *et al.* (1992) examined clinical and MRI findings in 24 demented and 20 non-demented stroke patients. The presence of dementia was best predicted by the total area of white-matter lesions, followed in order of utility by area of left-hemisphere white-matter lesions, VBR, right-hemisphere white-matter lesions, age, left cortical-infarct area, left parietal-infarct area and total infarct area. Overall, left-hemisphere areas were most strongly associated with the presence of cognitive deficit.

Longitudinal changes

Few, if any, neuroradiological studies have documented longitudinal changes in patients with vascular dementia.

Presymptomatic diagnosis

Several studies of late-life-onset depression and late-life-onset psychosis have documented an excess of WMH and subcortical white-matter abnormalities, even in patients who did not meet criteria for cognitive impairment. It is feasible that such individuals represent individuals at very high risk for the later development of vascular dementia. Similarly, the study of Boone *et al.* (1992) of normal controls documented that 25% of subjects had minimal or moderate white-matter lesions. Longitudinal radiological and cognitive follow-up of such individuals would be most helpful in documenting their risk-proneness for the later development of vascular dementia.

Huntington's disease

Characteristic changes

Huntington's disease (HD) is an inherited autosomally dominant, completely penetrant, neurodegenerative condition, resulting from an abnormal expansion of triplet base repeats on chromosome 4, and is frequently preceded by affective disorder. The illness has its usual clinical onset in middle age and is characterised by a 'subcortical' dementia and an involuntary choreiform movement disorder. Neuropathologically, there is striking atrophy and neuronal loss in the neostriatum (Bruyn, 1968). These changes are usually reported to occur most in the caudate and less so in the putamen and globus pallidus. Vonsattel *et al.* (1985) documented that the medial dorsal caudate is generally most affected in the earlier stages of the illness. In addition, there is neuropathological involvement of both frontal and occipital cortices (Bruyn, 1968) and amygdala. The pathology of HD is complex, and readers are referred to recent reviews (e.g. Roberts *et al.*, 1993).

Focal caudate atrophy with secondary ventricular anterior horn enlargement is often seen in moderately advanced HD. This can be quantified on both CT and MRI, using the *bicaudate ratio* (BCR) (see Aylward *et al.*, 1991; Fig. 13.8).

Most post-mortem cases of HD represent the end stage of the illness. The advent of MRI has provided an *in vivo* opportunity to extend our knowledge of the early neuroanatomical changes. With MRI, both patients and carriers of the gene marker can be examined early in the course of their illness. In one such study, Harris *et al.* (1992) showed a marked reduction in putamen volume, exceeding that of the caudate nucleus, in mild, early cases of HD.

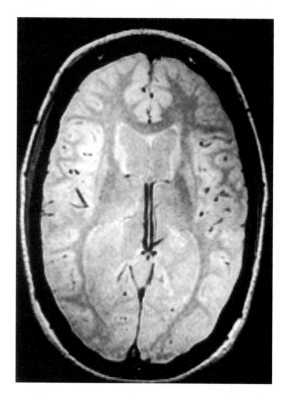

Fig. 13.8 A 37-year-old female with moderately severe Huntington's chorea (quantitative neurological examination score = 47). This axial MRI scan illustrates moderate caudate atrophy. Field = 1.5 T, TR = 3000, TE = 20, matrix = 256 × 256, field of view (FOV) = 24 cm, slice thickness = 3 mm.

Sensitivity and specificity

Severity of basal-ganglia atrophy measured by the BCR has been shown to correlate with the duration of the disease, as has bifrontal ratio. The BCR is a relatively specific and sensitive tool in diagnosing moderately advanced HD. Using BCR, however, there is poor discrimination on both CT and MRI between patients with *early* HD and healthy control subjects. In the Harris *et al.* (1992) paper, 15 patients with early HD were compared with 19 age- and sex-matched normal controls, using volumetric MRI assessments, including measures of basal-ganglia structures. Putamen volume normalised by brain area completely separated patient from control groups. Caudate volume normalised by brain area was a relatively poor diagnostic discriminator, yielding a net discrimination of less than 70%. Similarly BCR gave an overall discrimination of 82%. Hence volumetric measurements of putamen were a more sensitive indicator of abnormalities in mild HD than both direct and indirect measures of caudate atrophy.

Clinical–cerebral associations

Patients with the rigid subtype of HD may exhibit relatively more signal intensity in the putamen. In the Harris *et al.* (1992) study, putamen changes (unlike those in the caudate) correlated with neurological impairment, in accord with research indicating that relevant motor circuits involve putamen but not caudate, whereas regional cognitive circuits are thought to involve the caudate (Alexander *et al.*, 1986; DeLong *et al.*, 1990). This idea is also supported by prior CT studies in patients with HD (e.g. Starkstein *et al.*, 1988).

Thus, both MRI and CT studies of early-affected patients suggest that caudate atrophy is more associated with cognitive deterioration, while putamen shrinkage seems more linked to choreo-athetoid symptomatology.

Longitudinal changes

There are few longitudinal follow-up studies, especially with MRI. However, the previously mentioned studies of early HD can be contrasted with those of Jernigan *et al.* (1991b), using MRI, which examined severely demented patients with advanced HD (when marked subcortical and cortical atrophy is visible on CT and MRI scans). These investigators documented reduced caudate volume which exceeded atrophy of the lentiform nucleus (putamen plus globus pallidus), a finding consistent with the post-mortem work of Vonsattel *et al.* (1985) showing modest globus pallidus atrophy relative to caudate/putamen change. Vonsattel *et al.* (1985) also showed greater neuronal cell loss in early-stage HD in caudate than in putamen, but did not assess putamen volume. Lange *et al.* (1976) and De La Monte *et al.* (1988) reported equivalent post-mortem atrophy and neuronal loss of caudate and putamen in advanced cases of HD. Hence, structural putamen changes initially exceed those seen in caudate, but, as the disease evolves, severe and comparable volume reductions affect both structures.

Presymptomatic diagnosis

Aylward *et al.* (1993b) measured volumes of caudate, putamen and globus pallidus from MRI, in 10 gene-marker-positive and 18 gene-marker-negative asymptomatic individuals at risk for HD (Fig. 13.9). Volumes of all basal-ganglia structures were significantly reduced in the marker-positive group, even after controlling for age, total brain volume and presence of minor neurological signs. Percentage volume reductions in gene-marker-positive subjects were 31% for caudate, 29% for globus pallidus and 26% for putamen. Putamen volume was the single measure that best predicted marker status. Total brain volume was reduced by 7% in the marker-positive group, although group differences only approached statistical significance on this variable. These results indicate that basal-ganglia volumes are reduced even *before*

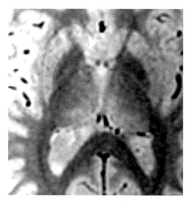 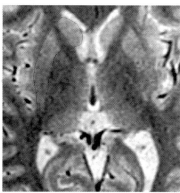

Fig. 13.9 Two individuals, matched on sex and age who were respectively positive (left) and negative (right) for the Huntington's-disease gene marker. The asymptomatic marker-positive individual can be seen to have reduced basal-ganglia size.

individuals with the HD gene become clinically symptomatic.

AIDS dementia complex

Human immunodeficiency virus (HIV)-associated dementia is the commonest infective dementia and an increasingly common cause of all dementias in young adults. Cognitive decline is not infrequently seen in cases of AIDS (see general review of De La Paz & Enzmann, 1988). The HIV virus has a predilection for the central nervous system (CNS) and there are reports of detectable cortical atrophy and ventriculomegaly even in HIV-positive, non-demented individuals. Many CNS complications are associated with HIV infection (see review of Kramer & Sanger, 1990). This chapter will discuss only the neuroradiological changes associated with *primary HIV-associated dementia* and not on the opportunistic CNS infections that commonly occur in immuno-compromised individuals, such as cytome-galovirus and toxoplasmosis. CNS tumours (mainly lymphomas) also occur in HIV-infected persons, but will not be further discussed here. It should be noted in passing, however, that both double-dose contrast CT and MRI are useful in the examination of cases in which one suspects such opportunistic infections and tumours (Fig. 13.10).

Characteristic changes

A relatively high proportion of AIDS patients suffer from the *AIDS dementia complex* (ADC), also referred to as HIV encephalopathy and HIV-associated dementia, which is due to direct brain involvement by the HIV virus, and can precede frank immunodeficiency. The high clinical prevalence of ADC is supported by neuropatho-logical evidence of frequent cerebral involvement in AIDS. As noted below, in ADC generalised white-matter pallor is often visible on MRI; it is not entirely clear what this represents neuro-pathologically. Post-mortem examination of the brain reveals a variety of changes, especially of white matter and subcortical grey matter and, less frequently, of cortical grey tissue.

Clinically, ADC manifests as a typical subcortical dementia of often insidious onset and variable natural history, with prominent motor, mood and cognitive abnormalities. As is typical of all subcortical dementias, psychomotor abnor-malities (including reduced psychomotor speed and especially marked problems on effortful cognitive tasks) are prominent. Sequencing problems (e.g. difficulties on trail-making tasks) are often prominent. The picture is variably accompanied by focal neurological symptoms and signs.

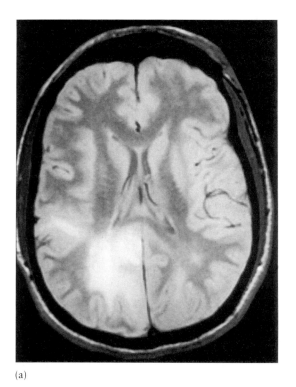

(a)

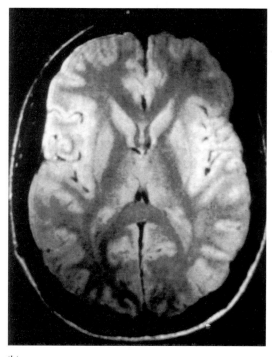

(b)

Fig. 13.10 (a) A 31-year-old HIV-positive male who presented clinically with rapid-onset dementia and focal neurological symptoms. T2-weighted MRI scan reveals posterior cerebral abnormalities. Diagnostic tests were consistent with cerebral toxoplasmosis. (b) Same individual as in (a) following treatment for toxoplasmosis and resolution of cognitive impairments.

Structural neuroimaging is important in the evaluation of any HIV-positive patient with neuropsychiatric abnormalities, and as part of the work-up of patients with suspected ADC. In ADC, in general CT shows mild to moderate cortical and subcortical atrophy, which evolves with the dementia, as well as low-density periventricular or deep white-matter lesions without mass effect. Occasionally, hypodensities may be seen in cortical grey matter. Typical MRI changes include white-matter abnormalities of various types, including increased signal in periventricular white matter on T2-weighted images that may evolve to diffuse subcortical white-matter changes as the ADC progresses (Figs 13.11 & 13.12). Bilateral, multiple, small, high-signal-intensity subcortical lesions are frequently observed, as are initially patchy and diffuse, later confluent, deep WMH. In the experience of Kramer and Sanger (1990), and also of our own hospital, although MRI is more sensitive than CT in detecting structural abnormalities associated with ADC, neuropathological examination almost invariably reveals more widespread abnormalities than detected by either imaging method. Using quantitative measures, Dal Pan *et al*. (1992) demonstrated that both overall cerebral atrophy and selective caudate shrinkage are associated with ADC.

Sensitivity and specificity

MRI is more sensitive than CT, especially for detection of focal lesions. Aylward *et al*. (1993a)

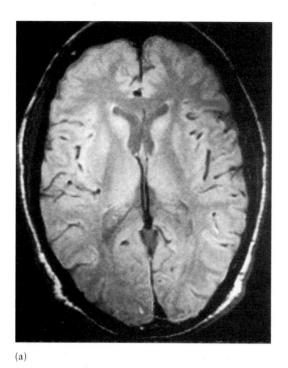

(a)

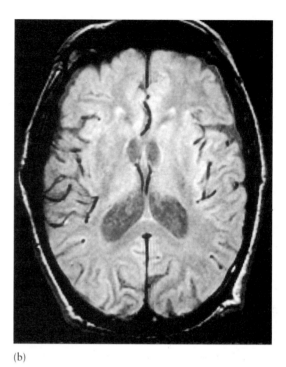

(b)

Fig. 13.11 (a) Cognitively normal 57-year-old HIV-positive individual with an essentially normal-appearing axial MRI scan. Field = 1.5 T, TR = 2500, TE = 20, matrix = 256 × 256, field of view (FOV) = 24 cm, slice thickness = 5 mm. (b) The same individual as in (a), 8 months after the onset of AIDS dementia complex (approximately 2 years after the first scan) Mild cortical and subcortical atrophy are evident. Field = 1.5 T, TR = 2500, TE = 20, matrix = 256 × 256, FOV = 24 cm, slice thickness = 5 mm.

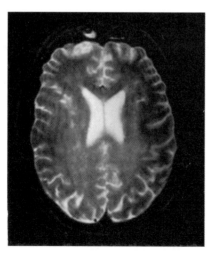

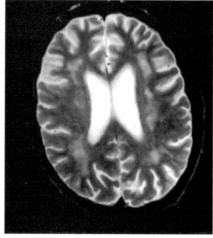

Fig. 13.12 Two T2-weighted axial 5 mm cuts through the brain of a 36-year-old male with AIDS dementia complex. Scans were taken 8 months apart. Progression of (i) bilateral/lateral ventricular enlargement, (ii) diffuse, patchy periventricular white-matter abnormalities, and (iii) deep white-matter hyperintensities are visible, which accompanied corresponding cognitive deterioration. Photo courtesy of Dr Justin McArthur, Neurology Service, John Hopkins Hospital.

found basal-ganglia volumes on MRI superior to more generalised atrophy measures in separating ADC from HIV-positive cognitively intact men.

ADC neuropathologically is accompanied by myelin pallor and loss, presumably corresponding to the white-matter changes seen on MRI, and by multifocal white-matter rarefaction and vacuolation. Reactive astrocytosis and perivascular infiltration are also seen post-mortem.

Clinical – cerebral associations

Clinicopathological correlation for MRI abnormalities in ADC is not clear-cut. Diffuse microgliosis is correlated with brain atrophy. Aylward *et al.* (1993a) measured volumes of basalganglia structures on MRI images in HIV-infected homosexual men with ADC, cognitively normal HIV-positive individuals and non-infected homosexual male controls. All groups were matched on age and years of education and the two HIV-positive groups were comparably immunosuppressed. Brain volumes decreased from the seronegative to the seropositive cognitively normal to the ADC group. Basal-ganglia volumes (even when corrected for intracranial volume) distinguished ADC patients from the other two groups. The authors concluded that, while HIV infection causes generalised brain atrophy, the clinical features of ADC developed in conjunction with selective basal-ganglia atrophy, consistent with the subcortical character of HIV dementia.

Further unpublished work from the same group assessed volumes of cerebrospinal fluid in grey and white tissue on MRI from the same three groups of individuals. Loss of white matter occurred with HIV infection and was most severe in seropositive patients with dementia, although those without had some reduction compared with seronegative controls. Some generalised grey-matter volume reductions were also detected in the ADC patients, which were significant in posterior cortical regions compared with both other groups.

Longitudinal changes

As summarised by Tien *et al.* (1993), progression of white-matter lesions in atrophy in general correlates with the evolution of cognitive decline in ADC. Antiviral therapy can cause some regression of the white-matter abnormalities.

Conclusions

In the diagnosis of dementing illnesses, structural brain-imaging methods are useful in conjunction with both clinical expertise and other laboratory investigations. Both CT and MRI are widely used for this purpose and offer different advantages. As commonly employed, neither is yet an ideal diagnostic method. There is still room for methodological refinement in improving sensitivity and specificity. A combination of neuroimaging with neurogenetic methods is likely to yield important information regarding preclinical changes in at-risk persons. Functional imaging with positron emission tomography (PET) and single-photon emission computed tomography (SPECT) often yields valuable additional information when used in conjunction with structural neuroimaging techniques.

Acknowledgements

The work was supported in part by the following National Institutes of Health (NIH) grants: MH43775, MH43326 and OP GCRC RR00722. Drs Elizabeth Aylward and Justin McArthur were most helpful in providing scans for the figures.

References

Agnoli, A. & Feliciani, M. (1987) Nuclear magnetic resonance imaging in the aging brain. *Gerontology* 33, 247–52.

Alexander, G.E., Delong, M.R. & Strick, P.L. (1986) Parallel organization of functionally segregated circuits linking basal ganglia and cortex. *Ann. Rev. Neurosci.* 9, 357–81.

Awad, I.A., Spetzler, R.F. & Hodak, J.A. (1986a) Incidental subcortical lesions identified on magnetic resonance imaging in the elderly, I: correlation with age and cerebrovascular risk factors. *Stroke* 17, 1084–9.

Awad, I.A., Johnson, P.C., Spetzler, R.F. & Hodak, J.A. (1986b) Incidental subcortical lesions identified on magnetic resonance imaging in the elderly, II: postmortem pathological correlations. *Stroke* 17, 1090–7.

Aylward, E.H., Schwartz, J., Machlin, S. *et al.* (1991) Bicaudate ratio as a measure of caudate volume on MR images. *Am. J. Neuroradiol.* 12, 1217–22.

Aylward, E.H., Brandt, J., Codori, A. *et al.* (1993a) Reduced basal ganglia volume in HIV-1-associated dementia: results from quantitative neuroimaging. *Neurology* 43, 2099–104.

Aylward, E.H., Brandt, J., Codori, A., Mangus, R.S., Barta, P.E. & Harris, G.J. (1993b) Reduced basal ganglia volume associated with the gene for HD in asymptomatic, at-risk persons. *Neurology* (in press).

Barboriak, D.P., Provencale, J.M. & Boyko, O.B. (1994) MR diagnosis of Creutzfeld–Jakob disease: significance of high signal intensity of the basal ganglia. *Am. J. Roentgenol.* 162, 137–40.

Bird, J.M., Levy, R. & Jacoby, R.J. (1986) Computed tomography in the elderly: changes over time in a normal population. *Br. J. Psychiatry* 148, 80–5.

Boone K.B., Miller, B.L., Lesser, I.M. *et al.* (1992) Neuropsychological correlates of white-matter lesions in healthy elderly subjects. *Arch. Neurol.* 49, 549–54.

Bowen, B.C., Barker, W.W., Loewenstein, D.A. *et al.* (1990) MR signal abnormalities in memory disorders and dementia. *Am. J. Neuroradiol.* 11, 283–90.

Bruyn, G.W. (1968) Huntington's chorea: historical, clinical, and laboratory synopsis. In Vinken, P.F. & Bruyn, G.W. (eds) *Handbook of Clinical Neurology*. North-Holland, Amsterdam, pp. 298–378.

Burns, A. & Pearlson, G.D. (1994) Computed tomography in Alzheimer's disease. In Burns, A. & Levy, R. (eds) *Dementia*. Chapman and Hall, London.

Burns, A., Jacoby, R. & Philpot, M. & Levy, R. (1991) CT in Alzheimer's disease—methods of scan analysis comparison with normal controls and clinical radiological correlations. *Br. J. Psychiatry* 159, 609–14.

Chui H.C., Victoroff, J.I., Margolin, D., Jagust, W., Shankle, R. & Katzman, R. (1992) Criteria for the diagnosis of ischemic vascular dementia proposed by the State of California Alzheimer's Disease Diagnostic and Treatment Centers. *Neurology* 42, 473–80.

Coffey, E.D. (1993) Anatomic imaging of the aging human brain. In Coffey, C.E. & Cummings, J. (eds) *Geriatric Neuropsychiatry*. American Psychiatric Press, Washington D.C.

Cummings, J.L. & Benson, D.F. (eds) (1992) *Dementia: a Clinical Approach*, 2nd edn. Butterworth-Heinemann, Boston.

Dal Pan, G.J., McArthur, J.H., Aylward, E.H. *et al.* (1992) Patterns of cerebral atrophy in HIV-1-infected individuals: results of a quantitative MRI analysis. *Neurology* 42, 2125–30.

Davis, P., Gado, M., Kumar, A. *et al.* (1989) *CERAD Neuroimaging Protocol for the Assessment of Alzheimer's Disease.* Consortium to Establish a Registry for Alzheimer's Disease, St Louis, MO.

DeCarli, C., Kaye, J., Horwitz, B. & Rapoport, S. (1990) Critical analysis of the use of CT to study human brain in ageing and dementia of the Alzheimer type. *Neurology* 40, 872–83.

De La Monte, S.M., Vonsattel, J.P. & Richardson, E.P. (1988) Morphometric demonstration of atrophic changes in the cerebral cortex, white matter and neostriatum in Huntington's disease. *J. Neuropathol. Exp. Neurol.* 47, 516–25.

De La Paz, R. & Enzmann, D. (1988) Neuroradiology of acquired immunodeficiency syndrome. In Rosenblum, M.L. *et al.* (eds) *AIDS and the Nervous System*. Raven Press, New York, pp. 121–53.

DeLeon, M.J., George, A.E, Reisberg, B. *et al.* (1989) Alzheimer's disease. *Am. J. Radiol.* 152, 1257–62.

DeLong, M.R., Alexander, G.E., Miller, W.C. *et al.* (1990) Anatomical and functional aspects of basal ganglia—thalamocortical circuits. In Franks, A.J., Ironside, J.W., Mindham, R.H.S. *et al.* (eds) *Function and Dysfunction in the Basal Ganglia*. Manchester University Press, New York, pp. 3–34.

Duara, R., Barker, W., Loewenstein, D., Pascal, S. & Bowen, B. (1989) Sensitivity and specificity of positron emission tomography and magnetic resonance imaging studies in Alzheimer's disease and multi-infarct dementia. *Eur. Neurol.* 29 (Suppl. 3), 9–15.

Earnest, M.P., Heaton, R.K., Wilkinson, W.E. & Manke, W.F. (1979) Cortical atrophy, ventricular enlargement and intellectual impairment in the aged. *Neurology* 29, 1138–43.

Erkinjuntti, T., Sulkava, R., Palo, J. & Ketonen, J. (1986) White matter low attenuation on CT in Alzheimer's disease. *Arch. Gerontol. Geriatr.* 8, 95–104.

Erkinjuntti, T., Ketonen, L., Sulkava, R., Vuorialho, M. & Palo, J. (1987) CT in the differential diagnosis between Alzheimer's disease and vascular dementia. *Acta Neurol. Scand.* 75, 262–70.

Erkinjuntti, T., Haltia, M., Palo, J., Sulkavya, R. & Paetau, A. (1988) Accuracy of the clinical diagnosis of vascular dementia: a prospective clinical and post-mortem neuropathological study. *J. Neurol. Neurosurg. Psychiatry* 51, 1037–44.

Erkinjuntti, T., Ketonen, L., Sulkava, R. *et al.* (1989) Do white matter changes on MRI and CT differentiate vascular dementia from Alzheimer's disease? *J. Neurol. Neurosurg. Psychiatry* 50, 37–42.

Faulstich, M.E. (1991) Brain imaging in dementia of the Alzheimer type. *Int. J. Neurosci.* 57, 39–49.

Gado, M., Hughes, C.P., Danziger, W. & Chi, D. (1983) Aging, dementia, and brain atrophy: a longitudinal computed tomographic study. *Am. J. Neuroradiol.* 4,

699–702.

Hachinski, V.C., Potter, P. & Merskey, H. (1987) Leuko-araiosis. *Arch. Neurol.* **44**, 21–3.

Harris, G.J., Pearlson, G.O., Peyser, C.E. *et al.* (1992) Putamen volume reduction on magnetic resonance imaging exceeds caudate changes in mild Huntington's disease. *Ann. Neurol.* **31**, 69–75.

Haug, G. (1977) Age and sex dependence of the size of normal ventricles in computed tomography. *Neuro-radiology* **14**, 201–4.

Inzitari, D., Diaz, F., Fox, A. *et al.* (1987) Vascular risk factors and leuko-araiosis. *Arch. Neurol.* **44**, 42–7.

Jacoby, R.J., Levy, R. & Dawson, J.M. (1980) Computed tomography in the elderly: I. The normal population. *Br. J. Psychiatry* **136**, 249–55.

Jernigan, T.L., Press, G.A. & Hesselink, J.R. (1990) Methods for measuring brain morphologic features on magnetic resonance images. *Arch. Neurol.* **47**, 27–32.

Jernigan, T.L., Archibald, S.L., Berhow, M.T., Sowell, E.R., Foster, D.S. & Hesselink, J.R. (1991a) Cerebral structure on MRI, I: localization of age-related changes. *Biol Psychiatry* **29**, 55–67.

Jernigan, T.L., Salmon, D.P., Butters, N. *et al.* (1991b) Cerebral structure on MRI, II: specific changes in Alzheimer's and Huntington's diseases. *Biol. Psychiatry* **29**, 68–81.

Kramer, E.L. & Sanger, J.J. (1990) Brain imaging in acquired immunodeficiency syndrome dementia complex. *Sem. Nucl. Med.* **20**, 353–63.

Lange, H., Thorner, G., Hopf, A. *et al.* (1976) Morphometric studies of the neuropathological changes in choreatic diseases. *J. Neurol. Sci.* **28**, 401–25.

LeMay, M., Stafford, J.L., Sandor, T. *et al.* (1986) Statistical assessment of perceptual CT scan ratings in patients with Alzheimer type dementia. *J. Comput. Assist. Tomogr.* **10**, 802–9.

Lim, K.O., Zipursky, R.B., Murphy, G.M.J. & Pfefferbaum, A. (1990) *In vivo* quantification of the limbic system using MRI: effects of normal aging. *Psychiatry Res. Neuroimaging* **35**, 15–26.

Liu, C.K., Miller, B.L., Cummings, J.L. *et al.* (1992) A quantitative MRI study of vascular dementia. *Neurology* **42**, 138–43.

Matsubayashi, K., Shimada, K., Kawanoto, A. & Ozawa, T. (1992) Incidental brain lesions on magnetic resonance imaging and neurobehavioral functions in the apparently healthy elderly. *Stroke* **23** 175–80.

Pearlson, G.D. & Marsh, L. (1993) MRI in psychiatry. In Oldham, J.M., Riba, M.B. and Tasman, A. (eds), *APA Annual Review of Psychiatry*. American Psychiatric Press, Washington, DC., 347–82.

Pearlson, G.D. & Petty, R.G. (1993) Late life onset schizophrenia. In: Coffey, C.E. & Cummings, J.(eds) *Geriatric Neuropsychiatry*. American Psychiatric Press, Washington D.C.

Pearlson, G.D., Warren, A., Starkstein, S.E. *et al.* (1990)

Brain atrophy in 18 patients with Down's syndrome. *Am. J. Neuroradiol.* **11**, 811–16.

Pearlson, G.D., Harris, G.J., Powers, R.E. *et al.* (1992) Quantitative changes in mesial temporal volume, regional cerebral bloodflow and cognition in Alzheimer's disease. *Arch. Gen. Psychiatry* **49**, 402–8.

Pearlson, G.D., Tune, L.E., Wong, D.F. *et al.* (1993) Quantitative D$_2$ dopamine receptor PET and structural MRI changes in late-onset schizophrenia. *Schizophrenia Bull.* **19**, 784–95.

Powell, A.L. & Benson, D.F. (1990) Brain imaging techniques in the diagnosis of dementia. *Neuropsychol. Rev.* **1**, 3–19.

Roberts, G.W., Leigh, P.N. & Weinberger, D.R. (1993) *Neuropsychiatric Disorders*. Wolfe Mosby, Baltimore.

Rusinek, H., de Leon, M.J., George, A.J. *et al.* (1991) Alzheimer's disease: measuring loss of cerebral gray matter with MR imaging. *Neuroradiology* **178**, 109–14.

Salerno, J.A., Murphy, D.G., Horwitz, B. *et al.* (1992) Brain atrophy in hypertension: a volumetric magnetic resonance imaging study. *Hypertension* **20**, 340–8.

Seab, J.P., Jagust, W.J., Wong, S.T.S., Roos, M.S., Reed, B.R. & Budinger, T.F. (1988) Quantitative NMR measurements of hippocampal atrophy in Alzheimer's disease. *Magnetic Resonance Med.* **8**, 200–8.

Soininen, H., Puranen, M. & Riekkinen, P.J. (1982) Computed tomography findings in senile dementia and normal aging. *J. Neurol. Neurosurg. Psychiatry* **45**, 50–4.

Starkstein, S.E. & Robinson, G. (1993) Neuropsychiatric aspects of stroke. In Coffey, C.E. & Cummings, J. (eds) *Geriatric Neuropsychiatry*. American Psychiatric Press, Washington, D.C., pp. 518–40.

Starkstein, S.E., Brandt, J. & Folstein, S.E. (1988) Neuropsychological and neuroradiological correlates in Huntington's disease. *J. Neurol. Neurosurg. Psychiatry* **51**, 1259–63.

Sullivan, P., Pary, R., Telang, F., Rifai, A.H. & Zubenko, G.S. (1990) Risk factors for white matter changes detected by magnetic resonance imaging in the elderly. *Stroke* **21**, 1424–8.

Tien, R.D., Feisberg, G.J., Ferris, M.J. & Osumi, A.K. (1993) The dementias: correlation of clinical features, pathophysiology, and neuroradiology. *Am. J. Roentgenol.* **161**, 245–55.

Verny, H., Duyckaerts, C., Pierot, L. & Hauw, J.J. (1991) Leuko-araiosis. *Developm. Neurosci.* **13**, 245–50.

Vonsattel, J.P., Meyers, R.H., Stevens, T.J. *et al.* (1985) Neuropathological classification of Huntington's disease. *J. Neuropathol. Exp. Neurol.* **44**, 559–77.

Zatz, L.M., Jernigan, T.L. & Ahumada, A.J. (1982a) Changes on computed cranial tomography with aging: intracranial fluid volume. *Am. J. Neuroradiol.* **3**, 1–11.

Zatz, L.M., Jernigan, T.L. & Ahumada, A.J.J. (1982b) White matter changes in cerebral computed tomography related to aging. *J. Comput. Assist. Tomogr.* **6**, 19–23.

14: Studies of Brain Ageing and Dementia Using Positron Emission Tomography and Magnetic Resonance Spectroscopy

D. G. M. Murphy, W. W. Hong, M. J. Mentis and C. L. Grady

The purpose of this chapter is to review studies of brain metabolism in dementia which used positron emission tomography (PET) and/or magnetic resonance spectroscopy (MRS). They will be dealt with in separate sections.

Positron emission tomography

In order to help understand studies of dementia, we shall first consider studies of brain metabolism in normal ageing.

Cerebral metabolism and ageing

Early studies of cerebral metabolism and ageing, using the Kety–Schmidt technique, generally reported a decrease in whole-brain blood flow and oxygen consumption with age (Kety, 1956; Dastur *et al.*, 1963; Gottstein & Held, 1979).

More recently, however, the finding of a consistent effect of age on cerebral metabolism has been elusive. Some studies have reported a 10–30% decrease in cerebral metabolism with age, while others have found no change (Table 14.1). Problems of subject selection, adequacy of health screening, differences in experimental conditions (e.g. eyes open vs. eyes closed), use of regional vs. global measures, resolution of the tomograph and use of atrophy correction all may have contributed to the variability of the published results.

Additionally, functional relationships between areas of the brain in ageing have been studied by applying a statistical correlation analysis (Clark *et al.*, 1984; Horwitz *et al.*, 1984; Metter *et al.*, 1984a). The assumption is that if two brain regions are functionally coupled so that activity in one depends on the activity in the other, an

Table 14.1 Summary of age-related changes in cerebral metabolism using positron emission tomography.

Authors	Year	$CMRO_2$	CMR_{glu}	Change (%)*
Kuhl *et al.*	1982		Decreased	−26
Duara *et al.*	1983		Unchanged	−17
Lebrun-Grandie *et al.*	1983	Unchanged		−32
Frackowiack & Gibbs	1983	Unchanged		−23
Pantano *et al.*	1984	Decreased		−17
Duara *et al.*	1984		Unchanged	−2
DeLeon *et al.*	1984		Unchanged	+2
Chawluk *et al.*	1987		Decreased	−16
Grady *et al.*	1990b		Decreased	−12
Leenders *et al.*	1990	Decreased		−19

* Percentage change over 20 – 80 years. (Some values estimated from published data.) $CMRO_2$, cerebral metabolic rate for oxygen; CMR_{glu}, cerebral metabolic rate for glucose.

increase or decrease in one brain region will be correlated with a similar increase or decrease in the other.

This approach was used to compare the regional intercorrelations of glucose metabolic rates in a group of young subjects and a group of older subjects (Horwitz *et al.*, 1986). The old group had the same general pattern of intercorrelations as the young group, but there were significantly fewer correlations in the old group between metabolic rates in the frontal and parietal regions and between regions within the parietal areas bilaterally. The reduced number of correlations within the parietal lobes and between the frontal and parietal areas were interpreted as a decrease in the integrated function between these areas and may be associated with some of the neuropsychological deficits that are seen in the elderly, specifically those that may depend heavily on the integrated function of anterior and posterior brain regions, such as tasks of attention (Mesulam, 1981).

However, hemispheric lateralisation of cognitive function is probably maintained during healthy ageing as demonstrated by asymmetries of cerebral metabolism during activation tasks. Berardi and colleagues (1990, 1991) had subjects perform continuous recognition tasks for both verbal and non-verbal visual stimuli, i.e. words and faces. Performance on these tasks was related to resting metabolic asymmetry in the parietal lobes in both age-groups such that those subjects with better verbal-memory performance had greater left than right parietal metabolism and those with better memory for faces showed greater right than left parietal metabolism (Fig. 14.1). Similarly, Miller *et al.* (1987) measured metabolism during performance of a verbal-memory task and found an increase in left temporal metabolism compared with baseline measures in healthy elderly subjects. These results suggest that relations between hemispheric lateralisation of cognitive function and asymmetries of cerebral metabolism can be demonstrated in healthy subjects, and that these correlations are maintained during the ageing process.

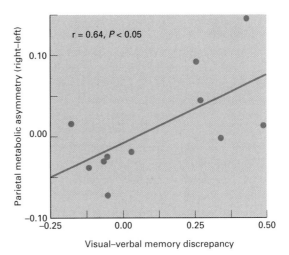

Fig. 14.1 The relation between parietal right–left metabolic asymmetry and visual–verbal differences in performance on memory tests for a sample of healthy elderly subjects. Points on the left of the graph represent subjects with better verbal memory and greater left than right parietal metabolic rates. Points on the right of the graph are subjects with better visual memory and greater right than left parietal metabolism.

Dementia of the Alzheimer type

Cerebral metabolism

The most common cause of dementia is Alzheimer's disease (AD), which acounts for 50–80% of patients with dementia (Chui, 1989; Evans *et al.*, 1989). According to current estimates, as much as 10% of the population over the age of 65 has AD (Evans *et al.*, 1989). Cerebrovascular disease accounts for 4–10% of cases, and other diseases, such as Pick's disease, account for an even smaller percentage. Each of these dementias has been studied in accord with its prevalence.

Post-mortem studies of the neuropathology of AD have shown that association neocortex, hippocampus and amygdala are more affected than primary neocortex (see Kemper, 1984, for a review), although there is disagreement about whether parietotemporal (Brun & Gustafson, 1976) or frontal (Jamada & Mehraein, 1968) neocortical regions are more damaged. One of the contributions of PET to the study of dementia has been to confirm this pattern of damage during life in patients with AD, i.e. hypometabolism is seen disproportionately in association neocortex with relative sparing of metabolism in primary cortical and subcortical regions. One early study (Ferris *et al.*, 1980) that used PET to examine regional cerebral metabolic rates for glucose (rCMRglu) in patients with AD reported equal degrees of metabolic reduction (about 35%) in both anterior and posterior association cortex compared with controls. Other reports have generally found that the parietal and temporal lobes show the most diminution of glucose or oxygen utilisation (Frackowiack *et al.*, 1981; Friedland *et al.*, 1983; Foster *et al.*, 1984; Duara *et al.*, 1986; McGeer *et al.*, 1986). These reductions were of the order of 30–40% for parietotemporal areas and 10–20% for frontal and occipital regions. Primary cortical and subcortical regions were reported to be relatively spared (Benson *et al.*, 1983; Metter *et al.*, 1984b;

Haxby *et al.*, 1988b). In addition, a significant relation between increasing dementia severity and decreasing metabolism was found by several groups (Ferris *et al.*, 1980; De Leon *et al.*, 1983; Foster *et al.*, 1984). Figure 14.2 shows the typical pattern of reduced glucose metabolism in association neocortex with relative sparing of primary cortical and subcortical regions in three AD patients compared with a healthy control.

Measurement of absolute metabolic rates may not provide the best way of assessing metabolic disturbances in AD. Duara *et al.* (1986) found that glucose metabolism in AD patients was most markedly reduced in parietal and temporal regions, compared with control values, but that these reductions were statistically significant only in severely demented patients, and were of the order of 35–45%. Normalised metabolic measures (such as ratios) are generally more sensitive to small differences between groups of subjects (Haxby, 1986), because of the smaller variance of these measures compared with the variance of absolute metabolic rates (coefficient of variation

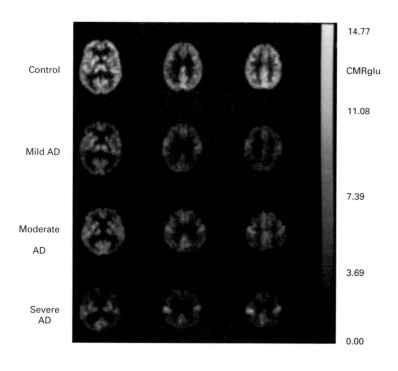

Control

Mild AD

Moderate
AD

Severe
AD

14.77

CMRglu

11.08

7.39

3.69

0.00

Fig. 14.2 PET scan images from a healthy control (age 69), a mildly demented patient (age 53), a moderately demented patient (age 63) and a severely demented patient (age 72). All patients and the control are women. Scans were obtained using a Scanditronix PC1024-7B positron tomograph (6 mm in-plane resolution). Three brain levels above the inferior orbitomeatal line are shown—45 mm on the left, 70 mm in the middle and 90 mm on the right-hand side of the figure. All the patients show reduced metabolism in association neocortex (predominantly in the right hemisphere), with relative sparing in the primary cortical and subcortical regions. The glucose metabolic scale on the right is in mg/100 g brain/min.

less than 10% vs. 20–30%). When normalised measures of metabolism (ratios of regional metabolism to whole-brain metabolism) were examined (Duara *et al.*, 1986), these were found to be reduced in parietal areas even in mildly affected patients, and also in frontal and temporal regions in both moderately and severely demented patients.

Much of the work on AD has focused on describing the early manifestations of the disease in order to discern which brain regions are most vulnerable to the disease, and to establish criteria for early diagnosis. In addition, emphasis has been placed on the interrelations between metabolic rates in various brain regions. For example, right/left asymmetries of metabolism in AD patients have received considerable attention. Although Benson *et al.* (1983) reported no metabolic asymmetry between right and left hemispheres in AD patients, Foster *et al.* (1983) examined patients chosen for either disproportionate aphasia or apraxia, and found that areas of reduced metabolism in these patients corresponded to the left and right hemispheres, respectively. In an unselected sample of patients with AD, an increase in asymmetry in either direction (right lower than left or vice versa) would cause an increase in the variance of left- vs. right-hemispheric metabolism in the patient group compared with control subjects. The variance of right/left-asymmetry indices was found to be increased in frontal, parietal and temporal association cortical regions in mildly to moderately demented patients compared with controls (Friedland *et al.*, 1985; Haxby *et al.*, 1985; Kumar *et al.*, 1991) (Fig. 14.3). Asymmetry was not significantly increased in primary occipital or sensorimotor cortex. In general, no directional tendencies in these measures have been reported, i.e. there are equal numbers of patients with disproportionate left-hemisphere abnormality and patients with disproportionate right-hemisphere reductions. Only Duara and colleagues (1988) have found a predominance of left-hemisphere abnormality in their patients.

In addition to interhemispheric heterogeneity,

intrahemispheric (anterior/posterior) heterogeneity is also found in AD patients (Chase, 1987; Haxby *et al.*, 1988b). When parietal/premotor and parietal/prefrontal metabolic ratios were calculated, an increased variance was demonstrated in AD patients compared with controls, similar to the increased variance seen in right/left measures. This increased variance was seen in mildly, moderately and severely demented patients, with some individuals showing greater reductions in parietal compared with frontal areas and others showing disproportionate frontal abnormality. One study used a type of cluster analysis to identify subgroups of patients with different metabolic patterns (Grady *et al.*, 1990a) and found four distinct patterns of abnormality (Plate 14.1, facing p.230): (i) bilateral parieto-temporal hypometabolism with relative sparing of frontal cortex (45% of the patient sample); (ii) metabolic deficit in paralimbic structures, including orbitofrontal and anterior cingulate (25%); (iii) left-hemisphere hypometabolism in frontal, parietal and temporal regions (15%); and (iv) frontal and posterior metabolic defect of equal severity (15%). Except for the fourth subgroup, which consisted of patients who were more severely demented, the patterns were not related to dementia severity, age at onset or duration of illness. These findings demonstrate that metabolic deficits in AD occur in a patchy distribution and are heterogeneous, both within and between hemispheres. In addition, frontal metabolism is not always spared in AD, in contrast to earlier reports (Foster *et al.*, 1984; Kuhl *et al.*, 1985), but can be found as the primary metabolic deficit, as can paralimbic association cortical abnormalities.

There is evidence that patients who have early onset of dementia have different clinical (Seltzer & Sherwin, 1983), neuropathological (Mountjoy *et al.*, 1983) and neurochemical (Rossor *et al.*, 1984) characteristics compared with those with later onset of dementia. The suggestion that early- and late-onset dementia represent two distinct diseases (Seltzer *et al.*, 1984) has been studied with imaging techniques. One study examined right/left metabolic asymmetries in early- vs. late-

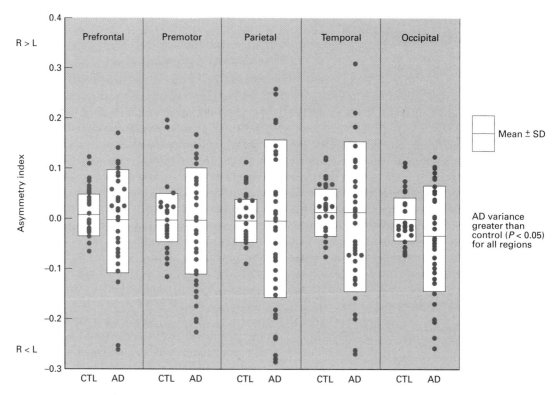

Fig. 14.3 Scatter plots of the metabolic-asymmetry indices for a group of mildly to severely demented AD patients and an age-matched control group (CTL) in five neocortical association regions. The asymmetry index is calculated as $(R - L)/((R + L)/2)$, where R is the metabolic value in a right-hemisphere region and L is metabolism in the homologous region on the left. Positive values indicate that right-hemisphere is greater than that in the left hemisphere and negative values represent right metabolism lower than left. All regions showed an increased variance of asymmetry in the AD patients compared with the control values.

onset AD patients and reported that the early-onset patients had a greater tendency toward disproportionate right-hemisphere diminution of glucose use, which was associated with poorer visuospatial performance (Koss *et al.*, 1985). Two other studies (Grady *et al.* 1987; Small *et al.*, 1989), found no relation between metabolic-asymmetry measures and age at onset. The early-onset patients did show significantly greater metabolic reductions in parietal regions, but these were not associated with greater reductions in performance on neuropsychological tests of parietal-lobe function. These data suggest that younger AD patients are better able to compensate cognitively for metabolic dysfunction than are older patients, but do not support the

view that early- and late-onset DAT are two distinct disease entities.

AD can be transmitted via autosomal dominant genes (Heston *et al.*, 1981; Berg *et al.*, 1986; St George-Hyslop *et al.*, 1987; Farrer *et al.*, 1989). Two studies have shown that familial patients have metabolic patterns that are indistinguishable from those of patients with sporadic disease (Friedland *et al.*, 1989; Hoffman *et al.*, 1989). Thus, the pattern of metabolic brain dysfunction in an individual patient does not seem to depend on whether or not the disease in that patient has a genetic component.

Intercorrelations of regional metabolic rates have also been examined in patients with AD. In one study that examined moderately to severely demented patients (Metter *et al.*, 1984b), interregional correlations were found to be elevated in the patients compared with controls, which may have been related to the diffuse nature of the hypometabolism seen in these patients, who were in the severe stages of the disease. When mildly to moderately demented patients were compared with age-matched controls, the patient group showed fewer significant correlations between frontal and parietal regions, the number of which was already reduced in the older controls compared with younger subjects (Horwitz *et al.*, 1987). In addition, the number of significant correlations between glucose metabolism in right/left homologous regions was significantly reduced in AD. This is of interest because these homologous correlations were among the largest correlations found in both the old and young healthy subjects (Horwitz *et al.*, 1986). Thus, in AD, there appear to be alterations in the functional coupling of brain regions that cannot be accounted for by ageing alone, i.e. further reductions in the number of frontal–parietal correlations and reduced homologous correlations.

Cerebral metabolism and cognitive function

The cerebral-metabolic patterns of AD patients are consistent with the types of neuropsychological impairments seen in these patients. For example, metabolic right/left-asymmetry measures in frontal and parietal cortices are significantly correlated with measures of right/left neuropsychological discrepancy, such that those patients with disproportionate left-hemisphere hypometabolism have greater language impairment compared with visuospatial function, and those with disproportionate right-hemisphere hypometabolism have more impairment of visuoconstructive abilities (Foster *et al.*, 1983; Friedland *et al.*, 1985; Haxby *et al.*, 1985). One study examined metabolic and neuropsychological patterns in mildly and moderately demented patients separately, and found that the mildly affected patients had abnormal memory performance, but

scored in the normal range on neocortically mediated cognitive tests of attention, language and visuospatial function (Haxby *et al.*, 1986). Moderately demented patients were significantly impaired on all neuropsychological tests. However, both mildly and moderately demented patients showed reductions in parietal/sensorimotor ratios of glucose metabolism, and had significantly increased metabolic asymmetry in frontal, parietal and temporal association cortex. There was a significant correlation between right/left metabolic asymmetry and neuropsychological discrepancy measures only for those patients that had impaired performance on the cognitive tests, i.e. the moderately demented patients. Thus, in mildly affected AD patients, metabolic changes in neocortex are seen prior to changes in neocortically mediated neuropsychological performance. In another study, parietal/frontal metabolic measures significantly correlated with cognitive measures, but again only in the moderately demented patients, not in the mildly demented patients (Haxby *et al.*, 1988b). Moderately demented patients with disproportionate parietal metabolic abnormality had more impairment on tests of calculations or visuoconstruction than on tests of sequencing or verbal fluency, whereas patients with disproportionate frontal metabolic defects showed the opposite pattern of neuropsychological impairments.

Furthermore, imaging studies have shown that right/left metabolic asymmetries in AD tend to be stable over periods of several years (Fig. 14.4), as are the correlations between these asymmetries and neuropsychological discrepancies (Grady *et al.*, 1986; Haxby *et al.*, 1990; but see Jagust *et al.*, 1988). For example, patients with a disproportionate left-hemisphere metabolic defect and poor language performance at the initial evaluation continue to show this pattern for long periods of time. In addition, these metabolic interhemispheric asymmetries are accentuated over time, but only in patients who are mildly affected at the initial evaluation (Grady *et al.*, 1988). The intrahemispheric measures of parietal/frontal heterogeneity are not only directionally stable, but

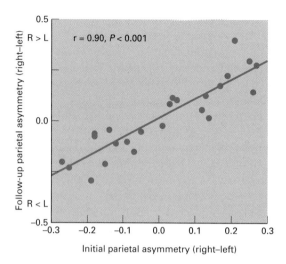

Fig. 14.4 Scatter plots of initial and follow-up parietal metabolic-asymmetry indices in a group of AD patients (mean follow-up period was 15 months; range 9–25 months). A significant correlation is shown, indicating that the initial pattern of glucose use in individual patients is maintained over time.

become more pronounced over time in mildly, moderately and severely demented patients (Haxby *et al.*, 1988b). These results suggest that metabolic patterns in individual patients are characteristic of the disease process in these patients and that these patterns are correlated with the clinical manifestations of disease progression. Also, the interhemispheric metabolic abnormalities appear to worsen in the early stages of the disease, whereas the intrahemispheric patterns continue to progress even in the later stages of AD.

Moreover, the location of the metabolic defects in mildly affected patients who suffer only memory loss predicts non-memory cognitive changes that develop later (Haxby *et al.*, 1987). Grady *et al.* (1988) showed that, in a group of mildly demented AD patients, neocortical metabolic abnormalities preceded the appearance of neocortically mediated neuropsychological impairment by as few as 8 or as many as 36 months. This relation between altered metabolic function and subsequent cognitive changes in AD is illustrated in Fig. 14.5, which shows the serial

evaluations of a patient who was first seen in the early stages of the disease (Grady *et al.*, 1988). This patient (age 45 years) presented initially with a progressive memory loss and a right parietal metabolic deficit, which became bilateral 6 months later. The first non-memory neuropsychological impairments were seen in the areas of abstract reasoning and complex attention more than a year after the first evaluation. Finally, impairments in language and visuospatial function were noted almost 2 years after the appearance of bilateral parietal metabolic changes. This patient demonstrates the typical finding in patients with AD, i.e. significant and stable neocortical metabolic deficits prior to the appearance of any neocortically mediated cognitive dysfunction (Haxby *et al.*, 1986; Grady *et al.*, 1988). In addition, the first non-memory impairments seen are in abstract reasoning and complex attention. These functions depend on the integrity of the frontal and parietal regions (Lezak, 1983) and probably involve the integrated function of these two brain areas (Mesulam, 1981). Changes in the functional connections between anterior and posterior brain regions early in the course of AD may impair the ability to attend to abstract and complex aspects of the environment. Thus, the longitudinal analysis of cerebral metabolic deficits in AD has been useful not only in identifying those brain regions that are affected at different stages of the disease, but also in predicting the course of cognitive deterioration.

Studies of divided attention have also shown the importance of attentional deficits in the early stages of AD. Performance on tests of dichotic listening, in which competing stimuli were delivered to the two ears simultaneously, was found to be deficient in AD patients and related to hypometabolism in the left temporal region (Grimes *et al.*, 1985). A subsequent study compared patients' performance on dichotic tests with performance on tests requiring discrimination of degraded monotic stimuli, and showed that dichotic performance was not only significantly more impaired than monotic performance, but that dichotic performance was again related

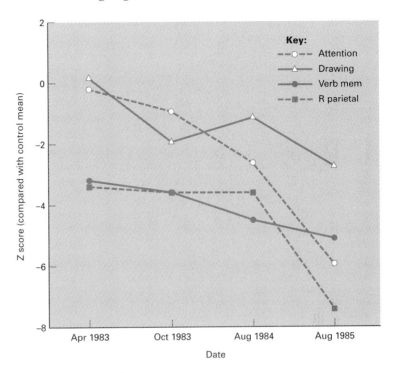

Fig. 14.5 Data from one AD patient seen over a period of $2\frac{1}{4}$ years. Scores on neuropsychological tests and the right parietal/sensorimotor metabolic ratio have been converted to Z scores based on the mean and standard deviation of an age-matched control group. The parietal metabolic measure and the memory score were significantly abnormal (Z score of –2 or less, $P < 0.05$) at the first evaluation and continued to deteriorate. Scores on tests of attention and drawing were not abnormal until over a year after the metabolic defect was first noted.

to temporal-lobe metabolism, whereas monotic performance was not (Grady *et al.*, 1989a). This suggests that the dichotic impairment was directly related to the divided attention demands of the task, and was not due to an inability to make a difficult auditory discrimination among degraded speech stimuli. In addition, AD patients are unable to attend selectively to either the right or the left ear during dichotic tasks, further indicating that the selective allocation of attention is impaired in this disease (Mohr *et al.*, 1990). A third study (Nestor *et al.*, 1991) examined reaction time for single-task and dual-task conditions during PET and found that subjects with AD had slowing of reaction time during dual-task but not during single-task conditions. Moreover, this slowing was correlated with reductions of brain metabolism in right premotor and right parietal association areas. In a fourth study, Parasuraman *et al.* (1992) found that reaction time to cue-directed shifts of spatial attention were correlated with right–left asymmetry in resting glucose metabolism of the

superior parietal lobe for subjects with mild to moderate AD but not for controls. These studies indicate that attentional mechanisms are disrupted in AD and that these disruptions are related to abnormal metabolism in association neocortex.

Two studies to date have used PET to examine the effect of pharmacological treatment of AD. Nordberg *et al.* (1992) used ^{18}F-2-fluoro-2-deoxy-D-glucose (FDG), ^{11}C-butanol, and ^{11}C-methylnicotine as tracers for glucose metabolism, blood flow and nicotine receptors, respectively, in three patients with AD who were being treated with tacrine, a cholinesterase inhibitor. Tacrine treatment appeared to increase the number of nicotine receptors and glucose metabolism in the most mildly affected patient. It was concluded that tacrine treatment might be most clinically effective early in the course of AD. Heiss *et al.* (1988) studied the effect of piracetam treatment on rCMRglu and found increases in frontal, auditory, parietal, occipital and cingulate cortex, as well as in basal ganglia and thalamus, in subjects with AD but not in subjects with non-Alzheimer's dementia after treatment compared with before. They concluded that treatment with piracetam might be of benefit in AD.

Other dementias

Cerebrovascular dementia

Cerebrovascular disease has long been known to cause dementia in older people (Hachinski *et al.*, 1975), and, indeed, most if not all studies of AD patients attempt to exclude a history of vascular disease in the patient sample. However, a history of vascular disease does not rule out the possibility of a mixed form of dementia involving AD and vascular disease. It is therefore important to examine the metabolic patterns in groups with different clinical diagnoses to try to differentiate among them and determine the specificity of the metabolic findings in AD.

An early ^{133}Xe study (Hachinski *et al.*, 1975) found reduced global cerebral blood flow (CBF) in patients with multi-infarct or cerebrovascular dementia (MID). A later PET study (Frackowiak *et al.*, 1981) compared MID patients with AD patients and controls and found that CBF and mean cerebral oxygen utilisation were negatively correlated with dementia severity, but that there was no increase in the global oxygen extraction ratio. This was thought to be inconsistent with a chronic ischaemic brain syndrome. Among MID patients, defects of oxygen utilisation were most marked in the parietal lobe. Benson *et al.* (1983) also compared MID and AD patients with controls and reported that, whereas the AD patients had reduced metabolism throughout the cortex and particularly in parietotemporal regions, the MID patients had reduced metabolism in parietotemporal regions, caudate and thalamus. In MID patients with evidence of infarcts on computed tomographic (CT) scans, areas of hypometabolism on PET images are reported to correspond well with the lesion sites on the CT images (Kuhl *et al.*, 1985).

More recently, interest has focused on white-matter lesions, evident on CT or magnetic resonance imaging (MRI), which are associated with vascular disease and possibly with vascular dementia. DeCarli and colleagues (1990) examined a group of patients with dementia, a history of vascular disease and white-matter lesions on MRI, and compared metabolic patterns in these patients with those of a group of AD patients. Whereas the AD patients showed metabolic reductions primarily in parietotemporal regions, the MID patients showed more sparing of parietal metabolism and significantly reduced metabolism in the basal ganglia and thalamus compared with the AD patients (Fig. 14.6). Duara *et al.* (1989) found no difference in metabolic pattern between MID and AD patients, but a significant fraction of

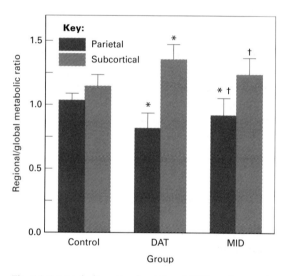

Fig. 14.6 Metabolic ratios for AD and MID patients and age-matched controls. The parietal ratio is the mean value for superior and inferior parietal regions referenced to global metabolism, and the subcortical ratio is the mean value for caudate, thalamus and putamen referenced to the global value. The AD patients show reduced parietal ratios compared with controls and increased subcortical ratios, reflecting the relative sparing of metabolism in subcortical regions. The MID patients also have reduced parietal ratios, but these are significantly less reduced than in the AD patients. In contrast, the MID patients have lower subcortical ratios than the AD patients, reflecting more involvement of these regions in MID. *Differs from control, $P < 0.01$; †differs from AD, $P < 0.01$.

their AD patients had evidence of white-matter disease on MRI. Interestingly, another study showed that AD patients with white-matter lesions had less metabolic deficit in parieto-temporal areas than did those patients without such lesions (de Leon *et al.*, 1988). This evidence suggests that vascular dementia is accompanied by cortical metabolic abnormality similar to, but less severe than, that seen in AD, but, unlike AD, is associated with metabolic dysfunction in basal ganglia and thalamus. This subcortical abnormality is probably secondary to white-matter demyelination and may contribute to some of the clinical features of MID.

Cerebrovascular disease is associated with hypertension. We have reported (Mentis *et al.*, 1994) functional neuronal connectivity loss primarily in the anterior watershed area in the brains of hypertensive subjects without neuropsychological impairment. However, as noted above, we have also reported that metabolic abnormalities may precede and predict cognitive abnormalities by a period of months to years (Haxby *et al.*, 1986; Grady *et al.*, 1988). Thus, hypertensive subjects, without obvious dementia, may also eventually manifest cognitive abnormalities.

Pick's disease

PET studies have examined glucose metabolism in Pick's disease. Salmon and Franck (1989) studied three patients with biopsy-proved Pick's disease, using FDG and PET. They found frontal and temporal hypometabolism in the two Pick's cases with frontal syndromes, and left perisylvian hypometabolism in one patient with a slowly progressive aphasia. Single case-studies, using FDG and PET, have also reported frontal hypometabolism (Kamo *et al.*, 1987) alone, and in combination with temporobasal cortex, hippocampus and caudate (Szelies & Karenberg., 1986).

Acquired immune deficiency syndrome (AIDS) dementia complex

Both single-photon emission tomography (SPET) and PET studies have been carried out in subjects with the AIDS dementia complex (ADC). Studies which employed FDG and PET to investigate glucose metabolism in ADC, have reported that early ADC is characterised by subcortical hypermetabolism, whereas, late in ADC, cortical and subcortical hypometabolism prevail (Rottenberg *et al.*, 1987). Brunetti *et al.* (1989) examined cerebral glucose metabolism in subjects with ADC before and after treatment with 3'-azido-2',3'-dideoxythymidine (AZT; zidovudine). Following treatment, one subject regained symmetry of frontal and occipital cortical regions, one normalised rCMRglu values for frontal, temporal and occipital regions and two showed generalised increases in cortical glucose metabolism. Costa *et al.* (1988) studied regional CBF (rCBF) in ADC with ^{99m}Tc-hexamethylpropylene-aminoxime (HMPAO) and SPET, and reported that subjects with ADC had decreased rCBF in temporal and parietal cortices—a pattern of regional hypometabolism similar to that of AD subjects. In contrast, Pohl *et al.* (1988) reported a generalised decrease in rCBF in ADC.

Magnetic resonance spectroscopy

As noted in previous chapters, there are a number of methods by which nuclear magnetic resonance (NMR) can be used to perform *in vivo* human studies. The more widely used is MRI, which employs the magnetic signal from the hydrogen atoms of water to generate images of anatomical structures of the human body (Budinger & Lauterbur, 1984). The second technique is MRS. Rather than images, spectra of the magnetic signals of such nuclei as phosphorus, carbon and hydrogen are obtained. Thus, NMR spectra can be used to measure relative concentrations of various nuclei and biochemicals.

Hydrogen (proton) spectroscopy

In MRS of hydrogen atoms, the number of metabolites that can be resolved in the spectrum obtained from a patient's brain depends upon the sequence used: longer echo times (TE) are used to measure N-acetyl-L-aspartate (NAA), creatine/phosphocreatine (Cr) and choline (Cho) (Weiner & Hetherington, 1989), whereas short-echo-time spectroscopy is also able to measure myoinositol (MI). NAA is thought to be a marker for viable neurons, and has been found to be decreased in disorders with neuronal death, including strokes (Bruhn *et al.*, 1989a), tumours (Bruhn *et al.*, 1989a; Gill *et al.*, 1990), infections (Menon *et al.*, 1990b) and demyelinating diseases (Wolinsky *et al.*, 1990). Cho is the precursor for acetylcholine, the neurotransmitter most widely implicated in the aetiology of AD, and is also a precursor of phosphatidylcholine (a major constituent of cell membranes). MI is a component of the polyphosphoinositol second-messenger cascade, which is thought to be pathophysiologically involved in AD. Creatine is converted by creatine kinase into phosphocreatine, which provides storage of high-energy phosphate in neurons. However, creatine's principal importance in MRS of AD is probably as a control value against which peak heights, or peak areas, of NAA, Cho and MI can be measured.

Numerous groups have reported decreases in NAA/Cr in the brains of patients with AD (Bruhn *et al.*, 1992; Ide *et al.*, 1992, Meyerhoff *et al.*, 1992; Schiino *et al.*, 1993). In addition, Miller *et al.* (1993) performed localised *in vivo* spectroscopy on 10–15 ml voxels in the parietal and occipital lobes of patients with probable AD and healthy age-matched controls, using a short TE (time to repetition (TR)/TE 1500/30 ms) sequence to resolve four peaks (MI, NAA, Cr and Cho). They reported significant elevations of MI/Cr and decreases in NAA/Cr in both the parietal and occipital lobes. The finding of elevated MI/Cr in the brains of patients with AD is consistent with previously reported abnormalities in AD of the inositol polyphosphate

system (Young *et al.*, 1988). However, as noted above, NAA is found to be decreased in other disorders with neuronal death, and so reductions of NAA/Cr may be a non-specific finding in AD. This suggestion is supported by the results of Shiino *et al.* (1993), who conducted an MRS and SPET study of patients with AD, Parkinson's disease with dementia, and dementia secondary to normal-pressure hydrocephalus. They found that the NAA/Cr ratio in their demented Parkinson's disease group was significantly lower than in the other two groups, which did not differ from each other in NAA/Cr. Further, some subjects had low ratios of NAA/Cr in the absence of gross brain atrophy on MRI and in spite of normal rCBF on SPET. Thus, reduction of NAA/Cr appears to be a sensitive (but not specific) marker for neuronal degeneration in AD.

Proton MRS has also been used to assess cerebral metabolic and cognitive dysfunction in AIDS. Reductions have been reported in NAA/Cho (Menon *et al.*, 1990b) and in NAA/Cr ratios in moderately to severely, but not in mildly, demented AIDS subjects (Menon *et al.*, 1992; Jarvik *et al.*, 1993). Elevations of Cho/Cr have also been reported (Menon *et al.*, 1992; Jarvik *et al.*, 1993), although these findings are difficult to interpret, because changes in Cho/Cr can reflect non-neuronal metabolic activity (Bruhn *et al.*, 1989a; Menon *et al.*, 1990b; Wolinsky *et al.*, 1990). However, all the above findings were reported in brain areas that appeared normal on structural MRI. Thus, proton MRS appears able to assess cerebral pathology in the absence of gross abnormalities on structural MRI. Significant reductions in NAA/Cho and NAA/Cr have also been found in the proton spectra obtained from the brains of patients with human immunodeficiency virus (HIV) infection and 'neurological signs', as well as elevations in Cho/Cr in patients with low CD4-lymphocyte counts and structural MRI abnormalities (Chong *et al.*, 1993).

Phosphorus spectroscopy

As reviewed in Chapter 6, MRS of phosphorus

(^{31}P) generates a spectrum from which information can be obtained about concentrations of ^{31}P, phosphomonoesters (PME), phosphodiesters (PDE), inorganic phosphorus (Pi), phosphocreatine (PCr) and adenosine triphosphate (ATP) (Prichard & Shulman, 1988). Phosphorus spectra are of interest because biological systems store energy in the form of phosphate compounds (PCr, ATP, adenosine diphosphate (ADP)). Also, because the position of the Pi peak changes as the acidity of the tissue is altered, pH can also be determined with this technique (Petroff *et al.*, 1985). PME and PDE spectra give information about phospholipids, the primary structural components of cell membranes and participants in second-messenger systems.

The PET FDG method measures the rate of phosphorylation of glucose, which is the primary substrate of the brain for energy metabolism. Ultimately, the energy content of glucose ends up in phosphate compounds, such as PCr and ATP. Concentrations of these metabolites provide information on steady-state energy stores in brain tissue, and ^{31}P spectroscopy is an appropriate tool to investigate this aspect of energy utilisation in AD.

Many ^{31}P spectroscopy studies of AD are in disagreement; this stems from differences in a number of factors, including study design, subject selection, medication effects and MRS techniques employed (i.e. surface coil vs. whole-head coil, volume of tissue studied, region of brain studied and use of ratio values vs. absolute quantification). Several *in vitro* ^{31}P NMR spectroscopy studies of AD, using brain tissue obtained by autopsy or biopsy, have reported differences from normal tissue in the PME and PDE regions of the spectrum (Pettegrew *et al.*, 1988a). In addition, Pettegrew *et al.* (1988b) reported that the number of senile plaques was correlated inversely with PME levels and directly with PDE levels. They suggested that initially in the course of AD there is an increase in PME levels (indicating perhaps regenerative processes), but later in AD the increases in both plaque count and PDE levels indicate that degeneration is dominant. In contrast, another *in vitro* study (Miatto *et al.*, 1986) found PME decreases in parietal, frontal and temporal brain matter. Thus, whether PME levels are elevated in ^{31}P NMR spectra of AD brain studied *in vitro* is not clear at present.

Post-mortem studies have several limitations, such as post-mortem delay, autolysis, fixation artefacts, patient-selection bias, incomplete medical information and inability to control patient medication, which *in vivo* imaging studies avoid. For example, the confounding effect of a non-specific 'disease factor' or of medications on *in vitro* measurement of PME and PDE is suggested by the fact that an elevated concentration of PME is not specific to AD. Thus, Pettegrew *et al.* (1988a) reported a significant elevation of PME in non-AD patients compared with controls and no significant difference between AD patients and non-AD patients with differing brain diseases.

There have also been several *in vivo* ^{31}P NMR spectroscopy studies of AD patients. One study, by Welch *et al.* (1988), found no difference between AD patients and controls in any phosphate ratio in the frontal or parietal lobes. In contrast, another *in vivo* study of AD (Brown *et al.*, 1989) appears to support some of Pettegrew's (1988a) *in vitro* results. Using a surface-coil MRS technique, it was reported that AD subjects had a larger area under the PME peak than did controls in the temporoparietal part of the brain, and that values of PCr/Pi distinguished AD patients from those with MID, using a bivariate classification method. However, the surface-coil technique allows no correction for relative amounts of brain and cerebrospinal fluid (CSF) in the region of analysis, and absolute concentrations of metabolites were not obtained (Brown *et al.*, 1989). Instead, the ratios of the areas of the corresponding peaks were used. Also, because the excitation field of a surface coil is non-uniform, the amount of partial saturation would have varied as a function of position in the sample, depending on the location of the signal sources relative to the detection coil. Further, AD and MID do not have similar histopathologies and affect different brain regions in varying degrees. Because of these neuropathological differences between AD and MID, ^{31}P signal sources would be expected to be systematically different distances from the detection coil. Thus, the combined effect of excitation-field inhomogeneity and group neuropathological differences may cause systematically different partial-saturation conditions in both patient and control populations, accounting (in part) for some of the reported differences in phosphate levels.

Bottomley *et al.* (1989) developed an MRS technique to obtain absolute concentrations of phosphorus metabolites, and our laboratory has published a technique for calculating the amount of brain matter and CSF in an MRI brain region of interest (ROI)—allowing correction for brain atrophy and partial voluming in patients and healthy controls (DeCarli *et al.*, 1992). Thus, we carried out a combined MRI, MRS and PET study (Murphy *et al.*, 1993) to determine: (i) if there are measurable differences between patients with AD and age/sex-matched healthy controls in brain concentrations or ratios of phosphorus metabolites; (ii) whether correlations exist between phosphorus-metabolite concentrations or ratios and disease severity in AD patients; and (iii) how glucose utilisation (measured by PET) is related to phosphorus energy stores and phospholipid metabolism in brain tissue (measured by MRS). This *in vivo* study of brain energy utilisation and storage in AD differed from previously published reports because we: (i) obtained absolute concentrations of phosphorus metabolites; (ii) calculated the amount of brain matter and CSF in the brain region from which phosphorus spectra were obtained, to correct for brain atrophy; (iii) evaluated the rCMRglu in the same brain region; and (iv) correlated concentrations of phosphorus metabolites with degree of dementia and with glucose metabolism (as measured by PET). We found that the AD patients had significantly ($P<0.01$) less brain matter and significantly ($P<0.01$) more CSF in the volume used for spectroscopy than did controls. Cerebral glucose metabolism was significantly

lower in the AD patients than in the controls, within the same volume used for MRS for whole volume (both atrophy-corrected and uncorrected), and also the right and left middle temporal, superior temporal, inferior parietal, posterior cingulate and right insula regions. However, although the brains of AD patients were significantly more hypometabolic than those of controls, no significant difference was found between the two groups in concentration or ratio of any phosphorus metabolite, and there was no correlation between severity of dementia or length of illness and any phosphorus-metabolite concentration or ratio. In summary, we found that within moderately impaired AD patients glucose metabolism per unit volume of tissue (as measured by PET) may be significantly reduced, but that phosphorus metabolism (as measured by MRS) is not significantly affected. Therefore, we suggested that: (i) in AD, glucose metabolism is affected early in the disease process (reflecting decreased basal synaptic functioning) and is not due to rate limitation in glucose delivery, abnormal glucose metabolism or an abnormal coupling between oxidation and phosphorylation; (ii) normal or near-normal levels of phosphorus metabolites may be maintained at all stages of the disease; and (iii) altered high-energy phosphate levels in AD are not a consequence of reduced glucose metabolism, nor do they play a major role in the neuropathology of the disorder, at least in whole-brain sections.

Finally, Bottomley *et al.* (1990) reported that subjects with ADC have significant reductions of PCr and nucleoside triphosphate (NTP). Also, Deicken *et al.* (1991) found significantly lower ATP/Pi and a trend toward lower PCr/Pi in subjects with HIV infection and neuropsychiatric impairments. Moreover, both ATP/Pi and PCr/Pi were significantly negatively correlated with the degree of neuropsychiatric deficit.

Future directions

PET

The majority of studies to date have examined cerebral metabolism and CBF in ageing and dementia in the resting or unstimulated state. Another approach is to examine metabolism under conditions of sensory or cognitive activation to determine the metabolic response to task performance (e.g. Fox *et al.*, 1987; Petersen *et al.*, 1989). This approach will become more important in the future, as the short-lived radioisotopes that make it possible become more widely available. Measurement of rCBF with ^{15}O-H_2O is particularly suited to this type of study since the 2-min half-life of ^{15}O-H_2O allows multiple studies to be performed on the same individual. The ability to measure blood flow under activation conditions will allow the study of age-related differences in structure–function relationships, as well as the deterioration of these relations in demented patients.

One activation paradigm that has been applied to the study of age-related changes in CBF is that of visual stimulation to examine the pathways involved in object discrimination and spatial location. These anatomically and functionally distinct pathways have been well defined in the extrastriate cortex of non-human primates (Ungerleider & Mishkin, 1982; Desimone & Ungerleider, 1989), and in humans have been studied using ^{15}O-H_2O to measure brain blood flow during face-matching (object) and dot-location-matching (spatial) tasks (Haxby *et al.*, 1988a). In young subjects, the face-matching task activates blood flow in occipitotemporal areas bilaterally and the dot-location task selectively activates flow in superior parietal regions (Haxby *et al.*, 1988a). Older subjects show a very similar pattern of activation in the two tasks, but have some parietal activation during the face-matching task that the young subjects do not show (Grady *et al.*, 1989b). Moreover, older subjects activate areas in prefrontal cortex and inferior and medial parietal cortex during location-matching more

than young subjects (Grady *et al.*, 1994). These results suggest that the functional dissociation of object and spatial vision in extrastriate cortex is preserved during ageing, but that subtle changes occur, making the two systems less efficient or less functionally separate. They further suggest that spatial vision may be affected to a greater degree by ageing than object vision.

Activation studies also yield information about synaptic integrity. Grady *et al.* (1993) found that the increase in blood flow to the extrastriate cortex of mild to moderately affected AD subjects during a face-matching task was not significantly different in magnitude from that in normal controls. Deutsch and Halsey (1990) also found a similar magnitude of activation in AD patients and controls during a mental rotation task. Duara *et al.* (1992) found that regional metabolic activation caused by a reading-memory task did not allow better discrimination of subjects with mild to moderate AD from normal controls, and noted that hypometabolic regions in AD subjects during rest showed metabolic activation during the task to the same degree as in the normals. This most probably represents a compensatory increase in the activity of remaining neurons in the context of progressive neurode-generation, which is known to affect association more than primary visual cortex (Lewis *et al.*, 1987). Work by DeKosky and Scheff (1990) has shown that, early in the course of AD, hypertrophy of surviving neurons is able to compensate for decrements of up to 30–35% in number of synapses, such that the net area of apposition remains stable, whereas later in AD hypertrophy of remaining synapses is insufficient to maintain normal levels of synaptic contact. Rapoport & Grady (1993) has proposed the use of drugs that have neurotransmitter effects at synapses as probes for studying specific neurotransmitter defects, synaptic efficacy and pharmacotherapeutic possibilities in AD. In conjunction with parametric cognitive-activation paradigms that employ stimuli of graded intensity, difficulty or complexity and single-subject analysis techniques, it should be possible in the future to assess the degree of synaptic failure in any given patient and the extent to which it can be ameliorated in that patient with a particular drug, during one scan session.

MRS

It is suggested that future MRS studies of dementia should attempt absolute quantification of metabolites, rather than ratio measures. This is of importance because two compounds may increase or decrease significantly in concentration but the ratios of their concentrations may remain unchanged. Further, wherever possible, MRS should not be used in isolation but should be combined with cognitive measures and other imaging techniques (MRI/PET/SPET), and sample from more than one brain area/volume. For example, proton MRS of one brain area may show a decrease in NAA, but without volumetric MRI it is unclear if this is because of changes in volume of total tissue or of grey or white matter, or if this change in NAA precedes loss of tissue volume. Further, longitudinal study designs, combined with measurement of more than one brain area (e.g. using chemical-shift imaging), will allow changes in metabolite concentrations over time to be correlated with each other and with cognitive decline, and effects of treatments on affected and unaffected brain areas can be measured.

Summary and conclusions

The results with PET in ageing have indicated that cross-sectional age-related changes in brain metabolism are relatively small in magnitude in healthy individuals. However, age-related reductions in the integrated activity among brain regions have been demonstrated and may be related to cognitive changes in the elderly. Nevertheless, preliminary comparisons of cognitive and metabolic relations in young and old subjects suggest that these relations are maintained in the elderly, with some alterations suggestive of reorganisation of functional networks.

This adds support of the notion that healthy ageing is, in general, accompanied by smaller age-related changes than are found in a less optimally healthy population.

The use of PET to examine cerebral metabolism in patients with AD has shown that the distribution of cortical metabolic abnormality seen during life is similar to that seen at post-mortem, i.e. the finding of larger numbers of neurofibrillary tangles in association neocortex than in primary cortex (Lewis *et al.*, 1987) is mirrored by the marked metabolic decreases seen in association cortex and the relative sparing of glucose metabolism in primary cortical regions. This is important information for identifying which brain areas are most susceptible to the disease process, and can lead to hypotheses about disease mechanisms. One such hypothesis (Rapoport, 1988) is that the rapid evolution of the human brain by various genomic processes has made the newest areas, specifically the association neocortices and connected amygdaloid, hippocampal and entorhinal areas, vulnerable to AD.

The use of PET has also shown that metabolic changes in the neocortex precede changes in the cognitive functions that depend on the integrity of the neocortex, sometimes by several years. This finding implies that there are cortical redundancies or compensatory mechanisms that allow cognitive processing to be maintained, despite considerable metabolic dysfunction. One such mechanism might be axonal sprouting to compensate for cell loss and dysfunction during the period of time before neocortically mediated neuropsychological impairments are seen (Horwitz, 1988).

PET has proved to be a sensitive tool for measuring cerebral metabolic changes, even in mildly demented patients. The ability to measure cerebral metabolism in AD patients has further increased our understanding of the heterogeneous nature of this type of dementia, by demonstrating both inter- and intrahemispheric differences in metabolic deficit that are related to different patterns of neuropsychological impairment.

Although it is probable that some variability is introduced from the inclusion of patients with diseases other than AD, due to the small but inevitable uncertainty in the clinical diagnosis, much of the heterogeneity may be inherent in the variable way the disease begins in the neocortex. The findings to date suggest that medial structures involved in memory, such as the hippocampus and amygdala, are affected first in most patients, given that memory loss is usually the first symptom (Rosen & Mohs, 1982; Haxby *et al.*, 1987; Grady *et al.*, 1988). After that, however, the particular area of association neocortex that is affected (i.e. right vs. left or frontal vs. parietal) may be random or due to regional differences in susceptibility or to different aetiologies. Whatever the cause of this heterogeneity in AD, a full understanding of how it affects both cognitive impairments and patients' responses to possible drug therapies will be important for the future. In addition, preliminary results suggest that other forms of dementia will be distinguishable from AD in terms of metabolic patterns, but more work needs to be done to determine the specificity of the PET findings for AD.

Finally, there are PET evidence (Deutsch & Halsey, 1990; Grady *et al.*, 1993) and neuro-pathological evidence (DeKosky & Scheff, 1990) to suggest that synaptic failure is reversible in mild to moderate AD. The use of neurotransmitter-specific drugs and parametric imaging techniques promise to make *in vivo* studies of synaptic efficacy in AD increasingly informative (Rapoport & Grady, 1993).

References

Benson, D.F., Kuhl, D.E., Hawkins, R.A., Phelps, M.E., Cummings, J.L. & Tsai, S.Y. (1983) The fluorodeoxy-glucose 18F scan in Alzheimer's disease and multi-infarct dementia. *Arch. Neurol.* 40, 711–14.

Berardi, A., Haxby, J.V., Grady, C.L. & Rapoport, S.I. (1990) Memory performance in healthy young and old subjects correlates with resting state brain glucose utilization in the parietal lobe. *J. Nucl. Med.* 31, 879.

Berardi, A., Haxby, J.V., Grady, C.L. & Rapoport, S.I. (1991). Asymmetries of brain glucose metabolism and memory in the healthy elderly. *Developm. Neuropsychol.* 7, 87–97.

Berg, G., Grady, C.L., Sundaram, M. *et al.* (1986) Positron emission tomography in dementia of the Alzheimer type: a brief review with a case study. *Arch. of Intern. Med.* 146, 2045–9.

Bottomley, P.A., Hardy, C.J., Cousins, J. Armstrong, M. & Wagle, W. (1989) Brain phosphate metabolite concentrations, not ratios, are reduced in AIDS dementia. *Abstr. 8th Ann. Meeting, Soc. Magnetic Resonance Med.*

Bottomley, P.A., Hardy, C.J., Cousins, J.P., Armstrong, M. & Wagle, W.A. (1990) AIDS dementia complex: brain high-energy phosphate metabolite deficits. *Radiology* 176, 407–11.

Brown, G.G., Levine, S.R., Gorell, J.M. *et al.* (1989) *In vivo* 31-P NMR profiles of Alzheimer's disease and multiple subcortical infarct dementia. *Neurology* 39, 1423–7.

Bruhn, H., Frahm, J., Gyngell, M.L., Merboldt, K.D., Hanicke, W. & Sauter, R. (1989a) Cerebral metabolism in man after acute stroke: new observations using localised proton NMR spectroscopy. *Magnetic Resonance Med.* 9, 126–31.

Bruhn, H., Frahm, J., Gyngell, M.L. *et al.* (1989b). Noninvasive differentiation of tumors with use of localised H-1 MR spectroscopy *in vivo*: initial experience in patients with cerebral tumors. *Radiology* 172, 541–8.

Bruhn, H., Stoppe, G., Merboldt, K.D., Michaelis, T., Hanicke, W. & Frahm, J. (1992) Cerebral metabolic alterations in normal aging and Alzheimer's dementia detected by proton MRS. *Abstr. Soc. Magnetic Resonance Med.* 752.

Brun, A. & Gustafson, L. (1976). Distribution of cerebral degeneration in Alzheimer's disease. *Arch. Psychiatr. Nervenkrankh.* 223, 15–33.

Brunetti, A., Berg, G., DiChiro, G. *et al.* (1989) Reversal of brain metabolic abnormalities following treatment of AIDS dementia complex with 3′-azido-2′,3′-dideoxy-thymidine: a PET–FDG study. *J. Nucl. Med.* 30, 581–90.

Budinger, T.F. & Lauterbur, P.C. (1984). Nuclear magnetic resonance technology for medical studies. *Science* 226, 288–98.

Chase, T.N. (1987) Cortical glucose utilization patterns in primary degenerative dementia of the anterior and posterior types. *Arch. Gerontol. Geriatr.* 6, 289–97.

Chawluk, J.B., Alavi, A., Jamieson, D.G. *et al.* (1987) Changes in local cerebral glucose metabolism with normal aging: the effects of cardiovascular and systemic health factors. *J. Cerebr. Blood Flow Metab.* 7 (Suppl. 1), S411.

Chong, W.K., Sweeney, B., Wilkinson, I.D. *et al.* (1993) Proton spectroscopy of the brain in HIV infection: correlation with clinical, immunologic, and MR imaging findings. *Radiology* 188, 119–24.

Chui, H.C. (1989) Dementia: a review emphasizing clinicopathologic correlation and brain–behavior relationships. *Arch. Neurol.* **46**, 806–14.

Clark, C.M., Kessler, R., Buchsbaum, M.S., Margolin, R.A. & Holcomb, H.H. (1984) Correlational methods for determining regional coupling of cerebral glucose metabolism: a pilot study. *Biol. Psychiatry* **19**, 663–78.

Costa, D.C., Ell, P.J., Burns, A., Philpot, M. & Levy, R. (1988) CBF tomograms with 99Tc-HM-PAO in patients with dementia (Alzheimer type and HIV) and Parkinson's disease—initial results. *J. Cerebr. Blood Flow Metab.* **8**, S109–S115.

Dastur, D.K., Lane, M.H., Hansen, D.B. *et al.* (1963) Effects of aging on cerebral circulation and metabolism in man. In Birren, J.E., Butler, R.N., Greenhouse, S.W., Sokoloff, L. & Yarrow, M.R. (eds) *Human Aging – A Biological and Behavioral Study*. US Department of Health, Education and Welfare, Publication no. 986, Bethesda, MD, pp. 59–76.

DeCarli, C.S., Grady, C.L., Clark, C.M. *et al.* (1990) Slowly progressive dementia with severe white matter changes (DWMC) on magnetic resonance imaging (MRI) —comparison to dementia of the Alzheimer type (DAT). *Neurology* **40** (Suppl. 1), 176.

DeCarli, C.D., Maisog, J., Murphy, D.G.M. *et al.* (1992) Method for quantitation of brain, ventricular, and subarachnoid CSF volumes from MR images. *J. Comput. Assist. Tomogr.* **16**, 274–84.

Deicken, R.F., Hubesch, B., Jensen, P.C. *et al.* (1991) Alterations in brain phosphate metabolite concentrations in patients with human immunodeficiency virus infection. *Arch. Neurol.* **48**, 203–9.

DeKosky, S.T. & Scheff, S.W. (1990). Synapse loss in frontal cortex biopsies in Alzheimer's disease: correlation with cognitive severity. *Ann. Neurol.* **27**, 457–64.

De Leon, M.J., Ferris, S.H., George, A.E. *et al.* (1983) Computed tomography and positron emission transaxial tomography evaluations of normal aging and Alzheimer's disease. *J. Cerebr. Blood Flow Metab.* **3**, 391–4.

De Leon, M.J., George, A.E., Ferris, S.H. *et al.* (1984) Positron emission tomography and computed tomography assessments of the aging human brain. *J. Comput. Assist. Tomogr.* **8**, 88–94.

De Leon, M.J., George, A.E., Klinger, A. *et al.* (1988) PET-11CDG studies of leukoencephalopathy in normal aging and Alzheimer's disease. *Neurology* **38** (Suppl. 1), 372.

Desimone, R. & Ungerleider, L.G. (1989) Neural mechanisms of visual perception in monkeys. In Boller, F. & Grafman, J. (eds) *Handbook of Neuropsychology*, Vol. 2. Elsevier, Amsterdam, pp. 267–99.

Deutsch, G. & Halsey, H. (1990) Cortical blood flow effects of mental rotation in older subjects and Alzheimer patients. *J. Clin. Exp. Neuropsychol.* **12**, 31.

Duara, R., Margolin, R.A., Robertson-Tchabo, E.A. *et al.* (1983) Cerebral glucose utilization, as measured with positron emission tomography in 21 healthy men between the ages of 21 and 83 years. *Brain* **106**, 761–75.

Duara, R., Grady, C.L., Haxby, J.V. *et al.* (1984) Human brain glucose utilization and cognitive function in relation to age. *Ann. Neurol.* **16**, 702–13.

Duara, R., Grady, C.L., Haxby, J.V. *et al.* (1986) Positron emission tomography in Alzheimer's disease. *Neurology* **36**, 879–87.

Duara, R., Loewenstein, D.A., Barker, W.W., Chang, J.Y. & Kothari, P. (1988) Evidence for predominant left hemisphere dysfunction in FDG/PET scans of patients with Alzheimer's disease and multi-infarct dementia. *J. Nucl. Med.* **29**, 912.

Duara, R., Barker, W., Loewenstein, D., Pascal, S. & Bowen, B. (1989) Sensitivity and specificity of positron emission tomography and magnetic resonance imaging studies in Alzheimer's disease and multi-infarct dementia. *Eur. Neurol.* **29** (Suppl. 3), 9–15.

Duara, R., Barker, W.W., Chang, J. Yoshii, F., Loewenstein, D.A. & Pascal, S. (1992) Viability of neocortical function shown in behavioral activation state PET studies in Alzheimer disease. *J. Cerebr. Blood Flow Metab.* **12**, 927–34.

Evans, D.A., Funkenstein, H., Albert, M.S. *et al.* (1989) Prevalence of Alzheimer's disease in a community population of older persons: higher than previously reported. *JAMA* **262**, 2551–6.

Farrer, L.A., O'Sullivan, D.M., Cupples, L.A., Growdon, J.H. & Myers, R.H. (1989) Assessment of genetic risk for Alzheimer's disease among first-degree relatives. *Ann. Neurol.* **25**, 485–93.

Ferris, S.H., de Leon, M.J., Wolf, A.P. *et al.* (1980) Positron emission tomography in the study of aging and senile dementia. *Neurobiol. Aging* **1**, 127–31.

Foster, N.L., Chase, T.N., Fedio, P., Patronas, N.J., Brooks, R.A. & DiChiro, G. (1983) Alzheimer's disease: focal cortical changes shown by positron emission tomography. *Neurology* **33**, 961–5.

Foster, N.L., Chase, T.N., Mansi, L. *et al.* (1984) Cortical abnormalities in Alzheimer's disease. *Ann. Neurol.* **16**, 649–54.

Fox, P.T., Miezin, F.M., Allman, J.M., Van Essen, D.C. & Raichle, M.E. (1987) Retinotopic organization of human visual cortex mapped with positron emission tomography. *J. Neurosci.* **7**, 913–22.

Frackowiack, R.S.J. & Gibbs, J.M. (1983) Cerebral metabolism and blood flow in normal and pathologic aging. In Magistretti, P.L. (ed.) *Functional Radionuclide Imaging of the Brain*. Raven Press, New York, pp. 305–9.

Frackowiack, R.S.J., Pozzilli, C., Legg, N.J. *et al.* (1981) Regional cerebral oxygen supply and utilization in dementia: a clinical and physiological study with oxygen-15 and positron tomography. *Brain* **104**, 753–78.

Friedland, R.P., Budinger, T.F., Ganz, E. *et al.* (1983) Regional cerebral metabolic alterations in dementia of the Alzheimer type: positron emission tomography with (18F)fluoro-deoxyglucose. *J. Comput. Assist. Tomogr.* **7**, 590–8.

Friedland, R.P., Budinger, T.F., Koss, E. & Ober, B.A. (1985) Alzheimer's disease: anterior–posterior and lateral hemispheric alterations in cortical glucose utilization. *Neurosci. Lett.* **53**, 235–40.

Friedland, R.P., Grady, C.L., Schapiro, M.B., Moore, A.M., Kumar, A. & Kinsel, V. (1989) Family history of dementia and regional cerebral glucose utilization in dementia of the Alzheimer type. *Neurology* **39** (Suppl. 1), 168.

Gill, S.S., Thomas, D.G.T., Van Bruggen, N. *et al.* (1990) Proton MR spectroscopy of intracranial tumours: *in vivo* and *in vitro* studies. *J. Comput. Assist. Tomogr.* **14**, 497–504.

Gottstein, U. & Held, K. (1979) Effects of aging on cerebral circulation and metabolism in man. *Acta Neurol. Scand.* **60**, (Suppl. 72), 54–5.

Grady, C.L., Haxby, J.V., Schlageter, N.L., Berg, G. & Rapoport, S.I. (1986) Stability of metabolic and neuropsychological asymmetries in dementia of the Alzheimer type. *Neurology* **36**, 1390–2.

Grady, C.L., Haxby, J.V., Horwitz, B., Berg, G.W. & Rapoport, S.I. (1987) Neuropsychological and cerebral metabolic function in early vs late onset dementia of the Alzheimer type. *Neuropsychologia* **25**, 807–16.

Grady, C.L., Haxby, J.V., Horwitz, B. *et al.* (1988) Longitudinal study of the early neuropsychological and cerebral metabolic changes in dementia of the Alzheimer type. *J. Clin. Exp. Neuropsychol.* **10**, 576–96.

Grady, C.L., Grimes, A.M., Patronas, N., Sunderland, T., Foster, N.L. & Rapoport, S.I. (1989a) Divided attention, as measured by dichotic speech performance, in dementia of the Alzheimer type. *Arch. Neurol.* **46**, 317–20.

Grady, C.L., Haxby, J.V., Horwitz, B. *et al.* (1989b) Mapping human visual systems for object recognition and spatial localization by measurement of regional cerebral blood flow. *J. Cerebr. Blood Flow Metab.* **9** (Suppl. 1), S574.

Grady, C.L., Haxby, J.V., Schapiro, M.B. *et al.* (1990a) Metabolic subgroups in dementia of the Alzheimer type identified using positron emission tomography. *J. Neuropsychiatry Clin. Neurosci.* **2**, 373–84.

Grady, C.L., Horwitz, B., Schapiro, M.B. & Rapoport, S.I. (1990b) Changes in the integrated activity of the brain with healthy aging and dementia of the Alzheimer type. In Battistin, L. & Gerstenbrand, F. (eds) *Aging Brain and Dementia: New Trends in Diagnosis and Therapy*. Wiley-Liss, New York, pp. 355–70.

Grady, C.L., Haxby, J.V., Horwitz, B. *et al.* (1993) Activation of cerebral blood flow during a visuoperceptual task in patients with Alzheimer-type dementia. *Neurobiol. Aging* **14**, 35–44.

Grady, C.L., Maisog, J.M., Horwitz, B. *et al.* (1994) Age-related changes in cortical blood flow activation during visual processing of faces and location. *J. Neurosci.* **14**, 1450–62.

Grimes, A.M., Grady, C.L., Foster, N.L., Sunderland, T. & Patronas, N. (1985) Central auditory function in Alzheimer's disease. *Neurology* **35**, 352–8.

Hachinski, V.C., Iliff, L.D., Phil, M. *et al.* (1975) Cerebral blood flow in dementia. *Arch. Neurol.* **32**, 632–7.

Haxby, J.V. (1986) Letter to the editor. *J. Cerebr. Blood Flow Metab.* **6**, 125–6.

Haxby, J.V., Duara, R., Grady, C.L., Rapoport, S.I. & Cutler, N.R. (1985) Relations between neuropsychological and cerebral metabolic asymmetries in early Alzheimer's disease. *J. Cerebr. Blood Flow Metab.* **5**, 193–200.

Haxby, J.V., Grady, C.L., Duara, R., Schlageter, N.L., Berg, G. & Rapoport, S.I. (1986) Neocortical metabolic abnormalities precede nonmemory cognitive defects in early Alzheimer's-type dementia. *Arch. Neurol.* **43**, 882–5.

Haxby, J.V., Grady, C.L., Friedland, R.P. & Rapoport, S.I. (1987) Neocortical metabolic abnormalities precede nonmemory cognitive impairments in early dementia of the Alzheimer type: longitudinal confirmation. *J. Neural Transmission* **24** (Suppl.), 49–53.

Haxby, J.V., Grady, C.L., Horwitz, B. *et al.* (1988a) Mapping two visual pathways in man with regional cerebral blood flow as measured by positron emission tomography and [^{15}O] water. *Abstr. Soc. Neurosci.* **14**, 751.

Haxby, J.V., Grady, C.L., Koss, E. *et al.* (1988b) Heterogeneous anterior–posterior metabolic patterns in Alzheimer's type dementia. *Neurology* **38**, 1853–63.

Haxby, J.V., Grady, C.L., Koss, E. *et al.* (1990) Longitudinal study of cerebral metabolic asymmetries and associated neuropsychological patterns in early dementia of the Alzheimer type. *Arch. Neurol.* **47**, 753–60.

Heiss, W.D., Hebold, I., Klinkhammer, P. *et al.* (1988) Effect of piracetam on cerebral glucose metabolism in Alzheimer's disease as measured by positron emission tomography. *J. Cerebr. Blood Flow Metab.* **8**, 613–17.

Heston, L.L., Mastri, A.R., Anderson, V.E. & White, J. (1981) Dementia of the Alzheimer type: clinical genetics, natural history and associated conditions. *Arch. Gen. Psychiatry* **38**, 1085–90.

Hoffman, J.M., Guze, B.H., Baxter, L.R. *et al.* (1989) Metabolic homogeneity in familial and sporadic Alzheimer's disease: an FDG/PET study. *Neurology* **39** (Suppl. 1), 167.

Horwitz, B. (1988) Neuroplasticity and the progression of Alzheimer's disease. *Int. J. Neurosci.* **41**, 1–14.

Horwitz, B., Duara, R. & Rapoport, S.I. (1984) Intercorrelations of glucose metabolic rates between brain regions: application to healthy males in a state of reduced sensory input. *J. Cerebr. Blood Flow Metab.* **4**, 484–99.

Horwitz, B., Duara, R. & Rapoport, S.I. (1986) Age differences in intercorrelations between regional cerebral metabolic rates for glucose. *Ann. Neurol.* **19**, 60–7.

Horwitz, B., Grady, C.L., Schlageter, N.L., Duara, R. & Rapoport, S.I. (1987) Intercorrelations of regional cerebral glucose metabolic rates in Alzheimer's disease. *Brain Res.* **407**, 294–306.

Ide, M., Naruse, S., Furuya, S. *et al.* (1992) Some investigations of senile dementia of Alzheimer type (SDAT) by 1H CSI. *Abstr. Soc. Magnetic Resonance Med.*

Jagust, W.J., Friedland, R.P., Budinger, T.F., Koss, E. & Ober, B. (1988) Longitudinal studies of regional cerebral metabolism in Alzheimer's disease. *Neurology* **38**, 909–12.

Jamada, M. & Mehraein, P. (1968) Verteilungsmuster der senilen Veranderungen im Gehirn. *Arkiv Psychiatr. Nervenkrankh.* **211**, 308–24.

Jarvik, J.G., Lenkinski, R.E., Grossman, R.I., Gomori, J.M., Schnall, M.D. & Frank, I. (1993) Proton MR spectroscopy of HIV-infected patients: characterization of abnormalities with imaging and clinical correlation. *Radiology* **186**, 739–44.

Kamo, H., McGeer, P.L., Harrop, R. *et al.* (1987) Positron emission tomography and histopathology in Pick's disease. *Neurology* **37**, 439–45.

Kemper, T. (1984) Neuroanatomical and neuropathological changes in normal aging and in dementia. In Albert, M. (ed.) *Clinical Neurology of Aging.* Oxford University Press, New York, pp. 9–52.

Kety, S.S. (1956) Human cerebral blood flow and oxygen consumption as related to aging. *J. Chronic Dis.* **3**, 478–86.

Koss, E., Friedland, R.P., Ober, B.A. & Jagust, W.J. (1985) Differences in lateral hemispheric asymmetries of glucose utilization between early- and late-onset Alzheimer-type dementia. *Am. J. Psychiatry* **142**, 638–40.

Kuhl, D.E., Metter, E.J., Riege, W.H. & Phelps, M.E. (1982) Effects of human aging on patterns of local cerebral glucose utilization determined by the [^{18}F]fluorodeoxyglucose method. *J. Cerebr. Blood Flow Metab.* **2**, 163–71.

Kuhl, D.E., Metter, E.J., Riege, W.H. & Hawkins, R.A. (1985) Patterns of cerebral glucose utilization in dementia. In: Greitz T. *et al.* (eds) *The Metabolism of the Human Brain Studied with Positron Emission Tomography.* Raven Press, New York, pp. 419–31.

Kumar, A., Schapiro, M.B., Grady, C.L. *et al.* (1991). High-resolution PET studies in Alzheimer's disease. *Neuropsychopharmacology* **4**, 35–46.

Lebrun-Grandie, P., Baron, J.-C., Soussaline, F., Loch'h, C., Sastre, J. & Bousser, M.-G. (1983) Coupling between regional blood flow and oxygen utilization in the normal human brain: a study with positron tomography and oxygen 15. *Arch. Neurol.* **40**, 230–6.

Leenders, K.L., Perani, D., Lammertsma, A. *et al.* (1990) Cerebral blood flow, blood volume, and oxygen utilization: normal values and effect of age. *Brain* **113**, 27–47.

Lewis, D.A., Campbell, M.J., Terry, R.D. & Morrison, J.H. (1987) Laminar and regional distributions of neurofibrillary tangles and neuritic plaques in Alzheimer's disease: a quantitative study of visual and auditory cortices. *J. Neurosci.* **7**, 1799–808.

Lezak, M. (1983) *Neuropsychological Assessment*, 2nd edn. Oxford University Press, New York.

McGeer, P.L., Kamo, H., Harrop, R. *et al.* (1986) Positron emission tomography in patients with clinically diagnosed Alzheimer's disease. *Can. Med. Assoc. J.* **134**, 597–607.

Menon, D.K., Sargentoni, J., Peden, C.J. *et al.* (1990a) Case report: proton MR spectroscopy in herpes simplex encephalitis: assessment of neuronal loss. *J. Comput. Assist. Tomogr.* **14**, 449–52.

Menon, D.K., Baudouin, C.J., Tomlinson, D. & Hoyle, C. (1990b) Proton MR spectroscopy and imaging of the brain in AIDS: evidence of neuronal loss in regions that appear normal with imaging. *J. Comput. Assist. Tomogr.* **14**, 882–5.

Menon, D.K., Ainsworth, J.G., Cox, I.J. *et al.* (1992) Proton MR spectroscopy of the brain in AIDS dementia complex. *J. Comput. Assist. Tomogr.* **16**, 538–42.

Mentis, M.J., Salerno, J., Horwitz, B. *et al.* (1994) Reduction of functional neuronal connectivity in long-term treated hypertension. *Stroke* **25**, 601–7.

Mesulam, M.M. (1981) A cortical network for directed attention and unilateral neglect. *Ann. Neurol.* **10**, 309–25.

Metter, E.J., Riege, W.H., Kuhl, D.E. & Phelps, M.E. (1984a) Cerebral metabolic relationships for selected brain regions in healthy adults. *J. Cerebr. Blood Flow Metab.* **4**, 1–7.

Metter, E.J., Riege, W.H., Kameyama, M., Kuhl, D.E. & Phelps, M.E. (1984b) Cerebral metabolic relationships for selected brain regions in Alzheimer's, Huntington's and Parkinson's diseases. *J. Cerebr. Blood Flow Metab.* **4**, 500–6.

Meyerhoff, D.J., MacKay, S., Gorssman, N. *et al.* (1992) Effects of normal aging and Alzheimer's disease on cerebral H-1 metabolites. *Abstr. Soc. Magnetic Resonance Med.*

Miatto, O., Gonzalez, G., Buonanno, F. & Growdon, J.H. (1986) *In vitro* ^{31}P NMR spectroscopy detects altered phospholipid metabolism in Alzheimer's disease. *Can. J. Neurol. Sci.* **13**, 535–9.

Miller, J.D., de Leon, M.J., Ferris, S.H. *et al.* (1987) Abnormal temporal lobe response in Alzheimer's disease during cognitive processing as measured by 11C-2-deoxy-D-glucose and PET. *J. Cerebr. Blood Flow Metab.* 7, 248–51.

Miller, B.L., Moats, R.A., Shonk, T., Ernst, T., Woolley, S. & Ross, B.D. (1993) Alzheimer disease: depiction of increased cerebral myo-inositol with proton MR spectroscopy. *Radiology* 187, 433–7.

Mohr, E., Cox, C., Williams, J., Chase, T.N. & Fedio, P. (1990) Impairment of central auditory function in Alzheimer's disease. *J. Clin. Exp. Neuropsychol.* 12, 235–46.

Mountjoy, C.Q., Roth, M., Evans, N.J.R. & Evans, H.M. (1983) Cortical neuronal counts in normal elderly controls and demented patients. *Neurobiol. Aging* 4, 1–11.

Murphy, D.G., Bottomley, P.A., Salerno, J.A. *et al.* (1993) An *in vivo* study of phosphorus and glucose metabolism in Alzheimer's disease using magnetic resonance spectroscopy and PET. *Arch. Gen. Psychiatry* 50, 341–9.

Nestor, P.G., Parasuraman, R., Haxby, J.V. & Grady, C.L. (1991) Divided attention and metabolic brain dysfunction in mild dementia of the Alzheimer's type. *Neuropsy-chologia* 29, 379–87.

Nordberg, A., Lilja, A., Lundqvist, H. *et al.* (1992) Tacrine restores cholinergic nicotinic receptors and glucose metabolism in Alzheimer patients as visualized by positron emission tomography. *Neurobiol Aging* 13, 747–58.

Pantano, P., Baron, J.-C., Lebrun-Grandie, P., Duquesnoy, N., Bousser, M.-G. & Comar, M. (1984) Regional cerebral blood flow and oxygen consumption in human aging. *Stroke* 15, 635–41.

Parasuraman, R., Greenwood, P.M., Haxby, J.V. & Grady, C.L. (1992) Visuospatial attention in dementia of the Alzheimer type. *Brain* 115, 711–33.

Petersen, S.E., Fox, P.T., Posner, M.I., Mintun, M. & Raichle, M.E. (1989) Positron emission tomographic studies of the processing of single words. *J. Cogn. Neurosci.* 1, 153–70.

Petroff, O.A.C., Prichard, J.W., Behar, K.L., Alger, J.R., denHollander, J.A. & Shulman, R.G. (1985) Cerebral intracellular pH by 31-P nuclear magnetic resonance spectroscopy. *Neurology* 35, 781–8.

Pettegrew, J.W., Moossy, J., Withers, G., McKeag, D. & Panchalingam, K. (1988a) 31-P nuclear magnetic resonance study of the brain in Alzheimer's disease. *J. Neuropathol. Exp. Neurol.* 47, 235–48.

Pettegrew, J.W., Panchalingam, K., Moossy, J., Martinez, J., Rao, G. & Boller, F. (1988b) Correlation of phosphorus-31 magnetic resonance spectroscopy and morphologic findings in Alzheimer's disease. *Arch. Neurol.* 45, 1093–6.

Pohl, P., Vogl, G., Fill, H., Rossler, H., Zangerle, R. & Gerstenbrand, F. (1988) Single photon emission computed tomography in AIDS dementia complex. *J. Nucl. Med.* 29, 1382–6.

Prichard, J.W. & Shulman, R.G. (1988) NMR spectroscopy of brain metabolism *in vivo*. In Boulton, A.A. & Baker, G.B. (eds) *Neuromethods*, Vol. 8: *Neurochemistry*. Humana Press, Clifton, NJ, pp. 233–63.

Rapoport, S.I. (1988) Brain evolution and Alzheimer's disease. *Rev. Neurol. (Paris)* 144, 79–90.

Rapoport, S.I. & Grady, C.L. (1993) Parametric *in vivo* brain imaging during activation to examine pathological mechanisms of functional failure in Alzheimer disease. *Int. J. Neurosci.* 70, 39–56.

Rosen, W.G. & Mohs, R.C. (1982) Evolution of cognitive decline in dementia. In Corkin, S., Davis, K.L., Growden, J.H., Usdin, E. & Wurtman, R.J. (eds) *Aging*, Vol. 19: *Alzheimer's Disease: A Report of Progress*. Raven Press, New York, pp. 183–8.

Ross, B., Kreis, R. & Ernst, T. (1992) Clinical tools for the 90's: magnetic resonance spectroscopy and metabolite imaging. *Eur. J. Radiol.* 14, 128–40.

Rossor, M.N., Iverson, L.L., Reynolds, G.P., Mountjoy, C.Q. & Roth, M. (1984) Neurochemical characteristics of early and late onset types of Alzheimer's disease. *Br. Med. J.* 288, 961–4.

Rottenberg, D.A., Moeller, J.R., Strother, S.C. *et al.* (1987). The metabolic pathology of the AIDS dementia complex. *Ann. Neurol.* 22, 700–6.

St. George-Hyslop, P., Tanzi, R., Polinsky, R. *et al.* (1987) The genetic defect causing familial Alzheimer's disease maps on chromosome 21. *Science* 235, 885–90.

Salmon, E. & Franck, G. (1989) Positron emission tomographic study in Alzheimer's disease and Pick's disease. *Arch. Gerontol. Geriatr.* 1 (Suppl.), 241–7.

Scheff, S.W., Dekosky, S.T. & Price, D.A. (1990) Quantitative assessment of cortical synaptic density in Alzheimer's disease. *Neurobiol. Aging* 11, 29–37.

Seltzer, B. & Sherwin, I. (1983) A comparison of clinical features in early- and late-onset primary degenerative dementia. *Arch. Neurol.* 40, 143–6.

Seltzer, B., Burres, M.J.K. & Sherwin, I. (1984) Left-handedness in early and late onset dementia. *Neurology* 34, 367–9.

Shiino, A., Matsuda, M., Morikawa, S., Inubushi, T., Akiguchi, I. & Handa, J. (1993) Proton magnetic resonance spectroscopy with dementia. *Surg. Neurol.* 39, 143–7.

Small, G.W., Kuhl, D.E., Riege, W.H. *et al.* (1989) Cerebral glucose metabolic patterns in Alzheimer's disease: effect of gender and age at dementia onset. *Arch. Gen. Psychiatry* 46, 527–32.

Szelies, B. & Karenberg, A. (1986) Disorders of glucose metabolism in Pick's disease. *Fortschr. Neurol. Psychiatr.* 54, 393–7.

Ungerleider, L.G. & Mishkin, M. (1982) Two cortical visual systems. In Ingle, D.J., Goodale, M.A. & Mansfield, R.J.W. (eds) *Analysis of Visual Behavior*. MIT Press, Cambridge, pp. 549–84.

Weiner, M.W. & Hetherington, H.P. (1989) The power of the proton. *Radiology* **172**, 318–20.

Welch, K.M.A., Gross, B., Licht, J. *et al.* (1988) Magnetic resonance spectroscopy of neurologic diseases. *Curr. Neurol.* **8**, 295–332.

Wolinsky, J.S., Narayana, P.A. & Fenstermacher, M.J. (1990) Proton magnetic resonance spectroscopy in multiple sclerosis. *Neurology* **40**, 1764–9.

Young, L.T., Kish, S.J., Li, P.P. & Warsh, J.J. (1988) Decreased brain [H3]inositol 1,4,5-trisphosphate binding in Alzheimer's disease. *Neurosci. Lett.* **94**, 198–202.

15: Functional Imaging
in the Neuroses

P. K. McGuire

Introduction

Conditions such as obsessive–compulsive disorder (OCD), generalised anxiety disorder (GAD) and panic have traditionally been described as neuroses, with the tacit implication that biological factors play a relatively minor role in their pathophysiology. However, the recent application of functional neuroimaging to these conditions has provided data which challenge this perspective.

Obsessive–compulsive disorder

Resting-state studies

Most imaging studies of OCD in the resting state have used positron emission tomography (PET) with ^{18}F-fluorodeoxyglucose (^{18}FDG) to examine regional glucose metabolism. In one of the first of these, Baxter *et al.* (1987) scanned 14 patients and compared them with equal numbers of patients with unipolar depression and healthy controls. Nine of the patients were also depressed, and five were on psychotropic medication. Most of the OCD patients were male and most of the unipolar group were female, while the gender ratio among the controls was equal. Differences between the first seven OCD patients and the control groups were examined with an analysis of variance (ANOVA) and regions which differed between the groups were selected for planned comparisons in the second half of the subjects. This analysis revealed increased absolute metabolism in the orbital gyri and the caudate nuclei bilaterally. Increases in metabolism relative to that in the ipsilateral hemisphere were restricted to the left orbital gyrus, and were not evident when patients with OCD were compared with those with unipolar depression.

Because of the potentially confounding effects of depression, medication and gender, the authors subsequently repeated this approach with 10 OCD patients who were medication-free, not depressed and matched to controls with respect to sex (Baxter *et al.*, 1988). This study again indicated that patients had higher absolute metabolic rates in the orbital gyri and the caudate nuclei, bilaterally, with higher orbital metabolism normalised to hemispheric metabolism. Other regions were not analysed. Men tended to have higher activity in the orbital gyrus on the right, whereas in women metabolism was higher on the left, an observation which applied to both patients and controls.

Nordahl *et al.* (1989) also sought to replicate Baxter *et al.*'s original findings in patients who were medication-free and not depressed. Eight patients and 30 healthy controls were scanned while performing an auditory continuous-performance task (CPT), using ^{18}FDG and PET. Sixty regions of interest were compared with t tests, without correction for multiple comparisons. Patients showed bilateral increases in metabolism (normalised to global grey-matter metabolism) in orbital–frontal regions bilaterally and in the midline, and decreases in right parietal and left occipitoparietal regions. It is unknown whether the neural correlates of the CPT differed in patients and controls, although there was no difference in their performance at a behaviour level.

PET with ^{18}FDG has also been used to examine patients with childhood-onset OCD. Swedo *et al.* (1989) compared 18 medication-free patients with an equal number of sex-matched controls. None of the patients were depressed, but nine had met DSM-III criteria for depression in the past, and another nine had done so for anxiety disorders. Eight patients also reported panic during the scanning procedure. Forty-six regions were delineated and compared with an ANOVA, without correction for multiple comparisons. A smaller subset of regions were also examined with planned comparisons. The exploratory analysis revealed increased absolute activity in prefrontal and anterior cingulate regions bilaterally, the left orbital–frontal and premotor cortex, the left paracentral region, the right sensorimotor and inferior temporal regions, the right cerebellum and the right thalamus. The planned comparisons identified increases normalised to cortical metabolism in the left anterior cingulate and right prefrontal cortex. There was a positive correlation between the clinical severity of OCD and metabolism in the right orbitofrontal cortex. Patients who resisted obsessive–compulsive (OC) phenomena during scanning showed greater right prefrontal activity than those who did not. There were no differences between patients who experienced compulsive urges and those who had obsessive thoughts.

In another PET study with ^{18}FDG, Martinot *et al.* (1990) compared 16 patients with OCD with eight controls. Patients with concurrent depression were excluded, but 10 were receiving psychotropic medication. The data were analysed with a bilateral regions-of-interest approach. The first eight patients were compared with the controls with an ANOVA and *post hoc t* tests, and then this analysis was repeated with the second eight. Only differences which were evident with both analyses were regarded as significant. Patients had lower absolute metabolism in all regions, but, when normalised to global metabolism, decreases were restricted to the dorsolateral prefrontal cortex. This study was unusual in that it found prefrontal *decreases*,

rather than the increases reported in most other studies. This might have been related to the fact that most of the patients were on medication, although there were no differences between the medicated and drug-free patients. Another factor may have been the patient's levels of anxiety, which were no different from those of the controls: in most other studies, patients with OCD have been rated as markedly anxious, and anxiety has been correlated with prefrontal metabolism in such patients (Swedo *et al.* (1989).

The first PET study of OCD to examine regional cerebral blood flow (rCBF), as opposed to glucose metabolism, was performed by Sawle *et al.* (1991). Six patients with obsessional slowness were compared with six controls, using ^{15}O-CO$_2$. The same subjects were also studied with ^{18}F-dioxyphenylalanine (DOPA), which was used to examine the dopaminergic system. Three of the patients were taking medication at the time of scanning, and one was depressed. The distribution of ^{15}O was examined in multiple regions of interest, without correction for multiple comparisons. Increased activity was evident bilaterally in orbitofrontal, dorsolateral pre-frontal and premotor regions and in the right sensorimotor cortex, with the most significant changes being in the right orbitofrontal cortex. There were no differences in DOPA uptake. Increased activity in the premotor region has not been a common feature of many other studies of OCD, and may have been a function of the extreme motor slowness and high prevalence of 'soft' neurological signs evident in the patients involved. The same may also apply to the increases seen in sensorimotor cortex, although changes in this area have also been reported in studies of patients with more typical OCD (Swedo *et al.*, 1989; Rubin *et al.*, 1992).

Resting brain activity in OCD has also been assessed with single-photon emission tomography (SPET). Machlin *et al.* (1991) used ^{99m}Tc-hexamethylpropyleneamineoxime (HMPAO) with a single rotating camera to measure rCBF in 10 non-depressed patients and eight normal controls. Only medial prefrontal/anterior cingulate and left and right orbitofrontal regions were analysed. Patients showed greater blood flow in the medial prefrontal/anterior cingulate cortex, and perfusion in this area was negatively correlated with Hamilton ratings of anxiety at the time of scanning. There were no correlations with ratings of OC symptoms. Rubin *et al.* (1992) compared rCBF in 10 patients without concurrent depression and 10 controls, using SPET with two different tracers, HMPAO and ^{133}Xe. Their respective distributions were analysed in several regions of interest, and between-group differences were examined with *t* tests, without correction for multiple comparisons. No differences were evident in the distribution of ^{133}Xe, but with HMPAO patients showed increased activity in the orbital surface of the frontal pole bilaterally, the temporoparietal region bilaterally and the left sensorimotor cortex. Reductions in activity were evident in the patients' caudate nuclei bilaterally. When regional activity was normalised to whole cortical activity, rather than that in the cerebellum, the temporoparietal differences disappeared. Although both tracers are thought to measure rCBF and their distribution was studied within subjects after administration in the same session, there was a worryingly poor correlation between their regional activities.

Changes in regional brain activity with treatment

After performing studies of patients in the resting state, many workers went on to rescan the same subjects after they had undergone treatment. In the first of these investigations, Baxter *et al.* (1987) examined 10 patients, most of whom were also depressed, with ^{18}FDG and PET before and after treatment with trazodone and/or tranylcypromine sulphate, with an interscan interval of 2–4 months. Analysis was restricted to the orbital gyri and caudate nuclei, regions where there had been increased activity prior to treatment. In the eight patients whose National Institute of Mental Health (NIMH) OCD and Hamilton depression scores markedly improved, there were no changes

in absolute metabolism, but an increase in left caudate metabolism when normalised to that in the ipsilateral hemisphere. However, the change in this region correlated with the improvement in the ratings for depressive, rather than OC, symptoms, and there was a strong correlation between the changes in the ratings of OC and depressive symptoms. These observations and the finding of similar increases in caudate metabolism in patients treated for unipolar depression (Baxter *et al.*, 1985) suggest that the results may have been confounded by the effects of treatment on mood.

Benkelfat *et al.* (1990) rescanned eight of 14 patients who had originally been studied in a PET examination of resting metabolism using ^{18}FDG (Nordahl *et al.*, 1989), following treatment with clomipramine for an average of 4 weeks. Patients with major depression were excluded, but five subjects had other psychiatric disorders, such as GAD, panic or atypical depression. Patients were scanned while performing an auditory CPT. Clomipramine treatment led to a reduction in ratings of OC symptoms, but not symptoms of depression or anxiety. There were decreases in metabolism (normalised to global grey-matter metabolism) in the left caudate and left inferomedial frontal cortex, and increases in the right anterior putamen, right hippocampus, left motor cortex and left parietooccipital region, although significance levels were not adjusted for multiple comparisons. No correlations were evident between regional changes in metabolism and changes in each of three different OC rating scales, but, when two of the latter (the NIMH global OC and the Comprehensive Psychiatric Rating Scale (CPRS)-OC-8) were combined, there was a correlation between changes in this composite scale and metabolic changes in the left caudate and the right posterior orbital–frontal cortex. When responders to treatment (four patients showing 50% or more improvement on the CPRS-OC-8 scale) were compared with non-responders, there was a greater decrease in left caudate metabolism in the former group, with a similar trend in the right caudate. Although task performance was not different before and after treatment, it is unclear whether the neural correlates of the CPT change with alterations in mental state.

Six patients who had participated in a resting-state study by Machlin *et al.* (1991) were rescanned after 3–4 months' treatment with fluoxetine, employing the same SPET methodology (Hoehn-Saric *et al.*, 1991). There was a significant improvement in ratings of OC phenomena (NIMH OC score, Yale–Brown Obsessive–Compulsive Scale (YB-OCS)) and of anxiety (Hamilton anxiety scale), and a reduction in activity in the medial prefrontal/anterior cingulate region. No correlations were evident between the change in clinical ratings and activity in this region or in the orbitofrontal cortex, the only other region examined.

Swedo *et al.* (1992) repeated a PET examination of resting metabolism with ^{18}FDG in 13 patients with childhood-onset OCD, a year or more after they had been scanned in an earlier study (Swedo *et al.*, 1989). Eight had been treated with clomipramine and two with fluoxetine, and three had not received pharmacotherapy. They were free of other medication for the 2 weeks prior to the scan, but may have taken other drugs during the rest of the interscan period. Four normal volunteers were also scanned twice, on average 2 years apart. The analysis was restricted to regions (orbitofrontal, prefrontal, anterior cingulate and caudate) which had shown increases in metabolism in patients before treatment. There were improvements in several different ratings of OC, depressive and anxiety symptoms, and bilateral decreases in orbitofrontal metabolism (normalised to mean cortical grey-matter metabolism) in the patients, but not in the controls. When patients were subdivided into responders (*n* = 7) and non-responders (*n* = 6, including three who did not receive pharmacotherapy) with respect to symptom severity at follow-up and symptomatic improvement, the former showed a greater reduction in left orbitofrontal metabolism than non-responders. However, this comparison may have been confounded by the inclusion in the latter group of

three patients (in a total of six) who had not received drug treatment. In patients who did receive pharmacotherapy, there was a correlation between the reduction in right orbitofrontal metabolism and the improvement in scores on the OC rating scale (OCRS).

In the only study which has examined the effects of psychological therapy and compared two different forms of treatment, Baxter *et al.* (1992) scanned two groups of nine patients, using ^{18}FDG and PET, before and after the administration of either fluoxetine or behaviour therapy. Four of those in the drug-treatment group had additional psychiatric disorders, including Tourette's and panic, as did three of those in the behaviour-therapy group. Four normal controls were also studied. Subjects were scanned twice, using the same methods as employed in earlier studies by the same authors (Baxter *et al.*, 1987). They had been drug-free for at least 2 weeks prior to the first scan and were rescanned an average of 10 weeks later. Patients chose which type of treatment they received. Fluoxetine was given in conjunction with supportive advice, while the behaviour therapy comprised exposure and response prevention facilitated by cognitive techniques, with some patients having additional therapist-assisted exposure or attending a cognitive-behavioural group. Brain metabolism before and after treatment was compared with a region-of-interest analysis and paired *t* tests. In those who responded (30% or more improvement in YB-OCS) to drug treatment (*n* = 7), there were reductions in metabolism (normalised to the ipsilateral hemisphere) in the right head of caudate, right anterior cingulate and left thalamus. In responders to behaviour therapy (*n* = 6), reductions were limited to the right head of caudate. Non-responders to treatment and healthy controls did not show significant reductions in right caudate metabolism, although it is unclear whether there were changes in other regions. There was a positive correlation between the percentage change in the YB-OCS score and the change in right caudate metabolism for those who received fluoxetine, and a trend for those who had behaviour therapy. When the responders to both treatments were grouped together, positive correlations were evident between metabolism in the orbitofrontal cortex and both the caudate and the thalamus of the same hemisphere before treatment, but not afterwards.

These findings compare with the decreases in metabolism in the left caudate and right orbitofrontal cortex (Benkelfat *et al.* 1990), right and left orbitofrontal cortex (Swedo *et al.*, 1992) and medial prefrontal/anterior cingulate cortex (Hoehn-Saric *et al.*, 1991) reported in other treatment studies. While changes in association with clinical improvement have thus been identified in a variety of regions, there is some overlap between studies, with reductions largely restricted to areas already implicated in the pathophysiology of OCD on the basis of resting-state investigations. Whether there are also changes in other areas is unclear, as the analyses in treatment studies have tended to focus on these latter regions. The variation in the precise location of the most significant changes may reflect differences in imaging methodology and analysis and in patient groups. In addition, fluoxetine and clomipramine, which have quite distinct receptor affinities, may have correspondingly different effects on cerebral metabolism which are independent of their effects on symptoms. The differences between the activity changes associated with fluoxetine and behaviour therapy in the study by Baxter *et al.* (1992) might be related to such direct pharmacological effects. The duration of treatment may also influence the pattern of regional change, and this varied across these studies. Only one investigation has reported *increases* in prefrontal or striatal regions with treatment (Baxter *et al.*, 1987). However, the results may have been confounded by the confounding effects of treatment on mood (see above).

Symptom-provocation studies

As the patients in all the above studies were scanned at rest, one cannot be certain whether the findings reflect the presence of OC symptoms or enduring features of the diagnosis, i.e. abnormalities of state or trait. The resolution of some regional increases in activity with treatment suggests an association with OC symptoms, but the relationship between functional changes and symptoms can be studied more directly when the latter are induced experimentally. Zohar *et al.* (1989) did this by playing 10 patients with OCD audiotapes with a spoken content reflecting their individual fears of contamination and by touching them with contaminants. These conditions were compared with listening to a tape with a relaxing content. Listening to the obsession-related tape elicited more OC symptoms and anxiety than the relaxing tape, and contact with contaminants elicited more OC symptoms and anxiety than the obsession-related tape, as measured by objective (Spielberger state-anxiety scale; Hamilton anxiety scale) and subjective (NIMH OCR, OC and anxiety analogue scales) instruments. Cortical rCBF was measured with SPET and ^{133}Xe, and the data were analysed in bilateral regions with a repeat-measures ANOVA and *post hoc* paired *t* tests. Listening to the obsession-related tape increased temporal perfusion relative to the relaxing tape, while exposure to contaminants led to *decreases* in temporal and parietal regions relative to the relaxation tape and in all cortical regions relative to the obsession-related tape. Although the conditions were performed in a set order, the authors addressed the issue of possible order effects by rescanning three of the subjects with a different sequence: this did not alter the results. There were no changes in respiratory rate or end-respiratory $P\text{CO}_2$ across conditions, making it unlikely that changes in ventilatory rate could have accounted for the findings. The authors interpreted the decreased rCBF with exposure relative to the other conditions as indicative of an inverse relationship between the presence of symptoms and cortical perfusion. However, the differences between the conditions could equally have represented *increases* in association with listening to words.

McGuire *et al.* (1994) also elicited symptoms

with exposure to contaminants, but employed a graded series of stimuli and a correlational, rather than a categorical, design. Four medication-free male patients with hand-washing compulsions and no other psychiatric diagnoses were scanned on 12 occasions in a single session with PET and intravenous ^{15}O-H_2O. Each scan was preceded by brief exposure to one of a series of 12 contaminants, with the series selected to elicit a range of urges to ritualise, from minimal to maximal. The contaminants varied between subjects, reflecting their own personal hierarchies of feared stimuli; e.g. minimal and maximal stimuli for one patient were perfume and rat poison, respectively, while for another they were salt and faeces. Contaminants were presented in a random sequence to control for order effects, and were held by the subjects during scanning in a sealed test tube, while their eyes were closed. The intensity of the urge to ritualise and of anxiety during scanning was rated by subjects on separate analogue scales. Patients were permitted to wash their hands between scans in order to bring their symptom levels back to baseline. Interscan head movement was corrected for by automatic realignment software. After correcting for variations in global blood flow with an analysis of covariance (ANCOVA), the data were analysed with statistical parametric mapping (SPM), which revealed pixels where there were correlations between the symptom scores and rCBF. There was a close correlation between the ratings of urges to ritualise and anxiety, precluding the identification of separate correlations with rCBF. Within the patients as a group, positive correlations were evident in the lower portion of the right inferior frontal gyrus, the right caudate, right putamen and right thalamus, and in the left hippocampus, left posterior cingulate and left cuneus (Plate 15.1, facing p. 230). Negative correlations were seen in the temporoparietal region, particularly on the right, and in the right superior frontal cortex. As 12 scans were performed in each patient, significant correlations were also evident within single subjects. While there were variations between individuals, the distribution in each

patient was broadly similar.

Rauch *et al.* (1994) employed a similar approach, but compared an activated state with a control condition. Eight patients with OCD (five male and three female), who were medication-free at the time of scanning, were scanned twice under two conditions, using PET with inhaled ^{15}O-CO_2. Both conditions involved exposure to a stimulus, the nature of which was determined by the content of each individual's obsessions and compulsions. Thus, one subject was shown a photograph of a serial killer prior to the activation condition and a photo of a pet dog before control scans; another was presented with a banknote said to have been used in the purchase of illicit drugs and a 'clean' banknote. These stimuli thus elicited responses which were heterogeneous with respect to their content, and whether subjects experienced urges to perform compulsive movements or obsessive thoughts was not specified. The intensity of OC and anxiety symptoms during scanning was rated by the patients on separate analogue scales. The two control scans were performed first, followed by the two activation conditions. The authors acknowledged the potential of thus introducing order effects, but felt that symptoms would persist too long to make an ABAB design practicable. Head movement between scans was assessed by visual inspection of the images, and was not considered significant. The data were analysed with a modification of the SPM technique (see above), whereby the significance of changes in regions of interest was estimated from the number of pixels showing differences beyond a threshold determined by the total number of pixels within each region and the smoothness of the image. Increases in rCBF were identified in the orbitofrontal cortex bilaterally, the right caudate nucleus and the left anterior cingulate cortex (Plate 15.2, facing p. 230). The provocation of symptoms was associated with increases in the ratings of both OC symptoms and anxiety.

In all of these studies, as the experimental induction of OC symptoms was accompanied by similar increases in anxiety, it is unclear to which of these phenomena the associated changes in brain activity were related.

Discussion

Despite considerable variations in methodology and imaging technology, comparisons of patients with OCD and controls in the resting state have produced fairly consistent results. Most studies have identified increased metabolism or blood flow in inferior prefrontal, anterior cingulate or striatal regions, and these do not seem to reflect a selection bias for the examination of such regions, as many investigations have included other areas in their analyses. The results are also consistent with those from treatment studies, which have usually shown reductions in activity in the same group of areas and a correlation between such reductions and clinical improvement. However, the analysis in treatment studies has largely been restricted to regions which showed abnormalities in the resting state, and, within a given patient population, the changes have tended to be in areas other than those which displayed increased activity before treatment. Nevertheless, studies in which OC phenomena have been experimentally induced have also found that these are associated with increased activity in inferior prefrontal, anterior cingulate and striatal regions. Overall, the findings from functional imaging studies are compatible with anatomical data which indicate that such areas are interconnected in a corticostriatal–thalamic 'loop' (reviewed in Alexander *et al.*, 1986), and clinical data which suggest that neurological conditions which are thought to involve the basal ganglia, such as Sydenham's chorea, post-encephalitic Parkinsonism (Jellife, 1932) and Huntington's disease (Cummings & Cunningham, 1992), and lesions in the basal ganglia or orbitofrontal cortex are associated with OC phenomena. Interruption of the subcortical projections from the prefrontal and anterior cingulate cortex is also claimed to alleviate such symptoms (Bridges, 1989; Jenike *et al.*, 1991), although this remains controversial.

While neuroimaging studies have thus implicated a number of areas in the pathophysiology of OCD, the correlates of specific symptoms await identification. Unfortunately, studies involving symptom provocation have consistently evoked OC phenomena and anxiety in parallel, and the dissection of their respective neural correlates will require the examination of OC symptoms which are not always accompanied by anxiety (such as some ruminations, or OC phenomena in patients with Tourette's syndrome) and of anxiety in the absence of obsessive phenomena. A further consideration in provocation studies is that, in addition to obsessive urges or thoughts, they may also involve a component of resistance and other phenomena, such as visual imagery (McGuire *et al.*, 1994). Resistance may be particularly relevant, as increases in orbitofrontal activity have been identified in non-obsessional subjects in situations where they are required to suppress motor responses to stimuli (Rosen *et al.*, 1993; Anderson *et al.*, 1994). Nevertheless, symptom-provocation studies permit the study of OC phenomena, as opposed to the condition itself, and may ultimately lead to the identification of the correlates of specific symptoms. The study of symptoms, as opposed to diagnoses, also permits the examination of the same phenomena in different conditions and in normal subjects, e.g. the neural correlates of persistent troubling thoughts, in patients with OCD or depression and in healthy people.

OCD may also be associated with activity in other areas, which have yet to be identified. The bulk of the literature comprises studies which employed region-of-interest analyses, and these are liable to lead to type I errors through multiple statistical comparisons, unless a limited subset of regions is selected for examination. Quite logically, this selection has been influenced by the results of early studies, so most analyses have focused on prefrontal and striatal areas, particularly when addressing the issue of the effects of treatment. Analyses which permit the examination of the entire data set, such as SPM, reduce the chance of missing significant change elsewhere, and studies which have employed such approaches may thus identify regions not previously associated with OCD.

Most imaging work in OCD has described regional increases in activity, but a number of studies have also identified *decreases*. Nordahl *et al.* (1989) found reductions in parietal cortex in patients at rest, both Zohar *et al.* (1989) and McGuire *et al.* (1994) reported decreases in temporoparietal activity in association with symptoms, and Benkelfat *et al.* (1990) found that the resolution of symptoms led to an increase in parieto-occipital activity. The significance of such reductions in activity has yet to be determined, but the visuospatial specialisation of the temporoparietal region and the superior prefrontal cortex (where decreases have also been identified) has led to the suggestion that diminished activity in such areas might reflect a shift in attention from the external to the internal environment, as patients become increasingly preoccupied with their symptoms (McGuire *et al.*, 1994). This would be consistent with neuropsychological data which indicate that patients with OCD exhibit deficits in visuospatial function (Hollander *et al.*, 1990; Hymas *et al.*, 1991). The observation that patients with panic disorder also show reduced parietal metabolism (Nordahl *et al.*, 1990) raise the possibility that these changes may be as much related to anxiety as to OC phenomena.

In addition to variability across studies in terms of the regional location of abnormalities, there have also been differences with respect to their laterality. Most studies have reported bilateral increases at rest (Baxter *et al.*, 1988; Nordahl *et al.*, 1989; Sawle *et al.*, 1991; Rubin *et al.*, 1992), while changes following treatment have been described on the right side (Baxter *et al.*, 1992), the left (Benkelfat *et al.*, 1990) and bilaterally (Swedo *et al.*, 1992), and symptom-provocation studies have identified unilateral changes in both hemispheres (McGuire *et al.*, 1994; Rauch *et al.*, 1994). Inconsistencies in the lateralisation of findings might reflect differences between patient groups with respect to psychopathology if different phenomena vary with respect to the lateralisation of their neural correlates. The observation that functional changes may be preferentially localised to different hemispheres in males and females (Swedo *et al.*, 1989) raises the passibility that between-study variations in gender composition might also have been a factor.

While the vast majority of functional imaging studies in OCD have examined regional brain activity, few have investigated the distribution of neurochemical ligands. The clinical efficacy of serotonergic reuptake inhibitors suggests that neuroimaging studies of 5-hydroxytryptamine (5-HT) receptors would be of considerable interest, and PET ligands have recently been developed for this purpose (Blin *et al.*, 1990; Nyberg *et al.*, 1993). The role of serotonergic inputs in modulating OC phenomena could also be investigated by examining the effects of serotonergic drugs on rCBF, and their interactions with cognitive activations (Friston *et al.*, 1992). Such studies should extend our understanding of the pathophysiology of OCD and provide insights into the normal functions of the neural systems involved in the disorder.

Anxiety

Perhaps the first report on the relationship between anxiety and cerebral function in humans *in vivo* was Kety's (1950) observation that cerebral blood flow increased in a subject who by chance experienced 'grave apprehension' during a study of blood flow using the nitrous oxide technique. Much of the subsequent literature has continued to deal with the relationship between anxiety and *global* cerebral perfusion (Gur *et al.*, 1987; Mathew & Wilson, 1988), and, while this is clearly of interest, it provides little information on the neural areas which may participate in the expression of anxiety. As this chapter aims to focus on the neural correlates of anxiety, the discussion will concentrate on studies of *regional* cerebral perfusion and metabolism.

Normal anxiety

Resting-state studies

Anxiety is experienced by normal individuals as well as those with anxiety disorders, and a number of neuroimaging studies have examined this phenomenon in healthy volunteers. Giordani *et al.* (1990) assessed resting anxiety at the time of scanning in 43 normal subjects, using the state–trait anxiety inventory (STAI), and examined its correlation with glucose metabolism, as determined with [18]FDG PET. There was no correlation between anxiety and regional or global brain metabolism. Wik and Wiesel (1991) adopted a similar approach, studying 10 normal volunteers with PET, using ^{11}C-glucose. They found several correlations between absolute regional metabolism and the subjects' anxiety immediately post-scanning, as rated by the investigators on an analogue scale. However, when the analysis was repeated after normalising the metabolic rates to global cerebral metabolism, these correlations largely disappeared. As the temporal resolution of PET with glucose isotopes is relatively poor (of the order of 30 min), and levels of state anxiety can fluctuate over short periods, it is difficult to precisely correlate cerebral metabolism with anxiety at a given point in time with this technique. Type II errors might also arise, because the variation in levels of anxiety in normal subjects at rest may be relatively small. One way to overcome this problem is to elicit high levels of anxiety experimentally and compare subjects in this state and at rest.

Symptom-provocation studies

Reiman *et al.* (1989b) employed this approach in a PET study of eight normal volunteers, using ^{15}O-H$_2$O to measure rCBF. Subjects were told that they would receive a painful electric shock within the next 2 min and that its intensity would rise as the delay increased, and were scanned under these conditions and at rest. Subjective (analogue scale, STAI) and objective (pulse rate and ectodermal response) measures of anxiety increased during the activation condition, confirming that anxiety had been elicited. After stereotactic transformation of the PET data into a standard brain shape, the rCBF in the active and resting conditions was compared, within subjects, on a voxel-by-voxel basis. A statistically significant overall change was indicated by the presence of a greater number of pixels which were 'outliers' than would have been expected by chance, while the significance of local changes was confirmed with *post hoc* paired *t* tests. Variations in global cerebral blood flow (CBF) were controlled for by multiplying each voxel by a correction factor, which adjusted the rCBF values to a standard global rate. The analysis revealed bilateral increases in the temporal poles in association with anticipatory anxiety. However, doubts about the anatomical localisation of these findings have led to their retraction (see below).

Changes with treatment

The effects of diazepam on anxiety and cerebral metabolism in normal subjects were assessed with PET and [18]FDG by De Wit *et al.* (1991). Eight subjects were scanned three times while performing a visual monitoring task, before and then after a low and then a moderate dose of diazepam. Both doses reduced anxiety, as rated by the profile of mood states, and reduced global metabolism. An ANOVA indicated that both doses decreased absolute metabolism in several regions, but these effects disappeared when the data were normalised to global metabolism.

Panic

Resting-state studies

Prior to their study in normal subjects (see above), Reiman *et al.* (1984) examined resting rCBF using PET and ^{15}O-H$_2$O in 10 patients with episodic panic and 10 controls. Patients were subdivided into those in whom the intravenous infusion of lactate reliably induced panic (*n* = 7) and those in whom it had no effect ($n = 3$). A region-of-interest analysis and an ANOVA failed to identify any differences between the groups, but the ratio of right:left rCBF in the parahippocampal region was markedly higher in patients who were susceptible to lactate-induced panic compared with the other patients and the controls (Plate 15.3, facing p. 230). It was unclear whether this represented an increase in the perfusion of the right parahippocampal gyrus in these patients or a decrease in the left, as the absolute values for both were within normal limits.

Nordahl *et al.* (1990) sought to replicate this finding in a PET study of 12 patients with panic disorder, using [18]FDG. Cerebral glucose metabolism while the subjects were performing an auditory CPT was compared with that in 30 controls performing the same task. A region-of-interest analysis indicated a strong trend towards higher metabolism in the right parahippocampal–hippocampal area in the patients, and a greater right:left ratio of metabolism in this region. The patients also showed reduced metabolism in the left inferior parietal region. Although somewhat confounded by the possibility of differential effects of a CPT on cerebral metabolism, the results are consistent with those of Reiman *et al.* (1984). However, in the latter study, the parahippocampal findings were restricted to patients susceptible to lactate-induced panic, whereas in this investigation the effects were seen in the patient group as a whole but not in a subset who experienced panic in response to caffeine.

Symptom-provocation studies

Reiman's group subsequently examined rCBF in patients with panic disorder, after panic had been experimentally induced by lactate (Reiman *et al.*, 1989a). Regional perfusion was measured in 17 patients and 15 controls. The images were analysed in the same way as in the authors' study of normal anxiety, with intrasubject comparisons of the activation state and a resting condition (see above). Compared with controls, patients who panicked during scanning ($n = 8$) showed bilateral increases in rCBF in the temporal poles, a region spanning the insula, claustrum and putamen, and in the superior colliculi, and left-sided increases in the anterior vermis. Comparison of patients who did not panic ($n = 9$) with controls showed that increases were limited to the superior colliculi and the vermis, suggesting that these changes were more related to a direct effect of lactate than being associated with panic. The most significant changes were in the temporal poles and, as these seemed to mirror the author's earlier findings in normal subjects (see above), they attracted great interest. A subsequent study using cholecystokinin (CCK) to induce panic found increases in similar regions, but, when the PET data were coregistered on to magnetic resonance (MR) images, the functional changes were localised to the extracranial muscle superficial to the temporal poles, rather than the temporal cortex itself. A further PET study then demonstrated that teeth clenching reproduced the temporal polar increases seen in the studies of anticipatory anxiety and lactate-induced panic by Reiman *et al.* (1989a,b), and MR coregistration again confirmed their localisation to the masseter muscles (Drevets *et al.*, 1992; Plate 15.4, facing p. 230). The association between evoked anxiety and temporal polar activity has thus been retracted, although this does not necessarily invalidate the association with the increases in the insula/claustrum/putamen.

The neural correlates of lactate-induced panic have also been investigated with SPET. Stewart *et al.* (1988) employed ^{133}Xe to examine rCBF in 10 patients with panic disorder, with or without agoraphobia, and five controls, after the infusion of lactate. Regional data were examined with an ANOVA, with activity normalised to hemispheric blood flow, and the activation condition was compared with rest or infusion of saline. Patients who experienced panic with lactate ($n=6$) differed from those who did not ($n=4$) and the controls in having greater right and left occipital activity. They also showed greater left-hemispheric perfusion than those who did not, which was attributed to the effect of panic-associated hyperventilation and consequent hypocapnia in the latter group. Controlling for the potentially confounding effects of hyperventilation is critical in studies of anxiety, particularly when high levels are elicited experimentally. One approach has been to measure respiratory P_{CO_2} and then use this to adjust CBF to that expected with a normal P_{CO_2} (Mountz *et al.*, 1989; see below). Other studies have normalised the global CBF for each scan to a standard level, using an ANCOVA, with global activity as the covariate and psychological task as the treatment, to control for interscan variations in overall perfusion.

Phobias

Mountz *et al.* (1989) measured rCBF with PET and ^{15}O-H_2O in seven patients with specific (animal) phobias during *in vivo* exposure to a feared animal, and compared this with rest. The animal concerned varied with the content of each individual's phobia. Although subjects experienced significantly increased anxiety following exposure, after controlling for the effects of hypocapnia there were no changes in either regional or global CBF.

Generalised anxiety disorder (GAD)

Resting-state studies

Wu *et al.* (1991) examined 15 patients with GAD with PET and ^{18}FDG while they were performing a visual vigilance task, and compared them with the same number of controls. A large number of regions were examined and then analysed in groups comprising functionally related areas and then cortical lobes, with ANOVAs and *post hoc t* tests. The former analysis indicated that patients had lower absolute metabolism than controls in an area comprising the caudate, putamen and globus pallidus, while the latter revealed higher normalised metabolism in a left occipital region, a right posterior temporal region and a right precentral region. However, these differences would not have been significant if the statistical threshold had been corrected for multiple comparisons, and the two methods of analysis gave quite different results. There was no evidence of asymmetry in metabolism in the parahippocampal region, as reported in patients with a susceptibility to lactate-induced panic (Reiman *et al.*, 1984).

Changes with treatment

Two studies have examined the effects of benzodiazepines on cerebral metabolism in patients with GAD. Buchsbaum *et al.* (1987) used PET with ^{18}FDG to study eight patients before and after treatment with clorazepate for 21 days, and 10 patients before and after administration of a placebo. During scanning, subjects performed a visual vigilance task. An ANOVA and *post hoc t* tests indicated that treatment with clorazepate, but not placebo, was associated with decreased activity in the occipital region. However, it is unclear whether the drug had any effect on anxiety levels, as these were not rated. Mathew and Wilson (1991) examined cortical blood flow in 15 patients with SPET and ^{133}Xe, before and after the administration of diazepam, ondansetron and placebo. Diazepam significantly decreased anxiety, as rated by the STAI, and reduced blood flow in both hemispheres, but had no regional effects. Neither ondansetron nor placebo altered anxiety ratings or cortical perfusion.

Symptom-provocation studies

In another study using ^{133}Xe and SPET, Mathew and Wilson (1988) attempted to compare the effects of CO_2-induced anxiety in patients with GAD and in controls. Unfortunately, the administration of CO_2 failed to elicit a significant increase in anxiety ratings. However, when patients and controls were pooled and then divided into those whose ratings had increased and decreased, the former group (who became anxious) showed a smaller increase in global perfusion than the latter (whose anxiety reduced).

Anxiety in other conditions

The neural correlates of anxiety have also been examined in patients with other psychiatric conditions, particularly following exposure to obsessional stimuli in OCD. Zohar *et al.* (1989) found that anxiety in response to exposure was associated with regional decreases in temporal and parietal regions relative to listening to relaxing speech, while 'imagined' exposure led to temporal increases compared with the same baseline. McGuire *et al.* (1994) identified positive correlations between the intensity of exposure-induced anxiety and rCBF in the left hippocampus and left posterior cingulate cortex, as well as with that in the inferior frontal gyrus, neostriatum, thalamus and cuneus. There were also negative correlations in the temporoparietal region, particularly in the right hemisphere, and in the right superior frontal cortex. Exposure in OCD patients has also been found to lead to increased activity in the orbitofrontal cortex, right caudate nucleus and left anterior cingulate (Rauch *et al.*, 1994). Unfortunately, in all of these studies, the close correlation between evoked anxiety and OC symptoms precluded dissection of their respective neural correlates.

Anxiety has also been examined in OCD patients in the resting state. Swedo *et al.* (1989) found positive correlations between Spielberger state-anxiety scale ratings and glucose metabolism in the right orbitofrontal cortex and the prefrontal cortex bilaterally. In a study of the effects of treatment with clomipramine on OCD patients, Benkelfat *et al.* (1990) reported a negative correlation between changes in Spielberger state-anxiety scale score and temporal-lobe metabolism bilaterally.

Bench *et al.* (1993) examined the relationship between ratings of anxiety in depressed patients and rCBF, using PET with ^{15}O-CO$_2$. A factor analysis of clinical ratings yielded a major factor with heavy loadings from items assessing anxiety and agitation. When the scores for this factor were correlated with resting rCBF, using SPM, positive correlations were evident in the inferior

parietal lobule and posterior cingulate cortex bilaterally. These regions also showed correlations with anxiety ratings in patients with OCD (McGuire *et al.*, 1994), but the correlation in the temporoparietal region in obsessional patients was negative rather than positive. This difference in polarity might reflect differences in the form of anxiety experienced in these two disorders, with that in OCD being internally focused and that in depression being directed externally.

Discussion

While there have been several studies of anxiety using functional imaging, its neural correlates remain uncertain. Although two investigations have identified asymmetry in parahippocampal gyral metabolism in patients with panic disorder (Reiman *et al.*, 1989b; Nordahl *et al.*, 1990), overall there has been little consistency across studies. This may partly reflect wide differences in the isotopes, scanners and experimental designs employed. Many investigations have studied global, rather than regional, perfusion, and have used imaging technology which, by today's standards, is relatively crude. For example, studies with ^{133}Xe have a poor spatial resolution and, as they can only measure perfusion on the brain surface, cannot examine the role of deep structures or those on the medial aspect of the hemispheres, where many of the regions presumed to participate in the expression of anxiety are located. More recent studies have employed activation paradigms with more sophisticated imaging technology, but some of the most promising work has been hampered by difficulties with the anatomical localisation of functional change.

Defining the neural correlates of anxiety is likely to require activation paradigms using state-of-the-art functional imaging technology, and the coregistration of functional and structural images. Provoking symptoms with *in vivo* exposure to natural stimuli may be preferable to eliciting them with chemicals, such as lactate, as the latter may have direct effects on brain activity which are unrelated to anxiety. Anxiety has been examined in several different subject populations, but whether the brain regions associated with anxiety in different disorders, and in healthy subjects are the same is still unknown. This is a key issue to be addressed in future studies. Another interesting task for future studies would be to dissect out the brain correlates of the cognitive, behavioural and autonomic components of anxiety. Despite evidence that gamma-aminobutyric acid (GABA) has an important role in its pathophysiology, there have been few imaging studies of the neuropharmacology of anxiety. Benzodiazepine receptor ligands, such as fluamazenil, are now available, and the effects of GABAergic drugs on experimentally induced anxiety could be explored with PET, as has been done with other pharmaceuticals (Friston *et al.*, 1992). The application of neuropharmacological techniques in this area should complement data from studies of CBF and metabolism.

Conclusion

PET and SPET studies in OCD have produced results which are among the most robust findings in psychiatric neuroimaging. They have made a significant contribution to the understanding of the condition's pathophysiology, particularly with respect to the role of the corticostriatal–thalamic loop, and have markedly elevated the profile of OCD research in general. In contrast, imaging studies of anxiety have provided less consistent data, and the results from what appeared to have been the most elegant studies have recently been retracted. Nevertheless, the current availability of sophisticated imaging technology, including the capacity to coregister functional and structural images, should permit comparable advances in the study of anxiety in the near future.

References

Alexander, C.E., Delong, M.R. & Strick, P.L. (1980) Parallel organization of functionally segregated circuits linking basal ganglia and cortex. *Ann Rev Neurosci* **9**, 357–81.

Anderson, T.J., Jenkins, I.H., Brooks, D.J. *et al.* (1994) Cortical control of saccades and fixation in man: a PET study. *Brain* **117**, 1073–84.

Baxter, L., Phelps, M.E., Mazziotta, J. *et al.* (1985) Cerebral metabolic rates for glucose in mood disorders. *Arch. Gen. Psychiatry* **42**, 441–7.

Baxter, L., Phelps, M.E., Mazziotta, J. *et al.* (1987) Local cerebral glucose metabolic rates in obsessive–compulsive disorder: a comparison with rates in unipolar depression and normal controls. *Arch. Gen. Psychiatry* **44**, 211–18.

Baxter, L., Schwartz, J., Mazziotta, J. *et al.* (1988) Cerebral glucose metabolic rates in nondepressed patients with obsessive–compulsive disorder. *Am. J. Psychiatry* **145**, 1560–3.

Baxter, L., Schwartz, J.M., Bergmann, K.S. *et al.* (1992) Caudate glucose metabolic rate changes with both drug and behaviour therapy for obsessive compulsive disorder. *Arch. Gen. Psychiatry* **49**, 681–9.

Bench, C.J., Friston, K.J., Brown, R. G. *et al.* (1993) Regional cerebral blood flow in depression measured by positron emission tomography: the relationship with clinical dimensions. *Psychol. Med.* **23**, 579–90.

Benkelfat, C., Nordhal, T.E., Semple, W. *et al.* (1990) Local cerebral glucose metabolic rates in obsessive–compulsive disorder. *Arch. Gen. Psychiatry* **47**, 840–8.

Blin, J., Sette, G., Fiorelli, M. *et al.* (1990) A method for the *in vivo* investigation of the serotonergic 5–HT$_2$ receptors in the human cerebral cortex using positron emission tomography and ^{18}F–labelled setoperone. *J. Neurochem.* **54**, 1744–55.

Bridges, P. (1989) Psychosurgery in the 1980s. *Prac. Rev. Psychiatry* **2** (5), 1–4.

Buchsbaum, M.S., Wu, J., Haier, R. *et al.* (1987) Positron emission tomography assessment of effects of benzodiazepines on regional glucose metabolic rate in patients with anxiety disorder. *Life Sci.* **40**, 2393–400.

Cummings, J.L. & Cunningham, K. (1992) Obsessive–compulsive disorder in Huntington's disease. *Biol. Psychiatry* **31**, 263–70.

De Wit, H., Metz, J., Wagner, N. *et al.* (1991) Effects of diazepam on cerebral metabolism in normal volunteers. *Neuropsychopharmacology* **5**, 33–41.

Drevets, W.C., Videen, T.O., MacLeod, A.K. *et al.* (1992) PET images of blood flow changes during anxiety: correction. *Science* **256**, 1696.

Friston, K.J., Grasby, P.M., Bench, C.J. *et al.* (1992) Measuring the neuromodulatory effects of drugs in man with positron emission tomography. *Neurosci. Lett.* **141**, 106–10.

Giordani, B., Boivin, M.J., Berent, S. *et al.* (1990) Anxiety and cerebral cortical metabolism in normal persons. *Psychiatry Res. Neuroimaging* **35**, 49–60.

Gur, R.C., Gur, R.E., Resnick, S.M. *et al.* (1987) The effect of anxiety on cortical cerebral blood flow and metabolism. *J. Cerebr. Blood Flow Metab.* **7**, 173–7.

Hoehn–Saric, R., Pearlson, G., Harris, G.J. *et al.* (1991) Effects of fluoxetine on regional cerebral blood flow in obsessive–compulsive patients. *Am. J. Psychiatry* **49**, 690–4.

Hollander, E., Schiffman, E., Cohen, B. *et al.* (1990) Signs of central nervous dysfunction in obsessive–compulsive disorder: *Arch. Gen. Psychiatry* **47**, 27–32.

Hymas, N., Lees, A., Bolton, D. *et al.* (1991) The neurology of obsessional slowness. *Brain* **114**, 2203–33.

Jellife, S.E. (1932) *Psychopathology of Forced Movements and the Oculogyric Crises of Lethargic Encephalitis.* Nervous and Mental Diseases Monograph No. 55, New York and Washington.

Jenike, M.A., Bear, L., Ballantine, H.T. *et al.* (1991) Cingulotomy for refractory obsessive–compulsive disorder: a long term follow up of thirty–three patients. *Arch. Gen. Psychiatry* **48**, 548–55.

Kety, S.S. (1950) Circulation and metabolism of the human brain in health and disease. *Am. J. Med.* **8**, 205–17.

McGuire, P.K., Bench, C., Frith, C.D. *et al.* (1994) Functional anatomy of obsessive–compulsive phenomena. *Br. J. Psychiatry* **164**, 459–68.

Machlin, S.R., Harris, G.J., Pearlson, G.D. *et al.* (1991) Elevated medialfrontal cerebral blood flow in obsessive–compulsive patients: a SPECT study. *Am. J. Psychiatry* **148**, 1240–2.

Martinot, J.L., Allilaire, J.F., Mazoyer, B.M. *et al.* (1990) Obsessive–compulsive disorder: a clinical, neuropsychological and positron emission tomography study. *Acta Psychiatr. Scand.* **82**, 233–42.

Mathew, R.J. & Wilson, W.H. (1988) Cerebral blood flow changes induced by CO_2 in anxiety. *Psychiatry Res.* **23**, 285–94.

Mathew, R.J. & Wilson, W.H. (1991) Evaluation of the effects of diazepam and an experimental anti-anxiety drug on regional cerebral blood flow. *Psychiatry Res. Neuroimaging* **40**, 125–34.

Mountz, J.M., Modell, J.G., Wilson, M.W. *et al.* (1989) Positron emission tomography evaluation of cerebral blood flow during state anxiety in simple phobia. *Arch. Gen. Psychiatry* **46**, 501–4.

Nordahl, T.E., Bankelfat, C., Semple, W.E. *et al.* (1989) Cerebral glucose rates in obsessive–compulsive disorder. *Neuropsychopharmacology* **2**, 23–8.

Nordahl, T.E., Semple, W.E., Gross, M. *et al.* (1990) Cerebral glucose metabolic differences in patients with panic disorder. *Neuropsychopharmacology* **3**, 261–73.

Nyberg, S., Farde, L., Eriksson, L. *et al.* (1993) 5-HT_2 and D_2 dopamine receptor occupancy in the living human brain. *Psychopharmacology* **110**, 265–72.

Rauch, S.L., Jenicke, M.A., Alpert, N.M. *et al* (1994) Regional cerebral blood flow measured during symptom provocation in obsessive-compulsive disorder using ^{15}O-CO_2 and positron emission tomography. *Arch. Gen. Psychiatry* **51**, 62–70

Reiman, E.M., Raichle, M.E., Butler, F.K. *et al.* (1984) A focal brain disorder in panic disorder, a severe form of anxiety. *Nature* **310**, 683–5.

Reiman, E.M., Raichle, M.E., Robins, E. *et al.* (1989a) Neuroanatomical correlates of a lactate-induced panic attack. *Arch. Gen. Psychiatry* **46**, 493–500.

Reiman, E.M., Fusselman, M.J., Fox, P.T. *et al.* (1989b) Neuroanatomical correlates of anticipatory anxiety. *Science* **243**, 1071–4.

Rosen, S.D., Paulesu, E., Frith, C.D. *et al.* (1993) Regional brain activation in acute myocardial ischaemia. *Circulation* **88**, I–647.

Rubin, R.T., Villanueva-Meyer, J., Ananth, J. *et al.* (1992) Regional xenon 133 cerebral blood flow and cerebral technetium 99m HMPAO uptake in unmedicated patients with obsessive–compulsive disorder and matched control subjects. *Arch. Gen. Psychiatry* **49**, 695–702.

Sawle, G., Hymas, N., Lees, A. *et al.* (1991) Obsessional slowness: functional studies with positron emission tomography. *Brain* **114**, 2191–202.

Stewart, R.S., Devous, M.D., Rush, A.J. *et al.* (1988) Cerebral blood flow changes during sodium lactate-induced panic attacks. *Am. J. Psychiatry* **145**, 442–9.

Swedo, S.E., Schapiro, M.B., Grady, C.L. *et al.* (1989) Cerebral glucose metabolism in childhood-onset obsessive–compulsive disorder. *Arch. Gen. Psychiatry* **46**, 518–23.

Swedo, S.E., Pietrini, P., Leonard, L.H. *et al.* (1992) Cerebral glucose metabolism in childhood-onset obsessive–compulsive disorder: revisualisation during pharmacotherapy. *Arch. Gen. Psychiatry* **49**, 690–4.

Wik, G. & Wiesel, F.-A. (1991) Regional brain glucose metabolism: correlations to biochemical measures and anxiety in patients with schizophrenia. *Psychiatry Res. Neuroimaging* **40**, 101–14.

Wu, J.C., Buchsbaum, M.S., Hershey, T.G. *et al.* (1991) PET in generalised anxiety disorder. *Biol. Psychiatry* **29**, 1181–99.

Zohar, J., Insel, T.R, Berman, K.F. *et al.* (1989) Anxiety and cerebral blood flow during behavioural challenge. *Arch. Gen. Psychiatry* **46**, 505–10.

16: Brain Imaging in Child and Developmental Psychiatry

A. Bailey and T. Cox

Introduction

It is now widely accepted that many major psychiatric disorders are the consequence of abnormalities in brain function and structure, and yet the underlying mechanisms remain largely elusive. Neuroimaging provides an important set of tools to help identify these mechanisms and the capacity to visualise cognitive operations and psychopathological processes seems particularly likely to aid the understanding of brain–behaviour links. While many conceptual and methodological issues are common to the study of psychiatric disorders of children and adults, it is the focus on *development* that distinguishes research in child psychiatry. Thus childhood psychiatric disorders are particularly common in individuals with abnormal brain development, and disorders such as autism and developmental language and reading disorders seem also to be associated with abnormal development of the brain.

Before the advent of neuroimaging, researchers largely formulated their hypotheses of brain–behaviour links on the basis of observations of patients with brain disorders and evidence from post-mortem and animal studies. With the capacity to visualise the brain, there has been an understandable temptation to assume that observable abnormalities underlie the disorder in question. Of course, that will occasionally be the case, but such assumptions sometimes either ignore the complexity of the phenomena that have to be explained or fail to acknowledge a lack of specificity. The development of new technologies has certainly not diminished the need for complementary approaches and convergent evidence for pathological mechanisms.

Several general limitations on neuroimaging research in child psychiatry merit brief mention. The study of children brings with it problems of cooperation and consequently many researchers have chosen to study adolescent and adult subjects. This may not present problems for the interpretation of structural studies, where there is an expectation that abnormalities in brain development will persist. Nevertheless, the anatomy and mechanisms underlying cognitive operations may change with development, and caution is needed in extrapolating from functional studies of adults. The desire to avoid radiation exposure in children has been a factor in restricting positron emission tomography (PET) and single-photon emission tomography (SPET) studies mainly to adult subjects. Consequently, the techniques of functional magnetic resonance imaging (FMRI) and magnetoencephalography (MEG) hold special promise for the investigation of childhood disorders. A final difficulty lies in the need to obtain convergent evidence for neuroimaging abnormalities. The major problem is the paucity of published post-mortem studies of childhood disorders. Such studies are an important source of convergent evidence for macroscopic abnormalities, in addition to identifying underlying microscopic pathology. When only a small number of cases have been studied, findings can be potentially misleading because of chance variation, a relatively narrow focus of study or substantial aetiological heterogeneity.

Mental handicap

High rates of psychiatric disorder are consistently found in studies of individuals with mental handicap. Although there are likely to be multiple factors mediating this relationship, it is generally accepted that abnormal brain function and structure are major risk factors. In terms of establishing brain–behaviour links, however, studies of mental handicap have been less productive than might have been expected. One reason is that many psychiatric disorders, such as hyperactivity, show no specific association with particular mental-handicap syndromes. Another is that some syndromes sometimes associated with mental handicap, such as cerebral palsy, may be aetiologically and pathologically heterogeneous. Researchers are tackling these difficulties in several ways. One approach has been to focus on those mental-handicap syndromes that have a behavioural phenotype (Flint & Yule, 1994) — that is, a distinctive behaviour or a collection of behaviours and cognitive strengths and weaknesses that appear to be associated with a particular aetiology. Such investigations are at a relatively early stage, but already a number of structural-imaging studies have been undertaken which illustrate the general approach.

Williams syndrome is a rare disorder diagnosed on the basis of a characteristic facies and a heart defect. Affected individuals usually have relatively preserved semantic and syntactic skills but diminished visuoperceptive functions (although processing of human faces appears relatively intact). MRI studies of a small number of affected individuals have been compared with those of subjects with Down's syndrome and with normal controls. Jernigan *et al.* (1993) found that total cerebral volume was reduced in both pathological groups compared with controls, but that there were differences between the two syndromes in cortical and subcortical volumes and in cerebellar vermal-lobule areas. Thus, the basal ganglia and thalamus were reduced in size in subjects with Williams syndrome, whereas individuals with Down's syndrome showed a relative reduction in frontal and medial temporal volumes. While replication of the subcortical findings is necessary, this study illustrates the potential of structural imaging to identify characteristic variations in brain morphology. In combination with identification of the single gene mutations that underlie some mental-handicap syndromes, imaging studies should contribute to the understanding of normal brain development. The apparent dissociation between impaired visuospatial skills and normal processing of faces in individuals with Williams syndrome also points to the potential of functional studies to identify the cognitive mechanisms underlying behavioural phenotypes.

A second disorder sometimes associated with a behavioural phenotype is the *fragile-X syndrome*. This is the commonest inherited cause of mental retardation, but only a few cases have come to post-mortem; consequently the scope for structural-imaging studies is considerable. Early claims of a strong association with autism have not been substantiated, but a proportion of affected individuals do show quite marked social avoidance (Cohen *et al.*, 1988). Unfortunately, because of the putative link with autism, most neuroimaging studies have focused exclusively upon the posterior fossa (see below). Reiss *et al.'s* (1991) MRI study of fragile-X males found a significantly smaller posterior cerebellar vermis and larger fourth ventricle compared with a mixed comparison group. The nature of the relationship between the posterior-fossa findings and social avoidance remains obscure. A recent report suggests that hippocampal volumes may be increased in individuals with the fragile-X mutation (Reiss *et al.*, 1994). As hippocampal abnormalities have not been noted in the published post-mortem cases, the significance of this finding is at present uncertain.

Another approach to identifying brain–behaviour links is the identification of homogeneous syndromes. Although cytogenetic and molecular genetic approaches are especially important, as illustrated by the fragile-X syndrome, neuroimaging also has a role. *Cerebral palsy* is associated with a high rate of psychiatric disorder, although there are no consistent associations with specific disorders. Recent structural-neuroimaging studies raise the possibility of correlating symptomatology with the nature, site, extent or timing of the underlying pathology. Thus, longitudinal imaging studies of preterm infants, initially using cranial ultrasound and then MRI later in infancy, have shown a relationship between the degree of periventricular leucomalacia, later MRI appearances and clinical outcome (de Vries *et al.*, 1993). This type of pathological process contrasts with that detected in some individuals with cerebral palsy who were born at term: Truwit *et al.* (1992) found that 55% had MRI findings suggesting intrauterine events, and nearly a third had neuronal migration anomalies. Rarely, individuals have very specific combinations of clinical and imaging features. Thus, Kuzniecky *et al.* (1993) have described the *congenital bilateral perisylvian syndrome*, in which affected individuals have pseudobulbar palsy, bilateral perisylvian abnormalities on imaging studies and usually mental handicap and epilepsy. These studies demonstrate the potential of structural imaging to aid in the recognition of more homogeneous syndromes. Nevertheless, pathology is not always visible on structural MRI, and complementary functional studies will also be needed to determine the extent of brain involvement in individuals with cerebral palsy.

Epilepsy

Children with epilepsy also have a high rate of non-ictal psychiatric disorder and, in part, this is mediated by psychosocial factors. Nevertheless, the rate of disorder is highest in individuals with associated neurological abnormalities, suggesting that underlying brain abnormalities have direct links with psychopathology. These links might be mediated by a number of different mechanisms. Thus, anatomically localised brain abnormality might be associated with specific symptomatology. Alternatively, particular behaviours might be linked with specific seizure types. A final possibility is that behavioural disturbance is linked with particular types of abnormality in brain function and structure. The difficulties to be overcome in establishing these links are similar to those described above: non-specificity of the associations and aetiological heterogeneity.

An example of a possible association between localised seizure activity and loss of specific skills is provided by the *Landau–Kleffner* syndrome. Affected children lose receptive and expressive language skills and some 70% develop seizures. Paroxysmal electroencephalographic (EEG) discharges occur in all cases, but computerised tomography (CT) and MRI studies have failed to show consistent structural lesions. A combination of functional-imaging approaches has pointed to a likely anatomical basis of the disorder. A PET study of three patients found metabolic abnormalities predominating over the temporal lobes (Maquet *et al.*, 1990); asymmetry of temporal glucose utilisation was found in two cases and bilateral temporal hypometabolism in a third. Another SPET study also found asymmetrical perfusion in four out of five cases, predominantly in the perisylvian cortex (O'Tuama *et al.*, 1992). An MEG study of one affected individual with complete auditory agnosia demonstrated an epileptogenic focus with limited spatial extent around the left auditory cortex (Paetau *et al.*, 1991); the authors suggested that unilateral discharges suppressed contralateral auditory function. In addition to these cases, various authors have reported an association between the syndrome and tumours or cysts in the perisylvian region. Language functions can sometimes return when these lesions are resected, or localised subpial transections are performed in idiopathic cases.

The difficulties in identifying the mechanisms that link a seizure type and specific psychopathology are illustrated by the putative relationship between *infantile spasms* and autism. Riikonen and Amnell (1981) found that 12.5% of children with infantile spasms had autistic behaviours, although these were transient in over half of the cases; other authors have also noted this association. In several individuals there was a history of birth injury, postnatal infection or a medical disorder such as tuberous sclerosis. The aetiological heterogeneity of the disorder is a significant problem in establishing the nature of any relationship with autism. Autopsy studies have found a wide range of pathology, while a study of cortical resections found the major abnormalities to be destructive lesions and varying degrees of dysplastic change (Vinters *et al.*, 1993). In some individuals, there were abnormalities in gyral formation; in others, dysplastic changes were more subtle, with grey–white matter boundary, cortical lamination, neuronal or astrocytic abnormalities. As might be expected, some structural abnormalities are detectable by MRI, whereas PET identifies additional areas of metabolic abnormality (in addition to those picked up on structural imaging); however, in some patients, no focal cortical abnormalities are seen (Chugani *et al.*, 1992). Relating symptomatology to type or site of pathology will require multimodal imaging approaches and collaborations with neuro-pathologists in cases that come to surgery.

Accurate delineation of underlying pathology is an important aspect of recognising aetiological heterogeneity, and neuroimaging has made a particularly useful contribution to this process. MRI has increased the detection of many structural lesions underlying some cases of epilepsy, in particular *neuronal migration disorders*. This group of conditions is charac-terised by an ectopic location of neurons in the cerebral cortex and includes *lissencephaly* (or agyria)—a smooth brain or brain with poor sulcation; *pachygyria*—a less severe form of lissencephaly with thick cortex and poor sulcation; double cortex or *band heterotopia*—grey matter underlying the cortical mantle and separated from it by white matter (Fig. 16.1); *hemimegalencephaly*—enlargement of all or part of a cerebral hemisphere; *schizencephaly*—grey-matter-lined clefts in the cerebral hemispheres, extending from the pia to the ependymal lining (Fig. 16.2); *polymicrogyria*—too many small, abnormal gyri; and *subependymal heterotopias*—

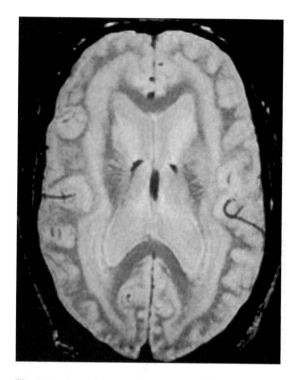

Fig. 16.1 Coronal magnetic resonance (MR) image showing band heterotopia. A second abnormal band of grey matter (shown as pale) can be seen interpolated between subcortical and periventricular white matter.

multiple smooth nodules of cortical grey matter lining the lateral ventricles (Kuzniecky, 1994). Individuals with severe disruption of cortical architecture are frequently mentally handicapped, although even lissencephaly can sometimes be associated with apparently normal early develop-ment (Barkovich *et al.*, 1991). Not all neuronal migration abnormalities are detectable by MRI, and PET can sometimes help to detect some small abnormalities by revealing focal increases or decreases in metabolic activity. It remains to be established whether there are specific associations with psychopathology.

Although detection of some neuronal migration disorders and hippocampal sclerosis, using MRI, is now well established, other morphological changes in epilepsy may be more subtle, leading to difficulties in establishing brain–behaviour links.

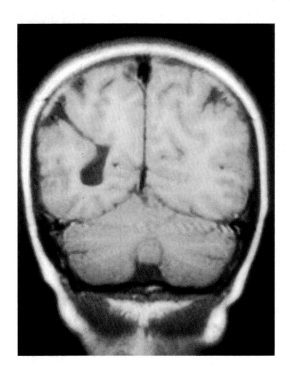

Fig. 16.2 Coronal magnetic resonance (MR) image of patient with schizencephaly. A full-thickness cleft can be seen extending from the surface of the cerebral hemisphere to the lateral ventricle.

Minor changes in gyral thickness or size and areas of focal cortical dysplasia may not be visualised even with MRI. Palmini *et al.* (1991) found that MRI did not detect macrogyria in four out of 12 surgical patients, and interictal epileptogenic abnormalities extended beyond the visible lesion boundary in over half of the cases. Imaging–histology correlations also suggest that visible dysplastic abnormalities are sometimes only the most abnormal structural area of a more extensive process (Palmini *et al.*, 1994). Surgery for epilepsy has also provided the opportunity to undertake cortical-stimulation studies, and several reports have noted anomalous localisation of language centres. Such studies are a reminder that functional studies are also needed to investigate the relationships between abnormal cortical organisation and cognitive impairment and psychopathology.

Autism

Autism is one of the most distinctive, best-validated and intensively investigated of childhood psychiatric disorders and holds considerable promise for establishing brain–behaviour links. That such links have not yet been convincingly demonstrated is partly a consequence of the rate of technological development. It also reflects, however, the influence that concepts of disorders have upon their investigation and the interpretation of findings.

Autism is characterised by impairments in social interaction and communication, restricted and repetitive patterns of behaviour and interests and an onset before 3 years of age. Three-quarters of sufferers are mentally handicapped and between a quarter and a third develop epilepsy. Since Kanner's original description, the prevailing view has been that autism is a psychological syndrome: a particular cluster of behaviours arising on the basis of diverse aetiologies. The association with mental handicap led to the notion of impairments in a specific brain system, usually, but not always, occurring in conjunction with widespread pathology (see, for instance, Frith, 1989). If this notion were correct, then autism might be associated with consistent localised abnormalities.

Several neuroimaging studies have identified localised parenchymal pathology in a small number of cases. What is striking about these findings is the diversity of sites at which pathology has been detected. For instance, Damasio *et al.* (1980) identified two patients with frontal-lobe lesions, dorsolaterally situated in one and in both the mesial and polar regions in the other. Gillberg and Svendsen (1983) identified a porencephalic cyst in the left parieto-occipital region in one individual and a defect near the right lateral geniculate body in another. Gaffney and Tsai (1987) observed heterotopic grey matter in the left occipital region in one individual, a ganglioglioma in the left temporal lobe in another and an area of increased signal in the parietal lobe of a third. Most recently, Piven *et al.* (1990)

observed a variety of cortical developmental malformations in seven patients; these were situated variously in the frontal, temporal, parietal and parietal–occipital lobes. In conclusion, there is no indication from these or other studies of any consistent localisation of parenchymal lesions.

Measurement of ventricular size has been undertaken by many investigators, and this provides an indirect approach to pathological localisation. These studies have been conducted across several decades, using different imaging modalities, slice orientations and thicknesses and widely differing methods of image analysis. Again, not only are the findings contradictory as to the presence of dilatation, but also there is no consistency in the site of putative abnormalities. The earliest claim of a specific abnormality was of left temporal-horn dilatation visualised using pneumoencephalography (Hauser *et al.*, 1975). Although not confirmed by subsequent CT studies, the finding has assumed some significance because of the strong claims by Bauman's group (Kemper & Bauman, 1993) and others that medial-temporal abnormalities underlie many autistic symptoms. This group found that post-mortem abnormalities were confined to the limbic system, cerebellum and brainstem, the neocortex being unaffected. The only relevant MRI study found volumes of the posterior hippocampus to be similar in autistic subjects and controls (Saitoh *et al.*, 1995).

Turning to the lateral ventricles, some of the early CT studies that included a heterogeneous group of subjects reported increased ventricular size in a subgroup (Damasio *et al.*, 1980; Gillberg & Svendsen, 1983). Increased lateral-ventricular size was also reported in a small proportion of autistic individuals in CT studies of individuals without concomitant neurological disorders (Campbell *et al.*, 1982), but subsequent CT studies have failed to replicate this finding (see, for instance, Jacobson *et al.*, 1988). Because the only MRI study to have examined lateral-ventricular area included two autistic subjects with neurofibromatosis (Gaffney *et al.*, 1988), the

significance of the reported increase in lateral-ventricular area is unclear. Again, there is little evidence of consistent change in lateral-ventricular measures.

A rather similar picture emerges with respect to the third ventricle. A subgroup of individuals in the study of Campbell *et al.* (1982) had enlarged third ventricles, and a significant increase in size was noted in the report by Jacobson *et al.* (1988); no difference in third-ventricular measurements was found, however, in the studies of Rosenbloom *et al.* (1984) or Creasey *et al.* (1986). Finally, the findings with regard to the fourth ventricle are clear. Only one group (Gaffney & Tsai, 1987; Gaffney *et al.*, 1987) has reported a statistically significant increase in fourth-ventricular size (although not consistently across different imaging planes). No significant increase in size has been found in at least six other studies.

Before concluding that there is no consistent localised macroscopic pathology in autistic individuals, the claims that autism is associated with specific cerebellar vermal lobules merit consideration. Courchesne *et al.* (1987) reported hypoplasia of the posterior cerebellar vermis in an MRI study of a high-functioning autistic individual. The finding was interesting because a decrease in cerebellar Purkinje cells had been noted in two post-mortem cases (Williams *et al.*, 1980; Bauman & Kemper, 1985). Subsequently, 18 autistic individuals and a group of normal controls were examined and a significant reduction in the size of cerebellar vermal lobules VI–VII was found in the autistic group, but no difference in the size of lobules I–V (Courchesne *et al.*, 1988). A subgroup of the patients were subsequently remeasured and the difference in size confirmed, although it was now reduced in magnitude.

Courchesne's group argue that there is concordant evidence that cerebellar abnormalities are the most consistent neuroanatomical lesion in autism (Courchesne *et al.*, 1994b) and that such abnormalities underlie some of the characteristic symptomatology. The significance of these claims is several-fold. Firstly, they are based on inductive logic: the cerebellar vermis has been afforded a central role in the pathophysiology of autism, not on the basis of an a priori hypothesis about the neurological basis of autism (Bailey, 1993), but on the basis of observations. Secondly, rather than attempting to disprove their own results, Courchesne's group have argued strongly for the superiority of their methodology over that of other groups (Courchesne *et al.*, 1994b) and latterly introduced an *ad hoc* hypothesis. The issues to address are whether these findings have been satisfactorily replicated; whether there is concordant evidence for cerebellar vermal involvement; and whether any putative finding is specific to autism.

Studies that have used a similar imaging approach to Courchesne's group have not replicated their findings (Holttum *et al.*, 1992; Kleinman *et al.*, 1992; Piven *et al.*, 1992). Courchesne *et al.* (1994a) argue that one reason for the failure to replicate is that the autistic population in fact comprises two subgroups: one with posterior vermal hypoplasia, the other with vermal hyperplasia. While the variance of posterior vermal areas may be increased in autistic individuals, the introduction of an auxiliary hypothesis of two subgroups reduces the falsifiability of the original claims. The recent MRI study of Hashimoto *et al.* (1995) has been cited in support of the cerebellar hypothesis, but this study is methodologically less rigorous than previous investigations and does not replicate the original claim of specific hypoplasia.

Furthermore, the argument that the post-mortem studies provide convergent evidence for the neuroimaging findings is not strongly supported by the evidence. First, none of the post-mortem studies have reported macroscopic vermal abnormalities (Williams *et al.*, 1980; Ritvo *et al.*, 1986, Kemper & Bauman, 1993). Secondly, Purkinje-cell loss in autistic individuals has been reported to occur in all areas of the cerebellum (Arin *et al.*, 1991). Thirdly, loss of Purkinje cells alone could not account for visible hypoplasia; the granule and/or molecular cell layers must also be reduced. Although a qualitative reduction in

granule cells has been noted in several cases (Kemper & Bauman, 1993), no granule-cell counts have been conducted, and there are no qualitative reports of regional variations in vermal granule-cell density.

If further imaging studies confirm vermal abnormalities in autistic individuals, are they likely to represent a basis for the autistic syndrome? That seems unlikely, as the finding of posterior vermal hypoplasia is not specific to autism. Thus, a reduction in posterior vermal area has been noted in individuals with the fragile-X syndrome (Reiss *et al.*, 1991), the vast majority of whom are not classically autistic. Older imaging and post-mortem studies noted other vermal abnormalities in patients with either schizophrenia or bipolar disorder. It seems probable that any vermal abnormalities in these diverse conditions are a consequence of abnormal brain development rather than aetiological factors.

The interest in the cerebellar vermis has focused attention on other posterior fossa structures but, as with the ventricular studies, the findings are at present inconsistent. In summary, a large number of structural studies, including many not dealt with here, have been unable to identify consistent localised abnormalities in autism. Of course, localised abnormalities may be detected in the future, but recent evidence suggests that the significance of such findings would have to be considered in a different conceptual framework from hitherto.

A number of recent twin and family studies suggest that autism is usually a specific genetic disease with variable phenotypic expression, rather than a homogeneous psychological disorder with many different medical and obstetric aetiologies. The same-sex twin studies all report much higher concordance for autism in identical than in non-identical twins and the British studies indicate that the genetic liability extends to a broader phenotype of milder impairments in communication and social interaction (Bailey *et al.*, 1995). A recent family genetic study has confirmed these findings (Bolton *et al.*, 1994). Identifiable medical disorders and obstetric hazards do not seem to be frequent aetiological factors (Bolton *et al.*, 1994; Rutter *et al.*, 1994; Bailey *et al.*, 1995).

If autism is usually a specific disease, the accompanying mental handicap is also likely to be a consequence of the disorder rather than a non-specific marker of brain damage. This view is supported by both the genetic findings (Bolton *et al.*, 1994) and the unusual psychological test profile found in many autistic individuals (for a description see Frith, 1989). Nevertheless, it is difficult to square the need to account for general cognitive impairments either with the notion of a localised brain abnormality or with the claims that post-mortem changes are confined to the limbic system, cerebellum and inferior olives (Kemper & Bauman, 1993). It appears, however, that the early post-mortem findings were probably misleading rather than the current conceptualisation of the disorder wrong. In a recent post-mortem study, we found that three out of four brains were large and megalencephalic. In one case, the cerebral cortex was increased in thickness and, in the other two, cortical neuronal density was high. These findings point to the possibility of a diffuse abnormality in cerebral-cortical development.

Of course, the findings from this small number of cases may be misleading, and independent replication is needed. There is, however, other evidence supporting the observation of increased brain size. First, the brains examined by Bauman's group are also reported to be considerably heavier than those in age- and sex-matched controls (M.L. Bauman, personal communication), although whether this is related to the causes of death is unclear. Secondly, head circumference appears to be increased in about a third of autistic individuals (Bailey, 1993; Woodhouse *et al.*, in press). Thirdly, two recent MRI studies found that the brains of autistic individuals were larger than those of controls (Filipek *et al.*, 1992; Piven *et al.*, 1995), although a number of earlier studies failed to find differences in various indices of brain size. Our own study of autistic twins and singletons (using siblings as controls) found no increase in total brain volume (A. Bailey and T. Cox, unpublished observations), raising the possibility that increased brain volume may be a familial trait.

There is an obvious need for further studies of total and regional brain volumes, taking into account variables such as sex, age, intelligence quotient (IQ) and socioeconomic status. Early CT studies suggested that autism was sometimes associated with abnormal hemispheric asymmetries, although later studies refuted this notion. If autism does involve abnormalities in cerebral-cortical development, a future finding of abnormal asymmetry would not be unexpected but may not represent the primary pathology underlying the syndrome. Similarly, the various localised cortical abnormalities detected by Piven *et al.* (1990) and others may be focal manifestations of a possibly diffuse pathological process. The finding of a number of subtle developmental brainstem abnormalities in our recent post-mortem cases points to the possibility that abnormal brain development may not be confined to the cerebral hemispheres.

These recent findings point to the importance of functional-imaging studies for establishing the mechanisms by which possibly widespread pathology leads to such distinctive psycho-pathology. The starting-point is to note that functional-imaging studies are generally supportive of the conclusions drawn so far. Because of the association between autism and not epilepsy, there have been many EEG studies. Seizures usually, but not always, occur in the most handicapped individuals, raising the possibility that they may be related to the severity of the underlying pathology. There are no strong associations between autism and any particular seizure type, and the anatomical localisation of epileptic foci is unremarkable. The EEG studies essentially confirm this pattern. Thus, studies conducted before the development of standardised diagnostic instruments suggest that EEG abnormalities are found in approximately 50% of autistic individuals. Tsai *et al.* (1985) found that in half of the individuals with an abnormal EEG there was evidence of bilateral diffuse abnormalities and, even when there were unilateral abnormalities, there was no predilection for any particular part of the brain. Small (1975) noted that abnormal EEGs were associated with lower IQ.

The EEG data are also supported by the findings from a small number of PET and SPET studies, conducted either at rest or during simple tasks. Thus, no consistent focal reductions or elevations in cerebral metabolism have been identified across studies. Although there were early claims of diffusely elevated cerebral metabolism (Rumsey *et al.*, 1985; Horwitz *et al.*, 1988), these have not been replicated. Rumsey *et al.* (1985) drew attention to greater variations in the findings in autistic subjects than in controls, with more autistic subjects showing extreme relative metabolic rates and asymmetries. Horwitz *et al.* (1988) subsequently examined the correlations between different regional metabolic rates and found these to be lower in autistic subjects than in controls.

There is general acceptance of the need to move towards specific activation studies, using PET and other paradigms. Unfortunately, the findings from existing event-related potential (ERP) studies do not provide many pointers for future studies. One reason is that the spatial localisation of neural events giving rise to electrical activity recorded from the scalp is poor. Thus, it is difficult to identify which areas of the brain contribute to changes in waveforms. Without anatomical information, clues about the likely significance of neural activity are lacking. Secondly, the choice of tasks studied in autistic individuals have generally been driven more by historical concepts of the field than by the nature of the disorder. Thus, human ERP work arose in part from animal studies of attentional mechanisms. These have consequently remained a major interest of neurophysiological investigators and, while autistic individuals do have attentional problems, it seems unlikely that autism can be reduced to attentional dysfunction. Additionally, much work in the area has been driven by observation of a particular

ERP and then postulating a construct which seems to describe the eliciting conditions. Thus, while autistic individuals may show ERP differences from normals on oddball tasks, there is difficulty linking these findings to autistic symptomatology. Finally, many of the findings are contradictory, probably in part because of differences in diagnosis and the occasional inclusion of cases with neurological conditions, but possibly also in part because of variations in the subject's level of ability. Of course, relating neuronal firing to cognitive activity is a major goal of neuroimaging research, and future possiblities are considered at the end of this chapter.

Developmental language and reading disorders

Articulation difficulties, delayed speech, problems with semantics, syntactics and pragmatics and reading and spelling difficulties are relatively common childhood problems, and the more severe disorders can persist into adulthood. There is evidence of continuities between these different difficulties, although heterogeneity is also likely.

Morphological research into developmental language and reading disorders had possible localising clues from the sites of acquired lesions in adults resulting in aphasias and alexia. The most significant motivation for the majority of structural-neuroimaging studies arose, however, from Geschwind and Levitsky's (1968) post-mortem study of normal subjects. These authors reported significant asymmetries in the supra-temporal plane. A subsequent small cytoarchitectonic study of the same region found asymmetry of an area of presumed auditory cortex (the planum temporale) and it was suggested that the larger area in the left hemisphere might represent the anatomical substrate of lateralised language functions (Galaburda *et al.*, 1978). Many researchers considered that damage or abnormal development of such left-sided structures might be implicated in the pathogenesis of language-related disorders. Consequently, a number of studies have sought to establish whether there are unusual patterns of morphological asymmetries in individuals with language-related disorders.

There have been many structural-neuroimaging studies, but only those that measured the planum temporale rather than larger regions are considered. Leonard *et al.* (1993) measured the length of the temporal and parietal banks of the sylvian fissure posterior to Heschl's gyrus in dyslexic subjects and controls. In autopsy studies of normal subjects, the temporal bank is about twice as long on the left as the right, and the relationship is reversed for the parietal bank, the overall length being roughly equal (Witelson & Kigar, 1992). Most subjects and controls demonstrated leftward asymmetry for the temporal bank and rightward asymmetry for the parietal bank. Most subjects and controls also had larger temporal than parietal banks in the left hemisphere. Five of the nine subjects, however, had larger parietal than temporal banks in the right hemisphere. Subjects and their relatives were also reported to have more minor cerebral anomalies, such as duplicated or missing gyri, in the planum and parietal operculum.

Larsen *et al.* (1990) measured the area of the planum temporale on coronal MRI scans. They reported more symmetrical plana in reading-disabled subjects than in controls and suggested, on the basis of planum lengths, that the symmetry resulted from larger plana on the right. Hynd *et al.* (1990) measured planum length (not defined) on extreme lateral sagittal slices in reading-impaired children, children with attention-deficit disorder and hyperactivity and normal children. The majority of the reading-impaired children had either symmetrical plana or right plana that were longer than the left; this appeared to be a consequence of a reduction in planum length on the left.

Although all three studies found differences in the plana temporale between subjects and controls, the nature of these changes was inconsistent. Variations in imaging and analytical protocols probably contributed to these differences and these may be resolved by further

studies. It is necessary to consider, however, whether structural studies should focus exclusively on this issue. The first point to note is that there is not a direct link between differences in planum size and language and reading disorders. Thus, nearly 40% of the normal population do not have larger left than right plana, and some individuals with language-related disorders have the normal pattern of asymmetry. Secondly, the presumed failure of the right hemisphere to compensate for putative left-sided abnormalities points to the likelihood of a bilateral disease process. Thirdly, functional-imaging studies of single-word reading in normal individuals indicate the involvement of widely distributed specific cortical areas. Fourthly, imaging studies have frequently been motivated by the search for localised abnormalities, based upon the assumption that affected individuals have a very narrow psychological deficit. It is well established, however, that some, but not all, affected children have concomitant cognitive and neurodevelopmental impairments which can persist into adult life (Kinsbourne *et al.*, 1991; Rutter & Mawhood, 1991), and theorists increasingly emphasise the possibility of basic processing deficits that are not confined to language (Bishop, 1992; Anderson *et al.*, 1993). Fifthly, other neuroimaging studies have found differences between subjects and controls that extend beyond the planum temporale. Again, the findings are not consistent, but they point to the possibility of more widespread abnormalities in cerebral-cortical development. Finally, the post-mortem findings do not provide unequivocal evidence of a highly localised abnormality. Galaburda *et al.* (1985) examined the brains of four males with developmental reading difficulties. They observed symmetry of the planum temporale in all cases, but also areas of minor focal cortical dysplasia (most severe in an individual who also had epilepsy) and neuronal ectopias. While many dysplastic lesions were in the left perisylvian region, this was not their exclusive location and every patient also had abnormalities in the inferior frontal gyrus. Abnormalities in the medial and lateral geniculate nuclei have subsequently been emphasised. The post-mortem findings do not support the notion of a localised abnormality and it is possible that both focal cortical abnormalities and unusual asymmetries are consequences of abnormal cortical development.

As with autism, developmental language disorders are associated with an elevated rate of seizures and there have been a number of EEG studies, particularly of individuals with reading difficulties. These were largely motivated by the search for EEG abnormalities specific to the disorder. Perhaps not surprisingly, claims of diagnosis-specific patterns of EEG activity have not been replicated. ERP studies have, however, not usually focused on tasks closely related to the central symptomatology. Investigators of normal language development and organisation have, however, made rather more thoughtful use of this technology. Thus many researchers have exploited the capacity of ERP to detect differences in neural activity elicited by stimuli whose psychological processing is thought to differ. The recent study by Dehaene-Lambertz and Dehaene (1994) nicely illustrates the application of ERP methodology to the study of syllable discrimination by infants. These developmental studies assume especial importance because of the genetic contribution to language and reading disorders and the consequent possibility of conducting prospective studies of language development in at-risk siblings.

The radioisotope studies of individuals with reading disorders have all used activation paradigms, but there have varied widely. Visually presented tasks have included reading single words aloud and semantic categorisation, whereas auditory tasks have included discrimination of phonemes, rhyme detection and detection of words containing four letters. Again, although every study found differences between subjects and controls, the nature of these differences varied. Some studies found differences in the amount of blood flow in a defined cortical region. While this might only reflect changes in the rate of neuronal activity, it is possible that in developmental disorders differences in cell density

might also be a contributory factor. Perhaps more interesting are the preliminary findings pointing to differences in the sites of cortical activation. Thus, Flowers *et al.* (1991) used the xenon technique to measure regional cerebral blood flow during a task in which subjects had to identify words of four letters in an auditorily presented list of nouns. This orthographic task activated a more posterior temporoparietal region of cortex in reading-disabled subjects than in controls. Rumsey *et al.* (1992) found less activation of left temporoparietal cortex in reading-impaired subjects than in controls using a rhyme-detection task, but noted activation of anterior temporal regions in some subjects. There is an obvious need for more detailed localisation studies of cognitive functions in individuals with language-related disorders. Work in normals indicates, however, that future studies will need to pay even greater attention to task variables (Price *et al.*, 1994) and the possibility of sex differences in the functional organisation of the brain for language (Shaywitz *et al.*, 1995).

Future directions

While there are obvious differences between the individual disorders and studies discussed in this chapter, a number of common themes emerge. One is the tremendous variability in findings when researchers have supposedly examined the same disorder. To achieve the full potential of new approaches it will be necessary to tackle the factors contributing to such variability, one of which is subject heterogeneity. The inclusion of individuals with recognised neurological causes of behavioural disorders introduces known heterogeneity. Unknown heterogeneity arises both because of variability in the application of diagnostic criteria and also because of unrecognised aetiological heterogeneity. The increasing use of standardised diagnostic instruments in child psychiatric research is likely to reduce, but not eliminate, diagnostic imprecision. Of course, the application of molecular genetic techniques to childhood disorders offers the promise of identifying aetiologically homogeneous subgroups of individuals for future study.

A second factor contributing to poor replic-ability is a lack of attention to methodological detail. Thus, in anatomical studies, structures have sometimes been visualised using suboptimal scan sequences. At other times, investigators have attempted to measure small or poorly defined structures in only one plane, or have been unable to replicate findings in another axis. While computer-assisted image analysis has improved the reliability of measurements, it is also important to ensure that the computer-derived measures are valid. The *post hoc* application of multiple correlational analysis to data has probably also contributed to spurious findings. Comparisons between studies have, of course, been hindered by the variability in the way that data are obtained. The increasing use of volumetric data acquisition in MRI studies offers the possibility of researchers reformatting their data for analysis in alternative ways. Such developments will increase the pressure for the development of standardised measurement protocols.

A second theme to emerge is the possibility that some structural abnormalities may be relatively non-specific consequences of abnormal brain development. Thus, minor cortical malformations are found in diverse disorders. Because cell division, differentiation and migration are com-plex and multistage events, it would not be surprising if different aetiological factors some-times resulted in apparently similar end-stage pathologies. A related theme is that of comor-bidity; various combinations of mental handicap, epilepsy, autism and language disorders can occur in different individuals. The critical issue is the meaning of these different associations. Thus, the association between language disorder and epilepsy in Landau–Kleffner syndrome seems in part a consequence of the anatomical location of the underlying abnormality, whereas the associa-tion between language disorders and other types of seizures is probably the result of a more pervasive abnormality in brain development with multiple sequelae. The apparent non-specificity of some structural abnormalities and the fact of comorbidity highlight the need for functional-imaging studies that identify specific pathological mechanisms.

Studies of normal cognitive processes in adults using PET have provided important insights into the localised nature of some cognitive functions and clarified the underlying nature of others. The rapid development of functional MRI using echoplanar and other fast imaging techniques offers the prospect of undertaking similar studies in children without radiation exposure. An understanding of normal development is neces-sary to interpret the pathological. The normal acquisition of language and reading skills seems likely to be an area of study using both MRI and other approaches.

Much of the recent success of PET studies has been attributable to the choice of subtraction paradigms. The approach assumes that cognitive processing is serial and non-interactive (see Sergent *et al.* (1992) for a fuller discussion of this issue). Interactive processes and those which are similar in their anatomical distribution but differ in their order or time course are not differentiated using the subtraction methodology. Fortunately, the continuing development of MEG and its associated analytical methods is likely to provide a complementary approach to PET and functional MRI. MEG detects the minute magnetic fields associated with dendritic currents (see Chapter 9) and, because the source space is sampled directly, spatial resolution is considerably better than with EEG (although gyri provide only weak signals). Coregistration with MRI and the use of distributed-image methods enables both localised and distributed current sources to be identified (Ioannides *et al.*, 1993). Millisecond time resolu-tion allows not only the sequence of activation to be determined, but also coherence of activity across spatially distributed regions (Plate 16.1, facing p. 230).

Utilising the full potential of these different approaches will require close collaboration between psychiatrists, psychologists, neuroscientists and neuroimagers. Cognitive tasks will need to be devised that not only differentiate between disorders but also expose underlying mechanisms. The challenges are substantial but the rewards will be an integrated understanding of the links between abnormal brain development and psychopathology.

References

Anderson, K.C., Brown, C.P. & Tallal, P. (1993) Developmental language disorders: evidence for a basic processing deficit. *Curr. Opin. Neurol. Neurosurg.* **6**, 98–106.

Arin, D.M., Bauman, M.L. & Kemper, T.L. (1991) The distribution of Purkinje cell loss in the cerebellum in autism. *Neurology* **47** (Suppl. 1), 307.

Bailey, A. (1993) The biology of autism. *Psychol. Med.* **23**, 7–11.

Bailey, A., Le Couteur, A., Gottesman, I. *et al.* (1995) Autism as a strongly genetic disorder: evidence from a British twin study. *Psychol. Med.* **25**, 63–77.

Barkovich, A.J., Koch, T.K. & Carrol, C.L. (1991) The spectrum of lissencephaly: report of ten patients analyzed by magnetic resonance imaging. *Ann. Neurol.* **30**, 139–46.

Bauman, M.L. & Kemper, T.L. (1985) Histoanatomic observations of the brain in early infantile autism. *Neurology* **35**, 866.

Bishop, D.V.M. (1992) The underlying nature of specific language impairment. *J. Child Psychol. Psychiatry* **33**, 3–66.

Bolton, P., McDonald, H., Pickles, A.R. *et al.* (1994) A case–control family history study of autism. *J. Child Psychol. Psychiatry* **35**, 877–900.

Campbell, M., Rosenbloom, S., Perry, R. *et al.* (1982) Computerized axial tomography in young autistic children. *Am. J. Psychiatry* **139**, 510–12.

Chugani, H.T., Shewmon, A., Sankar, R., Chen, B.C. & Phelps, M.E. (1992) Infantile spasms: II. Lenticular nuclei and brain stem activation on positron emission tomography. *Ann. Neurol.* **31**, 212–19.

Cohen, I., Fisch, G., Sudhalter, V. *et al.* (1988) Social gaze, social avoidance, and repetitive behaviour in Fragile X males: a controlled study. *Am. J. Mental Retardation* **92**, 436–46.

Courchesne, E., Hesselink, J.R., Jernigan, T.L. & Yeung-Courchesne, R. (1987) Abnormal neuroanatomy in a nonretarded person with autism. *Arch. Neurol.* **44**, 335–41.

Courchesne, E., Yeung-Courchesne, R., Press, G.A., Hesselink, J.R. & Jernigan, T.L. (1988) Hypoplasia of cerebellar vermal lobules VI and VII in autism. *N. Engl. J. Med.* **318**, 1349–54.

Courchesne, C., Yeung-Courchesne, R. & Egaas, B. (1994a) Methodology in neuroanatomic measurement. *Neurology* **44**, 203–8.

Courchesne, C., Townsend, J. & Saitoh, O. (1994b) The brain in infantile autism: posterior fossa structures are abnormal. *Neurology* **44**, 214–23.

Creasey, H., Rumsey, J., Schwartz, M., Duara, R., Rapoport, J.L. & Rapoport, S.I. (1986) Brain morphometry in autistic men as measured by volumetric computed tomography. *Arch. Neurol.* **43**, 669–72.

Damasio, H., Maurer, R.G., Damasio, A.R. & Chui, H.C. (1980) Computerized tomographic scan findings in patients with autistic behavior. *Arch. Neurol.* **37**, 504–10.

Dehaene-Lambertz, G. & Dehaene, S. (1994) Speed and cerebral correlates of syllable discrimination in infants. *Nature* **370**, 292–5.

de Vries, L.S., Eken, P., Groenendaal, F., van Haastert, I.C. & Meiners, L.C. (1993) Correlation between the degree of periventricular leukomalacia diagnosed using cranial ultrasound and MRI later in infancy in children with cerebral palsy. *Neuropediatrics* **24**, 263–8.

Filipek, P.A., Richelme, C., Kennedy, D.M. *et al.* (1992) Morphometric analysis of the brain in developmental language disorders and autism. *Ann. Neurol.* **32**, 475.

Flint, J. & Yule, W. (1994) Behavioural phenotypes. In Rutter, M., Taylor, E. & Hersov, L. (eds) *Child and Adolescent Psychiatry: Modern Approaches*, 3rd edn. Blackwell Science, Oxford, pp. 666–87.

Flowers, D.L., Wood, F.B. & Naylor, C.E. (1991) Regional cerebral blood flow correlates of language processes in reading disability. *Arch. Neurol.* **48**, 637–43.

Frith, U. (1989) *Autism: Explaining the Enigma*. Basil Blackwell, Oxford.

Gaffney, G.R. & Tsai, L.Y. (1987) Brief report: magnetic resonance imaging of high level autism. *J. Autism Developm. Disorders* **17**, 433–8.

Gaffney, G.R., Tsai, L.Y., Kuperman, S. & Minchin, S. (1987) Cerebellar structure in autism. *Am. J. Dis. Child.* **141**, 1330–2.

Gaffney, G.R., Kuperman, S., Tsai, L.Y. & Minchin, S. (1989) Forebrain structure in infantile autism. *J. Am. Acad. Child Adolescent Psychiatry* **28**, 534–7.

Galaburda, A.M., Sanides, F. & Geschwind, N. (1978) Human brain: cytoarchitectonic left–right asymmetries in the temporal speech region. *Arch. Neurol.* **35**, 812–17.

Galaburda, A.M., Sherman, G.F., Rosen, G.D., Aboitiz, F. & Geschwind, N. (1985) Developmental dyslexia: four consecutive patients with cortical anomalies. *Ann. Neurol.* **18**, 222–33.

Garber, H.J. & Ritvo, E.R. (1992) Magnetic resonance imaging of the posterior fossa in autistic adults. *Am. J. Psychiatry* **149**, 245–7.

Garber, H.J., Ritvo, E.R., Chiu, L.C. *et al.* (1989) A magnetic resonance imaging study of autism: normal fourth ventricle size and absence of pathology. *Am. J. Psychiatry* **146**, 532–5.

Geschwind, N. & Levitsky, W. (1968) Human brain: left–right asymmetries in temporal speech region. *Science* **161**, 186–7.

Gillberg, C. & Svendsen, P. (1983) Childhood psychosis and computed tomographic brain scan findings. *J. Autism Developm. Disorders* **13**, 19–32.

Hashimoto, T., Tayama, M., Murakawa, K. *et al.* (1995) Development of the brainstem and cerebellum in autistic patients. *J. Autism Developm. Disorders* **25**, 1–18.

Hauser, S.L., DeLong, G.R. & Rosman, N.P. (1975) Pneumographic findings in the infantile autism syndrome: a correlation with temporal lobe disease. *Brain* **98**, 667–88.

Holttum, J.R., Minshew, N.J., Sanders, R.S. & Phillips, N.E. (1992) Magnetic resonance imaging of the posterior fossa in autism. *Biol. Psychiatry* **32**, 1091–101.

Horwitz, B., Rumsey, J.M., Grady, C.L. & Rapoport, S.I. (1988) The cerebral metabolic landscape in autism: intercorrelations of regional glucose utilization. *Arch. Neurol.* **45**, 749–55.

Hynd, G.W., Semrud-Clikeman, M., Lorys, A.R., Novey, E.S. & Eliopulos, R.T. (1990) Brain morphology in developmental dyslexia and attention deficit disorder/hyperactivity. *Arch. Neurol.* **47**, 919–26.

Ioannides, A.A., Hellstrand, E. & Abraham-Fuchs, K. (1993) Point and distributed current density analysis of interictal activity recorded by magnetoencephalography. *Physiol. Measurement* **14**, 121–30.

Jacobson, R., Le Couteur, A., Howlin, P. & Rutter, M. (1988) Selective subcortical abnormalities in autism. *Psychol. Med.* **18**, 39–48.

Jernigan, T.L., Bellugi, U., Sowell, E., Doherty, S. & Hesselink, J.R. (1993) Cerebral morphologic distinctions between Williams and Down syndromes. *Arch. Neurol.* **50**, 186–91.

Kemper, T.L. & Bauman, M.L. (1993) The contribution of neuropathologic studies to the understanding of autism. *Neurol. Clin.* **11**, 175–87.

Kinsbourne, M., Rufo, D.T., Gamzu, E., Palmer, R.L. & Berliner, A.K. (1991) Neuropsychological deficits in adults with dyslexia. *Developm. Med. Child Neurol.* **33**, 763–75.

Kleinman, M.D., Neff, S. & Rosman, N.P. (1992) The brain in infantile autism: are posterior fossa structures abnormal? *Neurology* **42**, 753–60.

Kuzniecky, R. (1994) Magnetic resonance imaging in developmental disorders of the cerebral cortex. *Epilepsia* **35** (Suppl. 6), S44–S56.

Kuzniecky, R., Garcia, J.H., Faught, E. & Morawetz, R.B. (1991) Cortical dysplasia in temporal lobe epilepsy: magnetic resonance imaging correlations. *Ann. Neurol.* **29**, 293–8.

Kuzniecky, R., Andermann, F., Guerrini, R. & CBPS Multicenter Collaborative Study (1993) Congenital bilateral perisylvian syndrome: study of 31 patients. *Lancet* **341**, 608–12.

Larsen, J.P., Hoien, T., Lundberg, I. & Odegaard, H. (1990) MRI evaluation of the size and symmetry of the planum temporale in adolescents with developmental dyslexia. *Brain Lang.* **39**, 289–301.

Leonard, C.M., Voeller, K.K.S., Lombardino, L.J. *et al.* (1993) Anomalous cerebral structure in dyslexia revealed with magnetic resonance imaging. *Arch. Neurol.* **50**, 461–9.

Maquet, P., Hirsch, E., Dive, D. *et al.* (1990) Cerebral glucose utilization during sleep in Landau–Kleffner syndrome: a PET study. *Epilepsia* **31**, 778–83.

O'Tuama, L.A., Urion, D.K., Janicek, M.J., Treves, S.T., Bjornson, B. & Moriarty, J.M. (1992) Regional cerebral perfusion in Landau–Kleffner syndrome and related childhood aphasias. *J. Nucl. Med.* **33**, 1758–65.

Paetau, R., Kajola, M., Korkman, M., Hämäläinen, M., Granstrom, M.-L., & Hari, R. (1991) Landau–Kleffner syndrome: epileptic activity in the auditory cortex. *Neuroreport* **2**, 201–4.

Palmini, A., Andermann, F., Olivier, A. *et al.* (1991) Focal neuronal migration disorders and intractable partial epilepsy: a study of 30 patients. *Ann. Neurol.* **30**, 741–9.

Palmini, A., Gambardella, A., Andermann, F. *et al.* (1994) Operative strategies for patients with cortical dysplastic lesions and intractable epilepsy. *Epilepsia* **35** (Suppl. 6), S57–S71.

Piven, J., Berthier, M., Startstein, S., Nehme, E., Pearlson, G. & Folstein, S. (1990) Magnetic resonance imaging evidence for a defect of cerebral cortical development in autism. *Am. J. Psychiatry* **146**, 734–9.

Piven, J., Nehme, E., Simon, J., Barta, P., Pearlson, G. & Folstein, S.E. (1992) Magnetic resonance imaging in autism: measurement of the cerebellum, pons and fourth ventricle. *Biol. Psychiatry* **31**, 491–504.

Piven, J., Arndt, S., Bailey, J., Havercamp, S., Andreasen, N. & Palmer, P. (1995) An MRI study of brain size in autism. *Am. J. Psychiatry* **152**, 1145–9.

Price, C., Wise, R., Watson, J., Patterson, K., Howard, D. and Frackowiak, R. (1994) Brain activity during reading: the effects of exposure duration and task. *Brain* **117**, 1255–69.

Reiss, A.L., Aylward, E., Freund, L.S., Joshi, P.K. & Brian, R.M. (1991) Neuroanatomy of Fragile X syndrome: the posterior fossa. *Ann. Neurol.* **29**, 26–32.

Reiss, A.L., Lee, J. & Freund, L. (1994) Neuroanatomy of Fragile X syndrome: the temporal lobe. *Neurology* **44**, 1317–24.

Riikonen, R. & Amnell, G. (1981) Psychiatric disorders in children with earlier infantile spasms. *Developm. Med. Child Neurol.* **23**, 747–60.

Ritvo, E.R., Freeman, B.J., Scheibel, A.B. *et al.* (1986) Lower Purkinje cell counts in the cerebella of four autistic subjects: initial findings of the UCLA-NSAC Autopsy Research Report. *Am. J. Psychiatry* **143**, 862–6.

Rosenbloom, S., Campbell, M., George, A.E. *et al.* (1984) High resolution CT scanning in infantile autism: a quantitative approach. *J. Am. Acad. Child Psychiatry* **23**, 72–7.

Rumsey, J.M., Duara, R., Grady, C.L. *et al.* (1985) Brain metabolism in autism: resting cerebral glucose utilization rates as measured with positron emission tomography (PET). *Arch. Gen. Psychiatry* **42**, 448–55.

Rumsey, J.M., Andreason, P., Zametkin, A.J. (1992) Failure to activate the left temporoparietal cortex in dyslexia: an oxygen 15 positron emission tomographic study. *Arch. Neurol.* **49**, 527–34.

Rutter, M. & Mawhood, L. (1991) The long-term psychosocial sequelae of specific developmental dis-orders of speech and language. In Rutter, M. & Casaer, P. (eds) *Biological Risk Factors for Psychosocial Disorders* Cambridge University Press, Cambridge, pp. 233–59.

Rutter, M., Bailey, A., Bolton, P. & Le Couteur, A. (1994) Autism and known medical conditions: myth and substance. *J. Child Psychol. Psychiatry* **35**, 311–22.

Saitoh, O, Courchesne, E., Egaas, B., Lincoln, A. & Schreibman, L. (1995) Cross-sectional area of the posterior hippocampus in autistic patients with cerebellar and corpus callosum abnormalities. *Neurology* **45**, 317–24.

Sergent, J., Zuck, E., Levesque, M. & MacDonald, B. (1992) Positron emission tomography study of letter and object processing: empirical findings and methodological considerations. *Cerebr. Cortex* **2**, 68–80.

Shaywitz, B., Shaywitz, S., Pugh, K. *et al.* (1995) Sex differences in the functional organization of the brain for language. *Nature* **373**, 607–9.

Small, J.G. (1975) EEG and neurophysiological studies of early infantile autism. *Biol. Psychiatry* **10**, 385–97.

Truwit, C.L., Barkovich, A.J., Koch, T.K. & Ferriero, D.M. (1992) Cerebral palsy: MR findings in 40 patients. *Am. J. Neuroradiol.* **13**, 67–78.

Tsai, L.Y., Tsai, M.C. & August, G.J. (1985) Brief report: implication of EEG diagnoses in the subclassification of infantile autism. *J. Autism. Developm. Disorders* **15**, 339–44.

Vinters, H.V., De Rosa, M.J. & Farrell, M.A. (1993) Neuropathologic study of resected cerebral tissue from patients with infantile spasms. *Epilepsia* **34**, 772–9.

Williams, R.S., Hauser, S.L., Purpura, D.P., DeLong, G.R. & Swisher, C.M. (1980) Autism and mental retardation: neuropathologic studies performed in four retarded persons with autistic behavior. *Arch. Neurol.* **37**, 749–53.

Witelson, S.F. & Kigar, D.L. (1992) Sylvian fissure morphology and asymmetry in men and women: bilateral differences in relation to handedness in men. *J. Comparative Neurol.* **323**, 326–40.

Woodhouse, W., Bailey, A., Bolton, P., Baird, G., Le Couteur, A. & Rutter, M. (in press) Head circumference in autism and other pervasive developmental disorders. *J. Child Psychol. Psychiatry*.

Index